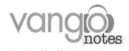

Hear it. Get It.

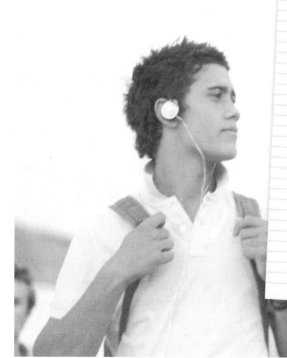

Study on the go with VangoNotes.

Just download chapter reviews from your text and listen to them on any mp3 player. Now wherever you are-- whatever you're doing--you can study by listening to the following for each chapter of your textbook:

Big Ideas: Your "need to know" for each chapter

Practice Test: A gut check for the Big Ideas-- tells you if you need to keep studying

Key Terms: Audio "flashcards" to help you review key concepts and terms

Rapid Review: A quick drill session -- use it right before your test

VangoNotes.com

Pearson Nursing Reviews & Rationales Series

SERIES EDITOR
MaryAnn Hogan, MSN, RN
Clinical Assistant Professor, University of Massachusetts, Amherst, Massachusetts

NURSING FUNDAMENTALS
Sara Bolten, RN, MSN
McKendree College
Louisville, KY

Mary Jean Ricci, MSN, RNBC
Good Shepherd Penn Partners
Philadelphia, Pennsylvania

Donna Taliaferro, RN, PhD
University of Missouri - St. Louis
St. Louis, MO

MEDICAL-SURGICAL NURSING
Joan Davenport, RN, PhD
University of Maryland
Baltimore, MD

Stacy Estridge, BSN, MN
Midlands Technical College
Columbia, SC

Dolores Zygmont, RN, PhD
Temple University
Philadelphia, PA

MATERNAL-NEWBORN NURSING
Vera Brancato, EdD, MSN, RN, BC
Kutztown University
Kutztown, PA

Rita Glazebrook, RNC, PhD, ANP
Minnesota Intercollegiate Nursing Consortium
Northfield, MN

Jean Rodgers, RN, MN
Hesston College
Hesston, KS

CHILD HEALTH NURSING
Vera Brancato, EdD, MSN, RN, BC
Kutztown University
Kutztown, PA

Kathleen Falkenstein, PhD, CPNP
Drexel University
Philadelphia, PA

Judy E. White, RNC, MA, MSN
Southern Union Community College
Opelika, AL

MENTAL HEALTH NURSING
Cory Gaylord, DNSc, ARNP
Palm Beach Community College
Lake Worth, FL

Rebecca Gruener, RN, MS
Louisiana State University at Alexandria
Alexandria, LA

Jean Rodgers, RN, MN
Hesston College
Hesston, KS

Kirstyn Kameg Zalice, MSN, CRNP
Robert Morris University
Moon Township, PA

COMMUNITY HEALTH NURSING
Mary Jean Ricci, MSN, RNBC
Good Shepherd Penn Partners
Philadelphia, Pennsylvania

HEALTH & PHYSICAL ASSESSMENT
Mary Jean Ricci, MSN, RNBC
Holy Family University
Bensalem, PA

FLUIDS, ELECTROLYTES, & ACID-BASE BALANCE
Margaret M. Gingrich, RN, MSN
Harrisburg Area Community College
Harrisburg, PA

Penny Overby, MSN, RN
Florence-Darlington Technical College
Florence, SC

Mary Jean Ricci, MSN, RNBC
Good Shepherd Penn Partners
Philadelphia, Pennsylvania

NUTRITION & DIET THERAPY
Evangeline DeLeon, RN
Delmar College
Corpus Christi, TX

Margaret M. Gingrich, RN, MSN
Harrisburg Area Community College
Harrisburg, PA

Kate Willcutts, MS, RD, CNSD
University of Virginia Medical Center
Charlottesville, VA

PATHOPHYSIOLOGY
Marcia Bower, CS, MSN, RN, CRNP
Holy Family University
Newton, PA

Karen Hill, RN, MSN, PhD
Southeastern Louisiana University
Hammond, LA

Kathleen S. Holm, RN, MSN, CNRN, FAAPM
Reading Area Community College
Reading, PA

PHARMACOLOGY
Geralyn Frandsen, EdD, MSN, RN
Maryville University
St. Louis, MO

Juanita F. Johnson, PhD, RN
Oklahoma Baptist University
Shawnee, OK

Lynn Warner, RN, DSNc
York College of Pennsylvania
York, PA

LEADERSHIP & MANAGEMENT
Donna M. Nickitas, RN, PhD, CNAA, BC
Hunter College
New York, NY

ANATOMY & PHYSIOLOGY
Barbara Carranti, MS, RN, CNS
Le Moyne College
Syracuse, NY

Pearson Nursing Reviews & Rationales

Health & Physical Assessment

MaryAnn Hogan, MSN, RN

Clinical Assistant Professor

University of Massachusetts-Amherst

Amherst, Massachusetts

Mary Jean Ricci, MSN, RNBC

Director of Corporate Clinical Support

Good Shepherd Penn Partners

Philadelphia, Pennsylvania

A Partnership between Good Shepherd and the Hospital of the University of Pennsylvania

Pearson

Boston   Columbus   Indianapolis   New York   San Francisco   Upper Saddle River

Amsterdam   Cape Town   Dubai   London   Madrid   Milan   Munich   Paris   Montréal   Toronto

Delhi   Mexico City   São Paulo   Sydney   Hong Kong   Seoul   Singapore   Taipei   Tokyo

Library of Congress Cataloging-in-Publication Data

Hogan, MaryAnn, MSN.
  Pearson nursing reviews & rationales : physical health & assessment / MaryAnn
Hogan, Mary Jean Ricci. -- 1st ed.
     p. ; cm.
  Other title: Nursing reviews & rationales
  Other title: Nursing reviews and rationales
  Includes bibliographical references.
  ISBN-13: 978-0-13-172052-7
  ISBN-10: 0-13-172052-X
  1. Nursing assessment--Examinations, questions, etc. 2. Nursing assessment--Exami-
nations,--Study guides. I. Ricci, Mary Jean. II. Title. III. Title: Nursing reviews & ratio-
nales. IV. Title: Nursing reviews and rationales.
  [DNLM: 1. Nursing Process--Examination Questions. 2. Nursing Assessment--meth-
ods--Examination Questions. 3. Nursing Care--methods--Examination Questions. WY
18.2 H714pa 2011]
  RT48.H64 2011
  616.07'5--dc22
                                  2010014474

Publisher: Julie Levin Alexander
Assistant to Publisher: Regina Bruno
Editor-in-Chief: Maura Connor
Editorial Assistant: Deirdre MacKnight
Development Editor: Danielle Doller
Media Product Manager: Travis Moses-Westphal
Director of Marketing: David Gesell
Marketing Coordinator: Michael Sirinides
Managing Editor, Production: Patrick Walsh
Production Editor: GEX Publishing Services
Production Liaison: Anne Garcia
Media Project Manager: Rachel Collett

Manufacturing Manager: Ilene Sanford
Design Coordinator: Maria Guglielmo-Walsh
Manager, Rights and Permissions: Zina Arabia
Manager, Visual Research: Beth Brenzel
Manager, Cover Visual Research & Permissions: Karen Sanatar
Image Permission Coordinator: Vickie Menanteaux
Composition: GEX Publishing Services
Printer/Binder: Edwards Brothers
Cover Printer: Lehigh-Phoenix Color/Hagerstown

Notice: Care has been taken to confirm the accuracy of information presented in this book. The authors, editors, and the publisher, however, cannot accept any responsibility for errors or omissions or for consequences from application of the information in this book and make no warranty, express or implied, with respect to its contents.

  The authors and publisher have exerted every effort to ensure that drug selections and dosages set forth in this text are in
accord with current recommendations and practice at time of publication. However, in view of ongoing research, changes in
government regulations, and the constant flow of information relating to drug therapy and reactions, the reader is urged to
check the package inserts of all drugs for any change in indications or dosage and for added warning and precautions. This is
particularly important when the recommended agent is a new and/or infrequently employed drug.

10 9 8 7 6 5 4 3 2 1

ISBN-13: 978-0-13-172052-7
ISBN-10: 0-13-172052-X

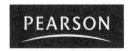

www.pearsonhighered.com

Contents

Welcome to the Pearson Nursing Reviews & Rationales Series!

This series has been specifically designed to provide a clear and concentrated review of important nursing knowledge in the following content areas:

- Anatomy & Physiology
- Pathophysiology
- Nursing Fundamentals
- Health & Physical Assessment
- Medical-Surgical Nursing
- Fluids, Electrolytes, & Acid-Base Balance
- Nutrition and Diet Therapy
- Pharmacology
- Maternal-Newborn Nursing
- Child Health Nursing
- Mental Health Nursing
- Community Health Nursing
- Nursing Leadership & Management

The books in this series are designed for use by current nursing students as a study aid for nursing course work or for NCLEX-RN® licensing exam preparation, or by practicing nurses seeking a comprehensive yet concise review of a nursing specialty or subject area.

This series is truly unique. One of its most special features is that it was developed and reviewed by a large team of nurse educators from across the United States and Canada to ensure that each chapter has been edited by a nurse expert in the content area under study. The series editor, MaryAnn Hogan, designed the overall series in collaboration with a core Pearson Education team to take full advantage of Pearson Education's cutting edge technology. The consulting editors for each book, also experts in that specialty area, then reviewed all chapters and test questions submitted for comprehensiveness and accuracy. Finally, MaryAnn Hogan reviewed the chapters in each book for consistency, accuracy, and applicability to the NCLEX-RN® Test Plan.

All books in the series are identical in their overall design for your convenience. As an added value, each book comes with a comprehensive support package, including a bonus *NCLEX-RN® Test Prep Companion Website* and a tear-out *NursingNotes* card for quick clinical reference.

Study Tips

Use of this book should help simplify your review. To make the most of your valuable study time, also follow these simple but important suggestions:

1. Use a weekly calendar to schedule study sessions.
   - Outline the timeframes for all of your activities (home, school, appointments, etc.) on a weekly calendar.
   - Find the "holes" in your calendar, which are the times in which you can plan to study. Add study sessions to the calendar at times when you can expect to be mentally alert and follow your plan!
2. Create the optimal study environment.
   - Eliminate external sources of distraction, such as television, telephone, etc.
   - Eliminate internal sources of distraction, such as hunger, thirst, or dwelling on items or problems that cannot be worked on at the moment.
   - Take a break for 10 minutes or so after each hour of concentrated study both as a reward and an incentive to keep studying.
3. Use pre-reading strategies to increase comprehension of chapter material.
   - Skim read the headings in the chapter (because they identify chapter content).
   - Read the definitions of key terms, which will help you learn new words to comprehend chapter information.
   - Review all graphic aids (figures, tables, boxes) because they are often used to explain important points in a chapter.

4. Read the chapter thoroughly but at a reasonable speed.
   - Comprehension and retention are actually enhanced by not reading too slowly.
   - Do take the time to reread any section that is unclear to you.
5. Summarize what you have learned.
   - Use questions supplied with this book and the *NCLEX-RN® Test Prep Companion Website* to test your application of chapter content.
   - Review again any sections that correspond to questions you answered incorrectly or incompletely.

Test-Taking Strategies

We provide test-taking strategies along with the rationales for every question in the series. These strategies will assist you to select the correct answer by breaking down the question, even if you don't know the correct response. Use also the following general strategies to increase your success on nursing examinations:

- Get sufficient sleep and have something to eat before taking a test. Take periodic deep breaths during the test. Remember, the brain requires oxygen and glucose as fuel. Avoid concentrated sugars before a test, however, to avoid rapid upward and then downward surges in blood glucose levels.
- Read each question carefully, identifying the stem, the options, and any critical words or phrases in either the stem or options.
  - Critical words in the stem such as "most important" indicate the need to set priorities, since more than one option is likely to contain a statement that is technically correct.
  - Remember that the presence of absolute words such as "never" or "only" in an answer option is more likely to make that option incorrect.
- Determine who is the client in the question; often this is the person with the health problem, but it may also be a significant other, relative, friend, or another nurse.
- Decide whether the stem is a true response stem or a false response stem. With a true response stem, the correct answer will be a true statement, and vice-versa.
- Determine what the question is really asking, sometimes referred to as the core issue of the question. Evaluate all answer options in relation to this core issue, and not strictly to the "correctness" of the statement in each individual option.
- Eliminate options that are obviously incorrect, then go back and reread the stem. Evaluate the remaining options against the stem once more.
- If two answers seem similar and correct, try to decide whether one of them is more global or comprehensive. If the global option includes the alternative option within it, it is likely that the more global response is the correct answer.

The NCLEX-RN® Licensing Examination

The NCLEX-RN® licensing examination is a Computer Adaptive Test (CAT) that ranges in length from 75 to 265 individual (stand-alone) test items, depending on individual performance during the examination. Upon graduation from a nursing program, successful completion of this exam is the gateway to your professional nursing practice. The blueprint for the exam is reviewed and revised every three years by the National Council of State Boards of Nursing according to the results of a practice analysis study of new graduate nurses practicing within the first six months after graduation. Each question on the exam is coded to a *Client Need Category* and an *Integrated Process*.

Client Need Categories   There are eight subcategories of client needs within four major categories of client needs. Each exam will contain a minimum and maximum percent of questions from each subcategory. The *Client Needs* categories and subcategories according to the NCLEX-RN® Test Plan effective April 1, 2010 are as follows:

- Safe, Effective Care Environment
  - Management of Care (16–22%)
  - Safety and Infection Control (8–14%)
- Health Promotion and Maintenance (6-12%)
- Psychosocial Integrity (6-12%)
- Physiological Integrity
  - Basic Care and Comfort (6–12%)
  - Pharmacological and Parenteral Therapies (13–19%)
  - Reduction of Risk Potential (10–16%)
  - Physiological Adaptation (11–17%)

Integrated Processes   The integrated processes identified on the NCLEX-RN® Test Plan effective April 1, 2010, with condensed definitions, are as follows:

- Nursing Process: a scientific problem-solving approach used in nursing practice; consisting of assessment, analysis, planning, implementation, and evaluation.
- Caring: client-nurse interaction(s) characterized by mutual respect and trust and that are directed toward achieving desired client outcomes.
- Communication and Documentation: verbal and/or nonverbal interactions between nurse and others (client, family, health care team); a written or electronic recording of activities or events that occur during client care.
- Teaching and Learning: facilitating client's acquisition of knowledge, skills, and attitudes that lead to behavior change

More detailed information about this examination may be obtained by visiting the National Council of State Boards of Nursing website at http://www.ncsbn.org and viewing the *2010 NCLEX-RN® Detailed Test Plan.*[1]

---

[1]Reference: National Council of State Boards of Nursing, Inc. *NCLEX Examination Test Plan for National Council Licensure Examination for Registered Nurses.* Effective April 1, 2010. Retrieved from the World Wide Web at https://www.ncsbn.org/2010_NCLEX_RN_TestPlan.pdf.

HOW TO GET THE MOST OUT OF THIS BOOK

Each chapter has the following elements to guide you during review and study:

- **Chapter Objectives** describe what you will be able to know or do after learning the material covered in the chapter.

Objectives

➤ Identify the anatomical structures of the neurological system.
➤ Identify the questions to ascertain information about health history, present history, and family history.
➤ Describe the assessment techniques for assessment of the nervous system.
➤ Describe the expected and unexpected findings in the assessment of the neurological system.
➤ Describe the considerations across the lifespan to be taken into account during assessment of the neurological system.
➤ Describe documentation of the assessment of the neurological system.

NCLEX-RN® Test Prep

Visit the Companion Website for this book at www.pearsonhighered.com/hogan to access additional practice opportunities and more.

Review at a Glance contains a glossary of key terms used in the chapter, with definitions provided up-front and available at your fingertips, to help you stay focused and make the best use of your study time.

Review at a Glance

belief something accepted as true, especially as a tenet or a body of tenets accepted by an ethnocultural group

cultural competency the awareness, knowledge and skills necessary to appreciate, understand and communicate with people of diverse cultural backgrounds

family a group of individuals related by blood, marriage, or mutual goals

family-centered maternity care maternity care that is family oriented and views childbirth as a vital, natural life event rather than an illness

scope of practice legally refers to permissible boundaries of practice for nurses and is defined by statute (written law), rules and regulations, or a combination of the two

Pretest provides a 10-question quiz as a sample overview of the material covered in the chapter and helps you decide in what areas you need the most—or the least—review.

PRETEST

1 The nurse performs a vaginal examination and determines that the fetus is in a sacrum anterior position. The nurse draws which conclusion from this assessment data?

1. The fetal sacrum is toward the maternal symphysis pubis.
2. The fetal sacrum is toward the maternal sacrum.
3. The fetal face is toward the maternal sacrum.
4. The fetal face is toward the maternal symphysis pubis.

Practice to Pass questions are open-ended to help stimulate critical thinking and reinforce mastery of the chapter information.

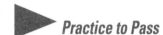

Practice to Pass

The client scheduled for a hysterosalpingogram reports an allergy to shellfish. What should the nurse do?

NCLEX Alert identifies concepts that are more likely to be on the NCLEX-RN® examination. Be sure to learn the information highlighted wherever you see this icon.

Case Study, found at the end of the chapter, provides an opportunity for you to use your critical thinking and clinical reasoning skills to "put it all together." It describes a true-to-life client case situation and asks you open-ended questions about how you would provide care for that client and/or family.

Case Study

A 14-year-old primigravida is admitted in early labor with severe preeclampsia at 42 weeks gestation. The client's blood pressure is 168/102.

1. What other assessment data would you obtain?
2. Describe the complications this client is at risk for.
3. Discuss the medications you expect to administer to this client.
4. What concerns do you have for this fetus? Why?
5. What would you teach this client and her family about her condition?

For suggested responses, see page 343.

Posttest provides an additional 10-question quiz at the end of the chapter. It provides you with feedback about mastery of the chapter material following review and study. All pretest and posttest questions contain comprehensive rationales for the correct and incorrect answers, and are coded according to cognitive level of difficulty and to the NCLEX-RN® Test Plan categories of Client Need and Integrated Process.

POSTTEST

1 A client who is a brittle diabetic is seeking to get pregnant. The nursing working in a primary care provider's office suggests that which of the following healthcare providers would be an optimal choice?

1. A certified nurse-midwife
2. A family nurse practitioner
3. An obstetrician
4. A maternal-fetal medicine specialist

NCLEX-RN® Test Prep Companion Website

For those who want to practice taking tests on a computer, the companion website that accompanies the book contains the pretest and posttest questions found in all chapters of the book. In addition, it contains 30 new questions for each chapter to help you further evaluate your knowledge base and hone your test-taking skills. We have also included some alternate format test items to give you valuable practice with different types of questions. Go to **www.pearsonhighered.com/hogan**.

Pearson Nursing Notes Card

These tear-out cards provide a reference for frequently used facts and information related to the subject matter of the book. They are designed to be useful in the clinical setting, when quick and easy access to information is so important!

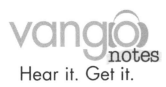

VangoNotes
Hear it. Get it.

Study on the go with VangoNotes. Just download chapter reviews from your text and listen to them on any mp3 player. Now wherever you are—whatever you are doing—you can study by listening to the following for each chapter of your textbook:

- **Big Ideas**: Your "need to know" for each chapter
- **Practice Test**: A gut check for the Big Ideas–tells you if you need to keep studying
- **Key Terms**: Audio "flashcards" to help you review key concepts and terms

VangoNotes are **flexible**; download all the material directly to your device, or only the chapters you need. And they're **efficient**. Use them in your car, at the gym, walking to class, wherever. So get yours today...and get studying.

About the Health & Physical Assessment Book

Chapters in this book cover "need-to-know" information about health and physical assessment. The first two chapters outline how to take a health history and the various techniques used in physical assessment. The next two chapters review mental health and nutritional assessment, which are integral to the health of every client. The remaining chapters in the book review health and physical assessment of specific body systems or anatomical areas, including cardiovascular, respiratory, gastrointestinal, neurological, musculoskeletal, breasts and axillae, female and male genitourinary systems, skin (including hair and nails), eyes, and ears, nose and throat. A firm knowledge base in health and physical assessment will serve you well as you care for clients in clinical practice.

Acknowledgments

This book is truly an effort of collaboration. Without the contributions of many individuals, this first edition of *Health & Physical Assessment: Reviews and Rationales* would not have been possible. A grateful acknowledgement goes to the reviewers who devoted their time and talents to this book. Their work will surely assist students to extend their knowledge in the area of physical assessment.

We owe a special debt of gratitude to the wonderful team at Pearson Nursing for their enthusiasm for this project, as well as their good humor, expertise, and encouragement as the series developed. Maura Connor, Editor-in-Chief for Nursing, was unending in her creativity, support, encouragement, and belief in the need for this series. Danielle Doller, Developmental Editor, devoted many long hours to coordinating different facets of this project, and tirelessly and cheerfully encouraged our efforts as well. Her high standards and attention to detail contributed greatly to the final "look" of this series. Editorial Assistants, Marion Gottlieb, Luz Costa, and Deirdre MacKnight, helped to keep the project moving forward on a day-to-day basis, and we are grateful for their efforts as well. A very special thank you goes to the designers of the book and the production team, led by Anne Garcia, Production Editor, and Mary Siener, Designer, who brought the ideas and manuscript into final form.

Thank you to the team at GEX Publishing Services, led by Project Manager Micah Petillo, for the detail-oriented work of creating this book. We greatly appreciate their hard work, attention to detail, and spirit of collaboration.

Finally, MaryAnn would like to acknowledge and gratefully thank her children, who helped with chores and sacrificed time that would have been spent with them, to bring this book to publication. Their love and support are the greatest gifts imaginable.

Contributors and Reviewers

Contributors

Joyce Welliver, MSN, RN, CRNP
Roxborough Memorial Hospital School
   of Nursing
Philadelphia, Pennsylvania
Chapters 1, 5, 13

Lee Murray, MSN, RN, CS, CADAC
Holyoke Community College
Holyoke, Massachusetts
Chapter 3

Reviewers

Joan Teague Bickes, MSN, APRN, BC
Wayne State University
Detroit, Michigan

Donna Cleary APRN, BC, AE-C
University of Texas at Arlington
Arlington, Texas

David J. Derrico, RN, MSN
University of Florida
Gainesville, Florida

Deovina N. Jordan, PhD, MSN, MPH, BSN, RN, BC
California State University Fullerton
Fullerton, California

James L. Jordan, PhD, MAdm, BSN, RN
Touro University Nevada
Henderson, Nevada

Sharon Redding, MN, RN, CNE
College of Saint Mary
Omaha, Nebraska

Rita K. Young MSN, RN, CNS
The University of Akron
Akron, Ohio

Health History

1

Chapter Outline

Introduction to Health
   Assessment

Interview Process

Components of a Health
   History

Objectives

➤ Define the purpose of a health history.
➤ Discuss the components of a health history.
➤ Describe the phases of the interview process and useful communication strategies.
➤ Identify communication barriers that can occur during a nurse–client interview.
➤ Relate developmental considerations when taking a history.
➤ Differentiate cultural expressions of health and illness.

NCLEX-RN® Test Prep

Visit the Companion Website for this book at www.pearsonhighered.com/hogan to access additional practice opportunities and more.

Review at a Glance

amenorrhea absence of menstruation

cataract diminished vision resulting from lens of eye becoming opaque or cloudy; usually occurring because of aging, trauma, or endocrine or intraocular disease

critical thinking a cognitive process including creativity, problem solving, and decision making

dysmenorrhea painful cramping or other discomfort associated with menstruation

dyspnea labored or difficult breathing, may also be accompanied by a sense of air hunger; may be described by client as a subjective feeling of shortness of breath

genogram a family map of three or more generations that records relationships, deaths, occupations, and history of health and illness

glaucoma an increase in intraocular pressure that can result in atrophy of the optic nerve or blindness if untreated

hydrocele a collection of serous fluid in the tunica vaginalis, surrounding the testis

oliguria condition of having abnormally small amounts of urine production, usually less than 30 mL/hr, or 0.5 mg/kg/hr

paresthesia an abnormal sensation described as burning or tingling

polydipsia condition of having excessive thirst

polyphagia eating abnormally large amounts of food

polyuria condition of having excessive urine production

tic a sudden spasmodic, painless, involuntary muscular contraction, most commonly involving the face, mouth, eyes, head, neck, or shoulder muscles

tinnitus a subjective ringing, buzzing, tinkling, or hissing sound in the ear

vertigo a sensation of tilting within stable surroundings or of being in tilting or spinning surroundings; sometimes described as dizziness

PRETEST

1 The nurse demonstrates the purpose of a health history by documenting which information about a client's respiratory system?

1. Perception of his or her respiratory health status
2. Tactile fremitus and breath sounds
3. Vital signs including respiratory rate and oxygen saturation
4. Respiratory excursion and respiratory effort

2 When obtaining information about a child's health history, the nurse would include which data? Select all that apply.

1. Past medical history
2. Present medical complaint
3. Review of systems
4. Physical assessment
5. Vital signs

3 When documenting subjective data for the cardiovascular system the nurse would include which of the following?

1. Vital signs
2. Peripheral pulses
3. Chest pain
4. Heart sounds

4 A client is admitted for evaluation of upper gastrointestinal symptoms. The nurse would document which statement as objective data in the client's medical record?

1. Client states, "I have a headache."
2. Client states, "I had chicken pox as a child."
3. Client has distended abdomen and active bowel sounds.
4. Client states, "I feel nauseated after eating."

5 A new nurse is employed on the pediatric unit of a hospital that uses problem-oriented charting. Which method of documentation should the nurse use?

1. Document findings on a flow sheet
2. Document only an abnormal finding
3. Document all findings using words, phrases, or sentences
4. Document subjective, objective, assessment, and planning data

6 The clinic nurse is conducting a health history. Place in proper sequence the questions the nurse would ask using the standard format for collecting health history information. All options must be used.

1. "Does anyone in your family have diabetes mellitus?"
2. "For what reason did you come to the clinic today?"
3. "What is your date of birth?"
4. "Can you tell me about your support systems?"
5. "Have you ever been hospitalized?"

7 After the nurse gathers health assessment data on a client admitted with pneumonia, the nurse would take which action?

1. Review the information gathered to analyze the data
2. Report all findings to the healthcare provider
3. Schedule an interdisciplinary planning meeting
4. Develop appropriate client goals for identified problems

8 The client is experiencing a headache that has lasted for 24 hours. Which of the following statements would be the most appropriate way for the nurse to document this complaint?

1. Client states, "I have a headache."
2. Client experiencing headache; states that it "has lasted 24 hours."
3. Client states, "I have had a headache for the last 24 hours."
4. Headache present without evidence of concurrent nausea

9 When responding to questions asked during a review of systems the client reports having a sore throat, which "happens all the time." The nurse should ask which question next?

1. "When did this sore throat begin?"
2. "What do you mean you have sore throats all the time?"
3. "Did you also have sore throats as a child?"
4. "Did you ever take antibiotics?"

10 The nurse is gathering a health history on an adult
female seeking healthcare because of recent onset
of leg pain when walking for two blocks. When gathering data on the family history the nurse should
include which item?

1. History of gallbladder surgery
2. Maternal history of diabetes
3. History of two pregnancies
4. History of performing self breast examinations monthly

➤ *See pages 12–13 for Answers and Rationales.*

PRETEST

I. INTRODUCTION TO HEALTH ASSESSMENT

A. Consists of health history and physical assessment

1. Health history: subjective data obtained during an interview
   a. Obtains client information not observable to healthcare providers
   b. Needs to be documented as accurately as possible, using the client's own words
   when doing a narrative recording (as opposed to using a checklist)

2. Physical assessment: objective data obtained by nurse or other healthcare provider
during a general survey and physical examination

B. Purposes

1. Obtain information about client's perception of his or her health

2. Obtain information about client's health status, health risks, and health promotion
activities using a systematic method to collect data

3. After this information is gathered, the nurse differentiates expected from unexpected findings using **critical thinking** (ability to sort through data to make a sound
judgment), which is integral to being able to accurately plan for and manage a
client's care

II. INTERVIEW PROCESS

A. Preparation for client interview

1. Provide private room or partitions for privacy

2. Maintain room temperature at a comfortable level

3. Provide adequate lighting

4. Reduce external stimuli such as noise or distractions and interruptions

5. Provide adequate seating, preferably at eye level

6. Maintain an appropriate distance from the client, approximately 4 to 5 feet

7. Provide a gown for the client if a physical examination will be performed

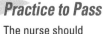

Practice to Pass

The nurse should
perform what actions
prior to interviewing
the client?

B. Phases of the interview process

1. Preinteraction phase
   a. Nurse collects data from medical record, health risk assessment, and health
   screenings
   b. Data is also collected from other healthcare professionals such as therapist, nutri-
   tionists, psychologists, and case managers
   c. Review new treatment procedures and prevention strategies from literature
   d. Choose appropriate settings and have all supplies, such as documentation materials, in the room
   e. Ensure adequate lighting and temperature
   f. Provide for privacy

2. Introduction phase
   a. Identify the client by using his or her surname
   b. Introduce self and state role (i.e., the nurse who will be working with you today)
   c. State reason for interview, and include the anticipated timeframe and that notes
   may be taken during the interview

Table 1-1   **Types of Interview Questions**

Type of Question	Description	Examples
Open-Ended	General question that encourages client to provide information; effective to use during initial phase of interview	"Can you tell me why you are here for treatment today?" "How would you describe the pain you are experiencing right now?"
Closed	Direct question that asks for specific information; requires "yes" or "no" response from client; effective to use to obtain specific data about client's health problem or when reviewing systems	"Do you have any allergies?" "Are you having any pain right now?"

      d. Encourage client to stop and ask for clarification if a question is not understood or client needs further clarification

      e. Assure client of confidentiality of data, and that client has the right to choose not to disclose some information, although a complete data base is most helpful in planning care

    3. Working phase

      a. Use a combination of open-ended and closed questions (see Table 1-1); initial questions are likely to be open-ended, with closed questions being used to clarify or gain specific information about the client's statements

      b. Gather data using a variety of effective communication techniques (see Table 1-2)

      c. Use effective non-verbal techniques (see Box 1-1)

      d. Be aware of barriers to effective communication

         1) False reassurance occurs when healthcare provider assures client of a positive outcome when there is no guarantee for that conclusion

Table 1-2   **Effective Communication Techniques**

Communication Techniques	Description	Examples
Active Listening	Listening to what client is saying while observing body language	Client states, "I'm okay" while nurse observes client crying
Facilitation	Response that encourages client to continue to share more data	"Go on." Nodding head
Empathy	Putting oneself in client's situation	Nurse: "This must be very difficult for you."
Reflection	Repeating client's own words back to him or her	Client: "I have a headache." Nurse: "You have a headache?"
Clarification	Asking for further clarification	Client: "I've been feeling strange lately." Nurse: "Can you describe what strange feels like?"
Paraphrasing	Using some of client's words and restating using own words	Client: "I am feeling anxious about having my surgery since my family expressed their concerns about my recovery." Nurse: "Your family's concerns have made you anxious about having the surgery?"
Confrontation	Focusing attention on specific situation where nurse observes client's non-verbal response to be in conflict with his or her verbal response	Nurse: "I noticed that when I was examining your abdomen you were guarding the area with your hands, but yet you said that you are not experiencing any pain."
Summarizing	Restating general themes that were discussed throughout interview	Nurse: "We identified some problem areas and will develop a health plan for you when you go home."

Box 1-1	**Professional Appearance**	**Facial Expressions**

Effective Non-Verbal Techniques

Professional Appearance
- Relaxed, open posture
- Seated at eye level
- Leaning slightly forward
- Appropriate touch

Facial Expressions
- Appropriate smiling
- Maintaining eye contact

Speech
- Moderate tone of voice
- Moderate rate of speech

        2) Changing the subject occurs when there is discomfort on caregiver's part about a topic; this demonstrates disregard toward the client's feelings

        3) Cross-examination occurs when caregiver asks multiple questions that cause the client fear or to feel threatened

    e. Actual content of the health history is gained during this phase of the interview (see section III to follow)

    4. Closing phase

        a. Summarize important aspects of the interview

        b. Encourage client to ask questions or express any feelings and any concerns

III. COMPONENTS OF A HEALTH HISTORY (BOX 1-2)

    A. Biographical data

        1. Categories may be pre-identified on the assessment form

        2. Consists of the following items of background information:

            a. Name, address, age

            b. Date of birth and location

            c. Gender, race, and ethnic origin

            d. Primary language

            e. Marital status

            f. Religion and spirituality

            g. Occupation

            h. Source of information and reliability

            i. Health insurance

            j. Authorized representative for health issues (if applicable)

    B. Present health status or history of present illness

        1. Comprehensive, chronological summary of current health situation, including chief complaint, history of present illness, health beliefs and practices, and medications (prescription, over-the-counter [OTC], herbal and vitamin supplements)

Practice to Pass

How should the nurse document the chief complaint?

        2. Chief complaint: statement in client's own words stating reason(s) for seeking healthcare at this time

            a. Ask a broad question initially such as, "What brings you to seek care today?"

            b. Document chief complaint using client's own words whenever possible

        3. History of present illness: an in-depth assessment of client's presenting problem

Box 1-2	

Components of the Health History

Biographical data
Present health status or history of present illness
Past history
Family history
Psychosocial history
Review of body systems

      a. Determine what symptom(s) the client is experiencing

      b. For each symptom determine the onset, location, duration, frequency, quality, alleviating and aggravating factors, and other associated symptoms

  4. Health beliefs and practices and health goals

      a. Health beliefs are influenced by cultural background, exposure to health information, and personal experience

      b. Health practices include measures that client uses to remain healthy (such as nutrition and adequate sleep) and includes the extent to which client follows recommendations for disease prevention, such as health screenings and staying current with immunizations

      c. Health goals include what the client hopes to achieve or maintain regarding health or to achieve as a result of obtaining healthcare

  5. Medications: prescription, OTC, and herbal and vitamin supplements

      a. For prescription and OTC medications, ask client the drug name, dosage, purpose, length (duration) and frequency of use, and desired and unintended effects

      b. Use of herbal supplements may be part of client's cultural heritage or acquired preference; assess type, dose and frequency of use, and intended purpose; inquire about effects and interactions with prescribed medications

      c. Determine type, dose, and purpose of vitamin supplements

C. Past medical history

  1. Purpose: to determine background health status of client

  2. Components include childhood diseases; immunizations; allergies; acute and chronic illnesses; hospitalizations; surgical procedures (planned and emergency); labor and deliveries (for adult females); injuries or accidents; blood transfusions; exposure to infectious/communicable diseases; mental health problems; and history of alcohol, tobacco, caffeine or other substance use; ask client if there were any complications associated with any of the above components

      a. Immunization history should include childhood immunizations if client is a child, and for adults should also include current status of tuberculosis (TB) screening, hepatitis B vaccine, tetanus toxoid, shingles vaccine, Gardasil vaccine, and influenza (flu) and pneumonia vaccines

      b. Allergy history should include the allergen (food, drug, latex, environmental), type of reaction, frequency and severity, treatment, and personal adaptation (avoidance of allergen)

      c. Acute and chronic illness history includes onset, frequency of exacerbations if appropriate, precipitating factors, signs and symptoms, methods of treatment, and long-term effects on lifestyle if appropriate

      d. Mental health history, if applicable, includes description of problem, type of care received (healthcare provider, support group, clergy, or other family or community resource), and description of therapy and its effectiveness

      e. History of substance use includes assessment of type, amount, and duration and frequency of use for each substance reported

D. Family history

  1. Includes data related to health status of client's blood relatives for purpose of trending any genetic or familial diseases; data should include age, chronic illnesses, current health status if living, and if deceased, cause of death if known

  2. Family members should include grandparents, parents, siblings, spouse, and children

  3. Ask about the following history data: hypertension, heart disease, blood disorders, diabetes, chronic respiratory problems, seizure disorders, cancer, infectious diseases, chronic kidney disease, alcoholism, and mental illness

  4. Construct a family tree, or **genogram** (a family map of three or more generations) that records relationships, deaths, occupations, and history of health and illness (see Figure 1-1)

Practice to Pass

What should the nurse include in the client's past medical history?

Practice to Pass

What should the nurse include when obtaining a family history?

Figure 1-1

Genogram

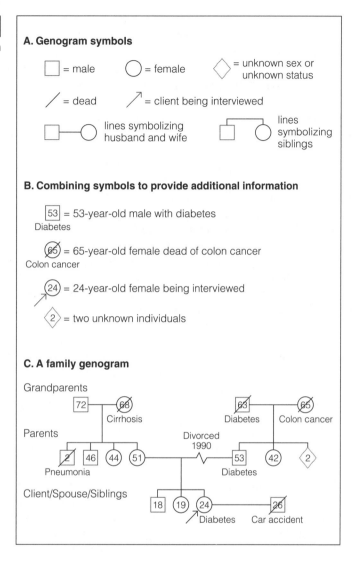

A. Genogram symbols

□ = male   ○ = female   ◇ = unknown sex or unknown status

╱ = dead   ╱ = client being interviewed

□—○ lines symbolizing husband and wife   □⌐○ lines symbolizing siblings

B. Combining symbols to provide additional information

53 = 53-year-old male with diabetes
Diabetes

65 = 65-year-old female dead of colon cancer
Colon cancer

24 = 24-year-old female being interviewed

2 = two unknown individuals

C. A family genogram

Grandparents

72 — 68   63 — 65
Cirrhosis   Diabetes   Colon cancer

Parents   Divorced 1990

2 46 44 51   53 42 2
Pneumonia   Diabetes

Client/Spouse/Siblings

18 19 24 — 26
Diabetes   Car accident

E. **Psychosocial history**

   1. Includes client's occupational history, educational level, financial ability to maintain health insurance or pay for healthcare, roles and relationships, ethnicity and culture, family, spirituality, and self-concept; evaluate client's travel history, which may provide information about malaria, parasites, or dysenteric diseases

   2. Information about occupation can reveal risk factors for certain health problems, such as cancer if exposed over time to harmful chemicals or radiation

   3. Educational level data may influence verbal communication during assessment and is also important when choosing client-teaching approaches and materials

   4. Data about roles and relationships, ethnicity and culture, family, spirituality, and self-concept help to identify support systems, family dynamics, and individual needs of the client

F. **The review of systems includes questions related to the following:**

   1. General health status: fatigue, weakness, fever, chills, night sweats, weight gain or loss

   2. Skin: history of pigment or color changes, changes in moles, excessive dryness or moisture, itching, bruising, rashes or lesions, skin care, and use of sun screens

   3. Hair: change in texture, hair loss

4. Nails: changes in color, shape, or contour
5. Head: vertigo, head injury or trauma, frequency and severity of headaches
6. Eyes: history of **glaucoma**, **cataracts**, eye surgery; changes in vision (double vision, blurring, blind spots), pain, redness, swelling, discharge; frequency and date of last eye exam and glaucoma testing, use of eyeglasses or contact lenses, maintenance of contact lenses, use of protective eyewear for sports or as occupational requirement, use of sunglasses or other ultraviolent light protection
7. Ears: changes in hearing, use of hearing aids, **tinnitus**, **vertigo**, infections, pain, discharge, exposure to environmental noise, method of cleaning ears, method used to prevent excessive sun exposure, method used with exposure to high noise levels at work (are protective noise coverings worn?)
8. Nose and sinuses: changes in smell, frequent colds, infections, pain, obstruction, allergies, hay fever, nosebleeds, discharge
9. Mouth and throat: changes in voice, hoarseness, frequent sore throats, pain, toothaches, bleeding gums, lesions in mouth, tongue, dysphasia (difficulty speaking), alteration in taste, patterns of daily dental hygiene, use of prostheses, last dental examination, use of dental appliances, use of dental night guards, use of dentures (how dentures are cared for), consumption of fluoridated water
10. Neck: limitation of movement, tenderness, swelling, enlarged nodes or lumps, goiter
11. Breast: breast changes for preadolescent and adolescent females and self-perception of development; self breast examination and routine mammogram screenings
12. Respiratory system: history of asthma, wheezing, difficulty breathing, cough, shortness of breath, **dyspnea**, and orthopnea
13. Cardiovascular system: history of congenital heart defects, murmurs, activity restrictions, cyanosis, hypertension, palpitations, decreased temperature and edema in the extremities, and sensitivity to cold
14. Gastrointestinal system: history of ulcer, pinworms, pattern and frequency of bowel movements noting color and characteristics, abdominal pain, nausea, occult blood and colonoscopy screenings
15. Urinary system: history of urinary tract infections, painful urination, color of urine, polyuria/**oliguria**, narrowed stream, toilet training, bedwetting
16. Male reproductive system: for preadolescent and adolescent any changes in penis and scrotum, nocturnal emissions; history of hernias or **hydrocele**, scrotum swelling, lesions, sores, pain in testicles or penis, descent of testes, sores, lesions, discharge; testicular self-examination
17. Female reproductive system: menstrual history (age at onset of menarche, last duration and description of last menstrual cycle, **amenorrhea** or **dysmenorrhea**, spotting, pain); menopausal history (age at onset, signs and symptoms, postmenopausal bleeding); vaginal itching, discharge (characteristics), last gynecological examination and Papanicolaou (Pap) smear
18. Sexual health: current sexual relations, use of contraceptives; history of sexually transmitted disease (gonorrhea, chlamydia, syphilis, herpes, venereal warts, HIV/AIDS), compliance with and use of treatment regimen
19. Musculoskeletal system: history of muscle weakness, cramping, pain, difficulty with gait or coordinated activities; history of arthritis, gout, pain, swelling, stiffness, deformity in joints; history of back pain, disk disease, stiffness, or limitation of motion; use of mobility aids; effects of limited range of motion on daily activities
20. Neurological system: history of seizures, stroke, motor weakness, coordination, **tics** or tremors, paralysis, sensory impairment such as numbness and **paresthesia** (tingling); changes in memory, orientation, mood, mental health, coping patterns
21. Hematologic system: history of blood transfusion and reactions; excessive bruising, bleeding tendencies, lymph node swelling, exposure to lead, carbon monoxide, paint fumes, pesticides, or radiation

22. Endocrine system: history of diabetic symptoms (**polyuria**, **polydipsia**, **polyphagia**), thyroid disease (intolerance to heat and cold), change in skin texture or pigmentation, excessive sweating, abnormal hair distribution, nervousness, tremors, weight gain or loss

G. Functional assessment

1. Measures ability to perform activities of daily living (ADLs) including eating, bathing, grooming, and toileting
2. Instrumental ADLs include ability to cook, clean, shop, pay bills, and get to healthcare provider appointments
3. Difficulties with any of these warrants follow-up and consultation with the interdisciplinary team (such as a social worker, occupational and physical therapist, home care personnel) for client assistance; it may also help determine whether client can live independently or needs assistance or supervision

H. Developmental considerations

1. Children and adolescents
   a. History of childhood illnesses, injuries, operations, hospitalizations
      1) What childhood illnesses has the child had?
      2) Has the child been hospitalized? If so, for what?
   b. History of immunizations, allergies, medications
      1) Is the immunization schedule up-to-date?
      2) Is there a history of allergies? If so, are they being treated?
      3) What current allergy medication is being used? Ask about compliance with medication use.
   c. Developmental history: includes milestones related to growth and development (gross and fine motor skills, language, social skills)
      1) Has the child achieved all milestones?
      2) Is the older child able to participate in the health history process?
2. Older adult
   a. Health measures: appropriate healthcare, alternative health practices used
      1) Does the client have health history issues treated immediately?
      2) Are spiritual healers or shamans used?
      3) Are any health or alternative health practices being used?
   b. Health history: presence of chronic illnesses, history of hospitalization, surgeries/procedures
      1) Are chronic illnesses under control?
      2) Is client taking medications? If not, can he or she afford medications?
      3) What was the cause of hospitalizations?
      4) What surgical procedure was performed?
      5) Was surgery successful?
   c. Functional ability: can client perform ADLs and participate in social activities?

I. Transcultural considerations

1. Cultural group: includes both racial affiliation and cultural group that client identifies with
   a. Where was client born?
   b. How long did client live there?
   c. How was client raised?
2. Values orientation: includes attitudes, values, beliefs about health/illness and birth/death
   a. What role is client assuming in healthcare?
   b. Is client active in care or does client rely on family to take care of his or her health?
   c. How is health and healthcare defined by client's culture?
   d. What does client believe has caused the illness?
   e. Does client use alternative health practitioners?

3. Practices and restrictions: include health practices, expectations, expression of beliefs, restrictions
   a. How much proximity does the client keep with people and the environment?
   b. How does the client respond to the nurse and the healthcare environment?
   c. What cultural objects are in the environment?

J. Documentation
1. Assessment is documented in the health record, which is a legal document
2. Record serves as a means to communicate among healthcare providers, achieve reimbursement for care, and as a database
3. Requires use of appropriate medical terminology; to avoid misinterpretation of data, do not use abbreviations during documentation
4. Documentation should be clear, concise, legible, timely, and confidential
5. Methods for documentation include narrative notes, problem-oriented charting, flow sheets, charting by exception, focused documentation, and computer documentation
   a. Narrative notes involve use of words in sentence form to document assessment or care given
   b. Problem-oriented charting includes SOAP and APIE methods of charting
      1) SOAP notes record subjective data (reported by client), objective data (nurse observes), assessment (conclusion nurse draws from data), and planning (action to resolve problem)
      2) APIE notes refer to assessment (subjective and objective data), problem (what is affecting the client), interventions (actions to resolve problem), and evaluation (client response to interventions)
   c. Flow sheets are check sheets used to document normal and abnormal findings; they may include space for narrative notes to fully document care not included on the checklist
   d. Focused documentation is a method of documenting specific symptoms, problems, or client needs
   e. Charting by exception is documentation limited to variances from normal findings to eliminate repetitive documentation
   f. Computer documentation includes any method of documentation previously discussed, except it is done utilizing a computer program; increases accuracy and is programmed to prevent nurse from omitting documentation, as the program does not allow the nurse to move away from essential documentation screens

Practice to Pass

What rules should the nurse follow when documenting?

Case Study

A 64-year-old female client is admitted to the hospital with a chief complaint of abdominal pain. The nurse prepares to complete the admission history and physical examination.

1. What actions should the nurse implement when preparing to interview the client?

2. What important considerations should the nurse include during the introduction phase of the interview?

3. During the working phase of the interview, what type of question would be most beneficial

   for the nurse to use in order to facilitate effective communication?

4. What questions would be important for the nurse to ask when obtaining data related to the client's chief complaint of abdominal pain?

5. How should the nurse end the nurse–client interview?

For suggested responses, see page 308

POSTTEST

1. The nurse is gathering present health practices data while taking a health history of a client admitted for back surgery. The nurse asks the client about alcohol use. The client angrily asks, "Why do you need to know?" What is the nurse's best response?

1. "If you consume alcohol then I will need to provide alcohol counseling."
2. "I need to know because alcohol can interact with many medications."
3. "You are very defensive and this suggests you probably have an alcohol problem."
4. "I can make a referral to alcohol self-help groups for you."

2. Prior to obtaining data for a health history the nurse should take which action?

1. Introduce self to client and position client comfortably in a chair
2. Bring in a family member to verify all data
3. Review medical record to validate client information
4. Tape record client information to avoid omissions

3. The nurse is gathering information about the health practices of an adult female client. The nurse should ask the client about which items related to health promotion?

1. Number of viable pregnancies and deliveries and number of pregnancies not resulting in a live birth
2. Allergies to medications
3. Performance of self breast examination
4. Results of the last Papanicolaou (Pap) test

4. The nurse is assessing a child and the mother states that the child just had a measles, mumps, and rubella (MMR) vaccine at age 12. Where would the nurse document this information in the health record?

1. Under past medical history
2. In review of systems
3. In health practices section
4. Under chief complaint

5. When completing the review of systems the nurse would ask which questions to gather information about past medical history? Select all that apply.

1. "Are you having any difficulty hearing?"
2. "Have you had any throat problems?"
3. "Tell me more about your eye surgery two years ago."
4. "Do you have a productive cough?"
5. "Can you please describe the pain in your neck?"

6. Which question would the nurse ask to gather information about the client's health beliefs?

1. "What is the name of the clinic you use for healthcare?"
2. "Can you tell me about your current abdominal pain?"
3. "What do you think it means to be healthy?"
4. "What type of health insurance do you have?"

7. When orienting a new nurse to a hospital unit, the nurse preceptor would reinforce which principles of appropriate documentation in the client record? Select all that apply.

1. Accurate
2. Complete
3. Computerized
4. Confidential
5. Completed according to professional standards

8. The nurse documents that the client has crackles bilaterally in the lower lobes of the lungs after completing a flow sheet for other assessment data. What format of documentation is this nurse most likely using?

1. Narrative notes
2. SOAP notes
3. Charting by exception
4. APIE notes

9. The adult male client is seeking care for a neurological health problem affecting his ability to carry out activities of daily living (ADLs). Which question during the assessment would be most appropriate for the nurse to ask to gather more data?

1. "Can you give more information about the previous treatment you had for the problem?"
2. "Have you ever had surgery?"
3. "Does the problem cause you discomfort?"
4. "Can you please tell me more about the problem?"

⑩ An adult male client has an appointment at a health clinic and the reason for the visit on the health record is listed as "leg pain." Which initial question would the nurse ask the client to begin the health history?

1. "What problem has brought you to the clinic today?"
2. "Do you have leg pain?"
3. "Can you tell me what kind of leg pain you are having?"
4. "Do you have burning leg pain?"

➤ *See pages 14–15 for Answers and Rationales.*

ANSWERS & RATIONALES

Pretest

① **Answer: 1** **Rationale:** The purpose of the health history is to document the client's perceptions of his or her health, which is subjective data. Tactile fremitus and breath sounds (option 2), vital signs (option 3), and respiratory excursion and effort (option 4) are objective data. They are part of the physical assessment, which is is the head-to-toe examination of the client.
Cognitive Level: Application **Client Need:** Health Promotion and Maintenance **Integrated Process:** Communication and Documentation **Content Area:** Adult Health: Respiratory **Strategy:** Differentiate between subjective and objective data in each option. A health history is subjective data yielding information in the client's own words and perceptions about biographical data, past and present health information, family history, review of systems, and health practices. For this reason, eliminate each incorrect option that focuses on objective data, which is measurable or observable to another person. **Reference:** D'Amico, D. & Barbarito, C. (2007). *Health & physical assessment in nursing.* Upper Saddle River, NJ: Pearson Education, Inc., p. 4.

② **Answer: 1, 2, 3** **Rationale:** The components of a health history include past and present medical history as well as a review of systems. Physical assessment and vital signs are components of the overall health assessment.
Cognitive Level: Application **Client Need:** Health Promotion and Maintenance **Integrated Process:** Nursing Process: Assessment **Content Area:** Child Health **Strategy:** Recall that a health history is composed of biographical data, perceptions of health, past and present history, family history review of systems, and health practices. Focus on the word *history* to choose items that are reported by the client rather than observed by the nurse. **Reference:** D'Amico, D. & Barbarito, C. (2007). *Health & physical assessment in nursing.* Upper Saddle River, NJ: Pearson Education, Inc., p. 4.

③ **Answer: 3** **Rationale:** Subjective data includes any information that the client experiences, such as perceptions of pain and other sensations within the body. Subjective data is that which can only be relayed to the nurse by the client. Vital signs (option 1), peripheral pulses (option 2), and heart sounds (option 4) are part of the objective data that the nurse identifies.
Cognitive Level: Application **Client Need:** Health Promotion and Maintenance **Integrated Process:** Communication and Documentation **Content Area:** Adult Health: Cardiovascular **Strategy:** Recall that subjective data is information the client verbalizes and objective data is information that the nurse can observe. Evaluate each option according to this criterion. **Reference:** D'Amico, D. & Barbarito, C. (2007). *Health & physical assessment in nursing.* Upper Saddle River, NJ: Pearson Education, Inc., pp. 4–5.

④ **Answer: 3** **Rationale:** Objective data is information the nurse can directly obtain and verify. The nurse can observe distention (using inspection) and active bowel sounds (using auscultation). The nurse cannot observe a headache (option 1), nausea (option 4), or a history of chicken pox (option 2). Subjective data is obtained during the review of systems, the aspect of the health history in which the nurse verbally gathers data from the client.
Cognitive Level: Application **Client Need:** Health Promotion and Maintenance **Integrated Process:** Communication and Documentation **Content Area:** Adult Health: Gastrointestinal **Strategy:** Eliminate options in quotations as they are subjective data, which is obtained from the client. Recognize that the only option containing information detectable by the nurse is option 3 (abdominal distention and active bowel sounds). **Reference:** D'Amico, D. & Barbarito, C. (2007). *Health & physical assessment in nursing.* Upper Saddle River, NJ: Pearson Education, Inc., pp. 4–5.

⑤ **Answer: 4** **Rationale:** The problem-oriented charting format is either the subjective, objective, assessment, and planning (SOAP) format, or the assessment, problem, intervention, and evaluation (APIE) format. Documenting on a flow sheet is a method of using checklists with space for clarifying data. Narrative charting uses words, phrases, and sentences. Charting by exception is where variations from predetermined standards are documented.
Cognitive Level: Comprehension **Client Need:** Safe Effective Care Environment: Management of Care **Integrated Process:** Communication and Documentation **Content Area:** Child Health **Strategy:** SOAP documentation involves

documenting a problem after drawing conclusions from the subjective and objective data gathered and planning interventions to correct the problem. This information will help you to systematically eliminate each incorrect option. **Reference**: D'Amico, D. & Barbarito, C. (2007). *Health & physical assessment in nursing.* Upper Saddle River, NJ: Pearson Education, Inc., pp. 6–7.

6 **Answer: 3, 2, 5, 1, 4** **Rationale**: Date of birth (option 3) is an item in the category of biographical data, which is gathered first. Why the client came to the clinic (option 2) is the chief complaint or reason for seeking care and is included in the category of present health or illness, which is gathered second. Assessment of prior hospitalizations (option 5) is part of the past history, which is gathered third. Family history of disorders (option 1) is the fourth category of assessment. Inquiring about support systems is part of the psychosocial history, which is assessed fifth. The sixth category, review of systems, is not assessed in this question.
Cognitive Level: Application **Client Need**: Health Promotion and Maintenance **Integrated Process**: Communication and Documentation **Content Area**: Fundamentals **Strategy**: Note the critical words *proper sequence* in the question. This tells you that there is a correct order in which the health history is collected and cues you to recall the categories of data to be collected and their order (biographical data, present health or illness, past history, family history, psychosocial history, review of body systems). Next, determine which health history category each option refers to. Finally, place the specific options in the sequence that matches the defined order for health history data collection. **Reference**: D'Amico, D. & Barbarito, C. (2007). *Health & physical assessment in nursing.* Upper Saddle River, NJ: Pearson Education, p. 167.

7 **Answer: 1** **Rationale**: After completing a health assessment the nurse systematically analyzes the data and then plans care for the client (option 1). Only abnormal findings are reported to the healthcare provider (option 2). Interdisciplinary care planning meetings (option 3) are a team approach to developing a plan to resolve problems. Goals (option 4) are developed to address health problems found on assessment once the nurse has completed the analysis phase of the nursing process, which leads to nursing diagnoses.
Cognitive Level: Application **Client Need**: Health Promotion and Maintenance **Integrated Process**: Nursing Process: Implementation **Content Area**: Adult Health: Respiratory **Strategy**: The nursing process is a systematic approach to provide care for clients based on assessment findings. Realize that the question is asking what to do with data once it has been obtained. Recall that these steps are assessment, analysis/nursing diagnosis, planning, implementation and evaluation. Select the option that best reflects the analysis/diagnosis phase. **Reference**: D'Amico, D. & Barbarito, C. (2007). *Health & physical assessment in nursing.* Upper Saddle River, NJ: Pearson Education, Inc., p. 11.

8 **Answer: 3** **Rationale**: If a client presents with a headache, the nurse documents it as a subjective complaint because the nurse cannot observe a headache. Option 1, "I have a headache," does not include the timeframe. Option 2 is incorrect because only the length of time is in quotations but the headache complaint should also be in quotations. Option 4 is incorrect because it does not include all the information the client has provided.
Cognitive Level: Application **Client Need**: Safe Effective Care Environment: Management of Care **Integrated Process**: Communication and Documentation **Content Area**: Adult Health: Neurological **Strategy**: Consider that in questions relating to documentation, the correct option is one that will most closely resemble the actual words of the client. With this in mind, evaluate each option and choose option 3 because it matches information in the question. **Reference**: D'Amico, D. & Barbarito, C. (2007). *Health & physical assessment in nursing.* Upper Saddle River, NJ: Pearson Education, Inc., p. 5.

9 **Answer: 1** **Rationale**: Knowing when the sore throat began may provide information as to whether it coincides with event, allergy, or illness (option 1). Option 2 sounds argumentative and is not therapeutic. Option 3 does not obtain useful information as children commonly have sore throats. Asking the client if he or she ever took antibiotics will not yield information about current medication use or further information about the sore throat (option 4).
Cognitive Level: Application **Client Need**: Health Promotion and Maintenance **Integrated Process**: Nursing Process: Assessment **Content Area**: Adult Health: Eye, Ear, Nose, and Throat **Strategy**: Eliminate options 3 and 4 as these questions do not produce information about current illness. Eliminate option 2 realizing that this is not therapeutic communication. Option 1 is question that allows the client to elaborate on the problem and provide needed information to the nurse. **Reference**: D'Amico, D. & Barbarito, C. (2007). *Health & physical assessment in nursing.* Upper Saddle River, NJ: Pearson Education, Inc., pp. 170–173.

10 **Answer: 2** **Rationale**: Family history is information about diseases that family members have experienced. The nurse should gather information about a family history of heart disease, hypertension, stroke, cancers, autoimmune diseases, mental health disorders, and diabetes. History of gallbladder surgery (option 1), two pregnancies (option 3), and performing self breast examinations (option 4) are part of the client history.
Cognitive Level: Application **Client Need**: Health Promotion and Maintenance **Integrated Process**: Nursing Process: Assessment **Content Area**: Adult Health: Cardiovascular **Strategy**: The critical words in the question are *family history*. This tells you that the focus of the question is on information about the client's family, not the client herself. Evaluate each of the options and choose option 2 because of the critical word *maternal*, indicating this information pertains to the client's mother. **Reference**: D'Amico, D. & Barbarito, C. (2007). *Health & physical assessment in nursing.* Upper Saddle River, NJ: Pearson Education, Inc., p. 173.

ANSWERS & RATIONALES

Posttest

1 Answer: 2 Rationale: Alcohol is a substance that may worsen many medical conditions and also interact with medications. Just because a client consumes alcohol does not mean that the client has an alcohol abuse problem or needs a referral for counseling or a self-help group. **Cognitive level:** Application **Client Need:** Health Promotion and Maintenance **Integrated Process:** Nursing Process: Assessment **Content Area:** Adult Health: Musculoskeletal **Strategy:** Eliminate option 3 as it would block communication by putting the client on the defensive. Options 1 and 4 are similar as one makes a referral for counseling and the other for a self-help group. Option 2 would reassure the client that the nurse is there to help and would keep the lines of communication open without upsetting the client. **Reference:** D'Amico, D. & Barbarito, C. (2007). *Health & physical assessment in nursing.* Upper Saddle River, NJ: Pearson Education, Inc., p.172.

2 Answer: 1 Rationale: Taking a health history takes time so it is important to place the client at ease by introducing oneself and making the client comfortable. To maintain confidentiality the nurse should not invite anyone into the examination room unless requested by the client. While the nurse may review information in the medical record, the nurse gathers data from the client during a health history. No information should be tape recorded to maintain confidentiality and also because it may make the client uncomfortable. The nurse may document the history as the client is revealing it. **Cognitive Level:** Application **Client Need:** Health Promotion and Maintenance **Integrated Process:** Nursing Process: Implementation **Content Area:** Fundamentals **Strategy:** Eliminate all options that do not make the client comfortable. Option 1 puts the client at ease and will enable the client to fully participate in the interview process. Recognize that the other options might make the client uncomfortable or put him or her on the defensive. **Reference:** D'Amico, D. & Barbarito, C. (2007). *Health & physical assessment in nursing.* Upper Saddle River, NJ: Pearson Education, Inc., pp. 165–166.

3 Answer: 3 Rationale: The health practice that promotes health in the female client is the performance of monthly self breast exam. Data about previous pregnancies, allergies, and the results of the last Pap smear are part of the previous medical history, not current health practices. **Cognitive Level:** Application **Client Need:** Health Promotion and Maintenance **Integrated Process:** Nursing Process: Assessment **Content Area:** Adult Health: Reproductive **Strategy:** Eliminate all options that do not promote health. Eliminate options that provide data related to the past medical history such as allergies, pregnancy history, and results of tests. **Reference:** D'Amico, D. & Barbarito, C. (2007). *Health & physical assessment in nursing.* Upper Saddle River, NJ: Pearson Education, Inc., pp. 171–172.

4 Answer: 1 Rationale: The immunization record is part of the past medical history (option 1). Review of systems is the component of the health history that reviews each system for diseases and problems (option 2). The health practice section documents cultural health practices and health promotion activities (option 3). The chief complaint is the problem that leads the client to seek healthcare (option 4). **Cognitive Level:** Application **Client Need:** Health Promotion and Maintenance **Integrated Process:** Communication and Documentation **Content Area:** Child Health **Strategy:** Recall that the chief complaint is the current problem to eliminate option 4. Note the word *systems* in option 2 (referring to body systems) to eliminate that option. Choose option 1 over option 3 after considering either that health practices may be health promotion activities or that immunizations are part of the past medical history. **Reference:** D'Amico, D. & Barbarito, C. (2007). *Health & physical assessment in nursing.* Upper Saddle River, NJ: Pearson Education, Inc., p. 172.

5 Answer: 2, 3 Rationale: A review of systems is a method to gather information about past medical history. Asking about throat problems (option 2) or talking about eye surgery from two years ago (option 3) provides past medical history data. Asking about trouble with the throat assesses the current health problem (option 1). Asking about a productive cough or pain in the neck assesses a current illness (option 5). **Cognitive Level:** Application **Client Need:** Health Promotion and Maintenance **Integrated Process:** Nursing Process: Implementation **Content Area:** Adult Health: Eye, Ear, Nose, and Throat **Strategy:** The critical word in the question is *past*. Eliminate options 1, 4, and 5 as these answers ask about a current problem rather than a past one. Recognize that options 2 and 3 ask about past medical history. **Reference:** D'Amico, D. & Barbarito, C. (2007). *Health & physical assessment in nursing.* Upper Saddle River, NJ: Pearson Education, Inc., p. 175.

6 Answer: 3 Rationale: When gathering information about present health the nurse would ask about the client's health beliefs and practices by asking for the definition of being healthy (option 3). Asking for the healthcare clinic name is part of the demographic information (option 1). Having the client describe abdominal pain is part of the present health history and does not provide data about health belief practices (option 2). Asking about health insurance is part of the demographic information (option 4). **Cognitive Level:** Application **Client Need:** Health Promotion and Maintenance **Integrated Process:** Nursing Process: Assessment **Content Area:** Fundamentals **Strategy:** Eliminate option 2 as it asks about abdominal pain as part of the present health information. Recognize that options 1 and 4 provide demographic information. Note that asking about the definition of health should provide information about health belief patterns and lead you to choose option 3. **Reference:** D'Amico, D. & Barbarito, C. (2007). *Health & physical assessment in nursing.* Upper Saddle River, NJ: Pearson Education, Inc., pp. 171.

7 **Answer: 1, 2, 4, 5** **Rationale:** The crucial elements of documentation are accuracy, completeness, maintaining confidentiality, and completion according to standards. The method of charting, such as a paper medical record or computerized medical record (option 3), is a health systems choice rather than a principle of documentation. **Cognitive Level:** Comprehension **Client Need:** Safe Effective Care Environment: Management of Care **Integrated Process:** Communication and Documentation **Content Area:** Fundamentals **Strategy:** Documentation of client information is a critical action in nursing. All information must be documented accurately, confidentially, appropriately, completely, and according to standards. **Reference:** D'Amico, D. & Barbarito, C. (2007). *Health & physical assessment in nursing.* Upper Saddle River, NJ: Pearson Education, Inc., p. 5.

8 **Answer: 3** **Rationale:** Charting by exception (option 3) is a form of documentation in which the institution has established a standard of "normal" parameters (often contained on a checklist) and the nurse only documents findings outside the established norm. Problem-oriented notes such as SOAP (subjective, data, objective data, assessment, and planning) or APIE (assessment, problem, intervention and evaluation) are problem-focused charting (options 2 and 4). Narrative notes (option 1) use phrases and sentences to describe client data and also client problems. **Cognitive Level:** Comprehension **Client Need:** Safe Effective Care Environment: Management of Care **Integrated Process:** Communication and Documentation **Content Area:** Fundamentals **Strategy:** Eliminate the two options that are similar. SOAP and APIE documentation are similar forms of documentation. Note that the term *narrative notes* implies lengthy documentation and not a form of charting by exception. **Reference:** D'Amico, D. & Barbarito, C. (2007). *Health & physical assessment in nursing.* Upper Saddle River, NJ: Pearson Education, Inc., p. 7.

9 **Answer: 4** **Rationale:** Asking the client to say more about the problem is an open-ended broad question to elicit data (option 4). Asking how the disease process is affecting him or her provides the nurse with functional ability of the client. Asking broad open-ended questions will obtain the most data about the problem. Asking about surgery, pain, and treatment each provide specific data, not comprehensive data, about the problem (options 1, 2, and 3). **Cognitive Level:** Application **Client Need:** Health Promotion and Maintenance **Integrated Process:** Communication and Documentation **Content Area:** Adult Health: Neurological **Strategy:** Open-ended questions promote discussion and provide the nurse with data. Recognize that options 1, 2, and 3 could all be answered by the client with a "yes" or "no" response, which would not provide the needed information to the nurse. **Reference:** D'Amico, D. & Barbarito, C. (2007). *Health & physical assessment in nursing.* Upper Saddle River, NJ: Pearson Education, Inc., p. 159.

10 **Answer: 1** **Rationale:** The nurse would first assess why the client is seeking treatment, which is called the chief complaint or reason for seeking care (option 1). The nurse would want to hear the client's own report of pain rather than asking directly about it from a prior chart notation (option 2). Asking the client about the characteristics of the pain would be follow-up questions after assessing why the client sought care at the clinic (options 3 and 4). **Cognitive Level:** Application **Client Need:** Health Promotion and Maintenance **Integrated Process:** Nursing Process: Implementation **Content Area:** Adult Health: Cardiovascular **Strategy:** Eliminate objective options 2, 3, and 4 as the chief complaint is subjective and the nurse would need to know what brings the client to the clinic today. The nurse should always ask the client to describe the problem for which treatment is sought, which is a broad question to gather the most data. **Reference:** D'Amico, D. & Barbarito, C. (2007). *Health & physical assessment in nursing.* Upper Saddle River, NJ: Pearson Education, Inc., p. 738.

References

Bickley, L. (2010). *Bates guide to physical examination and history taking* (10th ed.). Philadelphia: Lippincott Williams & Wilkins.

D'Amico, D. & Barbarito, C. (2007). *Health & physical assessment in nursing.* Upper Saddle River, NJ: Pearson Education, Inc.

Jarvis, C. (2008). *Physical examination and health assessment* (5th ed.). St. Louis, MO: Elsevier Saunders.

Zator Estes, M. (2009). *Health assessment and physical examination* (4th ed.). Clifton Park, NY: Delmar Cengage Learning.

2

Techniques of Physical Assessment

Chapter Outline

Preparation and Positioning
Equipment

Basic Techniques
Equipment Considerations

Assessment Procedure
Lifespan Considerations

Objectives

➤ Describe the four techniques used to perform a physical assessment.
➤ Describe the purpose and use of equipment utilized to perform a physical assessment.
➤ Identify measures to promote client comfort during a physical assessment.
➤ Describe methods to ensure client privacy and safety during a physical assessment.

Review at a Glance

auscultation the skill of listening to sounds produced by the body with or without equipment

inspection the skill of observing the client in a systematic manner

palpation the skill of assessing the client through the use of touch to determine characteristics of the body

percussion the skill of striking the body to produce a sound with or without an instrument to determine if the underlying structures are fluid-filled, air-filled, or solid

PRETEST

1 Prior to beginning a physical examination of a client, the nurse would carry out which activities? Select all that apply.

1. Wash hands
2. Provide for privacy of the client
3. Obtain a healthcare provider's order
4. Explain the procedure to the client
5. Position the client comfortably

2 The nurse performing a physical assessment is unable to palpate a pulse. What is the best action for the nurse to take at this time?

1. Ask another nurse to check for a pulse
2. Notify the healthcare provider about the finding
3. Page the nursing supervisor to try to palpate the pulse
4. Verify the finding with a Doppler

3 To assess vibration during a physical assessment, the nurse would use which part of the hand?

1. Ulnar aspect
2. Pointer finger
3. Palm
4. Dorsum

4 The nurse is preparing to conduct a physical assessment of a client's chest and will be utilizing all of the following examination techniques. Place the techniques in the correct order for use. All options must be used.

1. Percussion
2. Auscultation
3. Inspection
4. Palpation

5 The nurse has used percussion to assess the client's abdomen. The nurse documents which normal characteristic assessed over the liver in the right upper quadrant?

1. Tympany
2. Resonance
3. Dullness
4. Hyperresonance

6 During physical assessment, the nurse would palpate the skin for which characteristics? Select all that apply.

1. Temperature
2. Texture
3. Pigmentation
4. Moisture
5. Elasticity

7 To determine the quality and intensity of a cardiac murmur, the nurse would take which action?

1. Use a Doppler ultrasound device
2. Use the bell of the stethoscope
3. Percuss the thorax cavity
4. Palpate the chest wall to feel the intensity of the murmur

8 The client is admitted with hydronephrosis. To assess this client's kidneys, the nurse would use which examination technique?

1. Use light palpation
2. Use moderate palpation
3. Use deep palpation
4. Inspect to view edema over the flank

9 The nurse is preparing to assess the client's liver. Which examination technique would the nurse include in this assessment?

1. Inspect the left upper quadrant
2. Palpate the right upper quadrant
3. Percuss the left upper quadrant
4. Auscultate the right upper quadrant

10 In an effort to provide a comfortable environment for a client during a physical assessment, the nurse would take which action?

1. Drape the client prior to beginning the examination
2. Urge the client to have all abnormal findings treated promptly
3. Avoid wearing gloves so the client won't feel as though the nurse does not wish to touch the skin
4. Obtain a signed consent to perform a physical assessment

➤ *See pages 29–31 for Answers and Rationales.*

I. PREPARATION AND POSITIONING

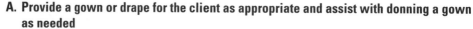

Practice to Pass

To provide privacy before beginning a physical examination, the nurse would implement which of the following actions?

A. Provide a gown or drape for the client as appropriate and assist with donning a gown as needed

B. Provide a comfortable, safe environment by offering the client a pillow or raising the head of examination table

C. Provide warmth by offering a blanket

D. Ensure the client's privacy by closing the door or drawing a curtain around the client

E. Ensure adequate lighting by turning on examination lighting or using a gooseneck lamp

F. Prevent exposing the client by exposing only the body part to be examined

G. Position the client near the bottom of the examination table; ensure the table is positioned to permit access to the client from three sides; elevate the head of the exam table or bed to 45 degrees

H. Explain the procedure to the client

II. EQUIPMENT

A. Examination table or bed: should be at a comfortable height to prevent strain on the examiner's back

B. Drape or blanket: used to prevent exposure of the client
   1. Keeping client warm will increase client comfort and enhance cooperation
   2. Draping client will increase feeling of privacy and prevent possible embarrassment

C. Sink: used to wash hands
   1. Handwashing is a critical preliminary step to each nursing procedure
   2. Standard precautions are used with every client contact to prevent transmission of disease

D. Stethoscope: used to auscultate body sounds; includes four parts: a pair of binaurals (earpieces), tubing, and a bell and diaphragm

E. Otoscope: a lighted instrument used to examine tympanic membrane and external ear

F. Ophthalmoscope: a lighted instrument used to examine internal eye structures

G. Reflex hammer: a tool used to elicit deep tendon reflexes

H. Sphygmomanometer: an instrument used to measure systolic and diastolic blood pressure

I. Tuning fork: a metal instrument used to evaluate auditory and vibratory sensation

J. Thermometer: an electronic instrument used to measure body temperature via the tympanic, axillary, oral, or rectal routes

K. Nasal speculum: a device used to examine nares

L. Tongue depressor: a wooden blade used to assess mouth and throat

M. Snellen eye chart: a standardized chart used to determine visual acuity

N. Examination gloves: vinyl gloves (preferably) used to maintain standard precautions and to protect client and nurse from pathogens; use of latex gloves has fallen into disfavor because of risk of latex allergies in clients

III. BASIC TECHNIQUES

A. *Inspection:* skill of observing client in a systematic manner to obtain data related to health status; begins with first contact with client; includes use of senses of smell and hearing to detect unusual body odors and sounds
   1. Observe client's appearance
   2. Look for data about mental and emotional status
      a. Is there any evidence of distress?
      b. What is client's tone of voice?
      c. Gather data about affect
   3. Compare sides of body for symmetry (normal finding)
      a. Observe for color, size, shape, texture, contour, movement, and drainage
      b. Inspect skin for lesions, scars, masses, pulsations

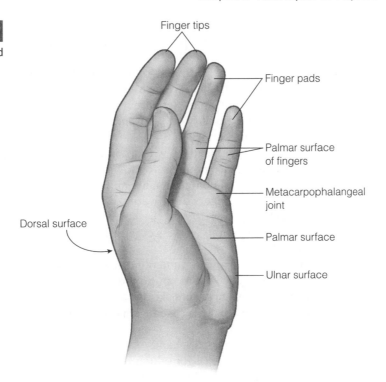

Figure 2-1

Sensitive areas of the hand

Finger tips

Finger pads

Palmar surface
of fingers

Metacarpophalangeal
joint

Palmar surface

Ulnar surface

Dorsal surface

4. When inspecting a large body area, such as the arm, look at entire arm first and then focus on component parts or areas, such as shoulder, upper arm, elbow, forearm, hand, and then fingers

B. *Palpation*: a skill that uses sense of touch to obtain information about characteristics of body parts, such as size and shape, position and mobility, location, pulsation or vibration, texture, moisture, temperature, and swelling (see Figure 2-1)

1. Use fingertips to determine swelling, texture, and pulsation
2. Use finger pads to feel for vibration
3. Grasp with thumb and fingers to feel size and location of organs or masses
4. Use dorsa of hands and fingers to assess temperature of client's skin; when palpating extremities, palpate bilaterally to compare the two sides
5. Use light palpation first (see Figure 2-2a)
   a. This determines skin surface characteristics

Practice to Pass

The nurse understands that what type of palpation will need to be employed to assess the liver?

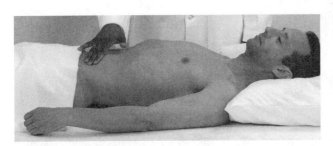

A. Light palpation

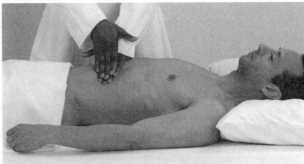

B. Deep palpation

Figure 2-2

    b. To use this technique, place finger pads of dominant hand on skin surface

    c. Move hand slowly and depress finger pads to a depth of 1 centimeter (0.39 inch) to form circles on skin

    d. Use palmar surface of fingers of dominant hand and press downward 1 to 2 centimeters (cm) (0.25 to 0.5 inch) while rotating fingers in a circular or dipping motion to determine pain, tenderness, and pulsations, as well as size, depth, shape, consistency, and mobility of organs near skin surface

6. Proceed to deep palpation

    a. Detects organs that lie deep within a body cavity (e.g., abdominal cavity)

    b. Place palmar surface of fingers of dominant hand on skin surface, and then place extended fingers of non-dominant hand over fingers of dominant hand

    c. Press and guide fingers downward to a depth of 2 to 4 cm (0.75 to 1 inch) (see Figure 2-2b)

7. Use bimanual palpation to assess organs that lie deep within body such as kidneys, uterus, or adnexa

8. Perform palpation in an intermittent manner (not continuous) to prevent pain or injury to organs; remember to use a gentle approach with warm hands, short fingernails

C. *Percussion:* **skill of tapping client's skin to assess underlying structures; tapping produces sounds that are characteristic to specific organs and provides information about location, size, and density of these organs**

    1. Procedure using a stationary hand

        a. Hyperextend middle finger of non-dominant hand and place phalanx (distal portion of finger) against client's skin

        b. Remove all other fingers from client's skin; using dominant second finger, rapidly strike hyperextended finger of non-dominant hand (see Figure 2-3a)

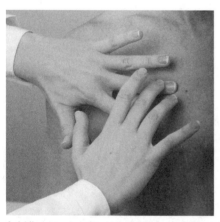

A. Indirect percussion

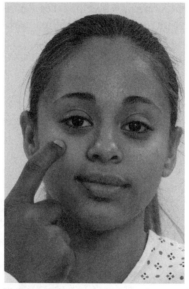

B. Direct percussion

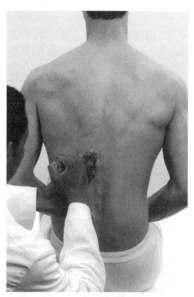

C. Blunt percussion

Figure 2-3

Practice to Pass

The nurse would expect to hear what sound when percussing an empty bladder?

2. Procedure for using one hand: directly strike client's skin (see Figure 2-3b)
3. Procedure for using blunt percussion involves placing non-dominant hand against body surface and striking non-dominant hand with dominant fist to assess pain and tenderness of organs (see Figure 2-3c)
4. Percussion notes (sounds elicited using percussion) will vary depending on tissue density (amount of air or fluid present, or whether solid masses and organs)
5. Penetrates about 5 cm below skin so it's not useful for deep masses
6. May be used to assess pain in underlying structures
7. Use of a hammer may determine deep tendon reflexes
8. Components of sounds produced during percussion:
   a. Amplitude: intensity of sound, described as loudness or softness
   b. Pitch: tone of vibrations described as high- or low-pitched
   c. Quality: differences in sound
   d. Duration: length of time during which a sound takes place
9. Characteristics of percussion sound
   a. Resonance: medium to loud amplitude, low-pitched with clear hollow quality in moderate duration (may hear over lungs)
   b. Hyperresonance: very loud amplitude, low-pitched with a booming quality in long duration (may hear over lung with chronic obstructive pulmonary disease [COPD])
   c. Tympany: very loud amplitude, high-pitched with musical-like sound of very long duration (may hear over stomach and throughout abdomen)
   d. Dull: soft amplitude, high-pitched thud of short duration (may hear over dense organs such as liver or spleen)
   e. Flat: very soft amplitude, high-pitched sound of very short duration (may hear over muscle or bone)

D. *Auscultation:* **skill of listening to sounds produced by body using a stethoscope (does not amplify sound, but rather blocks out extraneous noise in environment)**
   1. Position stethoscope so earpieces are pointed toward nurse's nose; earpieces should be comfortable and fill the ear canal, blocking extraneous environmental noise
   2. Stethoscope tubing should be of heavy duty construction with a length of 12 inches
   3. Stethoscope should have a bell for listening to low-pitched sounds; in some models, the examiner may need to twist the bell to be able to hear sounds; apply using light pressure to auscultate low-pitched sounds; if the bell is held firmly against the skin it will function as a diaphragm
   4. Stethoscope should have a diaphragm for listening to high-pitched sounds
   5. Clean stethoscope with alcohol prep or other cleaning agent between clients
   6. Warm stethoscope prior to placing on client's skin
   7. *Never* listen to client's body through clothing
   8. Become familiar with normal sounds to be able to differentiate abnormal sounds from normal sounds

Practice to Pass

How should the earpieces of a stethoscope be positioned to maximize sound?

IV. EQUIPMENT CONSIDERATIONS

A. **Ophthalmoscope**
   1. Instrument used to illuminate internal eye structures; consists of lens and mirrors to examine eye through the pupil at fundus
   2. Components include a viewer with five apertures, aperture selector dial, mirror, lens selector, lens indicator
      a. Aperture selection is chosen based on intended use
         1) Large aperture is used for dilated pupils
         2) Small aperture is used for undilated pupils

        3) Red free filter is a green light that permits examination of optic disc for hemorrhage (will appear black) and melanin deposits (will appear gray)

        4) Grid aperture is used to assess a fixation pattern and to determine size or location of lesions

        5) Slit is used to examine anterior portion of eye and to assess elevation or depression of lesions on fundus

     b. Lens indicator shows number of lens in examining position

        1) Black numbers indicate a positive lens from 0 to 40; this lens compensates for farsightedness

        2) Red numbers indicate a negative lens from 0 to negative 20; this lens compensates for nearsightedness

B. Otoscope

    1. Instrument that directs light into ear canal to view internal ear structures

    2. Choose largest speculum that will fit into ear so tympanic membrane may be assessed

C. Nasal speculum

    1. An attachment that is placed on an otoscope to examine nares

    2. Choose shortest, broadest speculum that will permit full viewing of nares

D. Automatic blood pressure cuff or sphygmomanometer and stethoscope are used to obtain systolic and diastolic blood pressure

E. Snellen eye chart for visual acuity

    1. Have client stand 20 feet from chart

    2. Ask client to read down chart to last line he or she can see clearly

V. ASSESSMENT PROCEDURE

A. Maintain infection control practices

    1. Clean all equipment used to examine client to prevent nosocomial infection

    2. Use standard precautions to minimize transmission of disease

    3. Remember to wash hands for 15 seconds before and after assessing client

    4. Wear gloves and protective attire including eyewear when needed

    5. Dispose of all equipment and waste in proper receptacle

B. Initiation and approach to assessment

    1. Proceed in a confident unhurried manner

    2. When performing an assessment, take into account the client's culture so as not to offend client or violate his or her health practices (see Table 2-1)

    3. Reduce client's anxiety and provide reassurance when necessary

    4. Begin by taking vital signs as this is a familiar procedure and is usually non-threatening

    5. Permit client to undress in private if not already undressed; offer assistance with undressing and donning a gown and/or drape as needed

    6. Explain each step of the assessment

    7. Always begin with inspection; inspecting skin of exposed body part is usually noninvasive

    8. Proceed in a systematic manner (head to toe)

    9. Do not expose the client unnecessarily

    10. During assessment it may be appropriate to educate client about assessment findings or his or her body, and may be an opportunity to establish trust and rapport; do not explain every aspect of the assessment or every finding in case there is an abnormal finding that requires further investigation prior to discussing it with the client

    11. Document findings appropriately

    12. Summarize findings with client

Practice to Pass

The nurse should begin a physical assessment of the client with what assessment technique?

Table 2-1 Cultural Phenomena Impacting Healthcare

Cultural Group	Communication	Temporal Relations	Dietary Concerns	Family Patterns	Health Beliefs	Health Practices
African Americans	Primary language is English. May use Black English, Pidgin, or Gullah. Highly verbal. Open communication about personal health and feelings with friends and family. Use touch readily with family and friends. Demonstrative facial expressions.	Relaxed about time. Present oriented.	High-fat, fried food diet. Early introduction of solids to infants. Muslims—no pork. Approximately 75% of African Americans are lactose intolerant.	Matriarchal. Value elders. Extended family closeness.	Sickness is a separation between God and humans. Health is harmony with nature. Illness is a disruption in harmony due to "bad spirits."	Religious and spiritual activities, especially prayer. Use home remedies, folk healers, and Western care. Often decreased access to healthcare.
Appalachians	English is the dominant language. May use Elizabethan or Chaucerian English. Pronunciation and word usage are generally local, not standard English. Concrete and direct in response to questions. Physical distancing in all settings during communication. Direct eye contact viewed as impolite.	In touch with rhythms of the body, not the clock. Present oriented.	Introduce foods including grease, coffee, and sugar to infants at early age. Snacks replace meals in adolescents. Limited knowledge of nutrition in health promotion and disease prevention.	Patriarchal. Older women preserve culture and impact healthcare decisions. Elders are respected. Obligation to family outweighs all other obligations.	Health includes body, mind, and spirit. Disease is not a problem unless it interferes with functioning. Fatalism—what happens is God's will.	Use folk remedies and self-medication. Seek help only when folk remedies fail and when condition becomes severe.
Arab Americans	Dominant language is Arabic. Colloquial language is used in everyday living. English is common second language. Use repetition, exaggeration, and gesturing. Outward display of emotion is demonstration of concern. Resist revelation of personal information. Sensitive to authority. Respond best to courtesy and initiating encounters with social conversation or "small talk." Touch between nonmarried individuals of the opposite sex is not acceptable.	Belief in predestination. Both good and evil are "God's will." Nonchalant about time.	Diet reflects USDA pyramid. Muslims eat no pork. Bread is served at every meal. Lamb and chicken are main meats. Muslims fast during month of Ramadan. No foods or fluids including water during daylight hours.	Patriarchal and hierarchical. The senior male member is the decision maker. Male role is to protect the women and family. Respect elders. Hijab—the covering of all but hands and face—provides protection for females.	Associate good health with good eating and fasting to cure disease. Good health means one has the ability to fulfill one's roles. Illness is attributed to diet, hot-cold shifts, exposure of the stomach during sleep, spiritual distress, envy, or the evil eye. Some belief in supernatural agents as the cause of disease.	Combine prayer with conventional medicine. Seek care for problems, not very involved in prevention. Not self-directive. The family oversees care. Disability and mental illness are social stigmas. Most respect is given to male physicians.

(continued)

23

Table 2-1 Cultural Phenomena Impacting Healthcare (Continued)

Cultural Group	Communication	Temporal Relations	Dietary Concerns	Family Patterns	Health Beliefs	Health Practices
Chinese Americans	Official language is Mandarin. Many dialects are spoken. Direct questions, instructions given in order, and simple sentences are best understood. May say they understand to avoid "loss of face." Share information when a trusting relationship is established. Dislike touch by strangers.	Time is cyclic as with the cycle of life. Two concepts regarding time: In "Chinese time," lateness is expected. In second view, punctuality is a sign of respect.	Regional differences exist. Rice is a staple in diet. Meat is included in diet but predominance is of vegetables and fruits. Genetic predisposition to lactose intolerance.	Male dominance. Children are highly valued, especially male children. Elders are venerated. Extended family is important, commonly with strong bonds and interdependence.	Two forces, yin and yang, are in balance to maintain health. Traditional concept of Qi as the vital force of life. Some is inherited; some is from the environment.	Traditional Chinese medicine, Western medicine, or both. Do not always provide information about all healthcare treatments and practices. Share medications with others. Herbal treatments common. May distrust Western practitioners because of the pain and invasiveness of care.
Cuban Americans	Dominant language is Spanish. First generation prefers Spanish over English. Second generation uses English or Spanglish (mixing of the two languages). Value courtesy and respect. Speech is rapid and loud in volume.	Present oriented. Cuban time is followed in which there is a flexible period of 1 to 2 hours after a scheduled time for events to begin or for individuals to arrive at appointments.	High fat, starch, and calorie diet. Root crops (yams, yucca, malanga, plantains) are a large part of diet. Foods include rice, beans, beef, and pork. Meats are generally fried.	Patriarchal. Family is the most important social unit.	Health is associated with overweight. Fatalistic—believe they lack control over their lives. Santeria: folk practice with the use of herbs, rituals, and ceremonies to diagnose and cure illness.	Use of botanica to obtain traditional teas, potions, or poultices from plants. Family is the primary source of advice for healthcare. In the U.S.— accept Western medicine and seek primary provider and preventive services when accessible via insurance.
European Americans	Language: English. Insist on personal space. Tolerate embraces from close friends. In public, maintain neutral facial expression.	Future oriented.	Food types associated with holidays and social occasions (hot dogs at ball games, turkey at Thanksgiving). Influenced by ancestry. Rituals influence intake (coffee break).	Nuclear family is "professed" norm. Egalitarian power in family.	Health is individual responsibility. Believe in germ theory. Illness results from pathology or injury that can be prevented or dealt with.	Self-care practices. Use healthcare system for all aspects of healthcare. Use resources to learn about health and illness. Want to be involved in decision making regarding health and treatment.

Table 2-1 Cultural Phenomena Impacting Healthcare (Continued)

Cultural Group	Communication	Temporal Relations	Dietary Concerns	Family Patterns	Health Beliefs	Health Practices
Filipino Americans	National language is Filipino or Tagalog with 8 distinct dialects. English is second national language. Cadence and inflection are influenced by the ethnic language dialect. Contextual in communication. "Actions speak louder than words." Eye contact varies—some avoid with elders to show respect. Nodding is common during conversation but does not always indicate understanding—may mean simply listening.	Relaxed outlook on life. Filipino time means one can be 1 to 2 hours late for social appointments. In America, demand respect for punctuality.	Fish, chicken, and pork are primary sources for protein. Somewhat lactose intolerant. Salt and vinegar are used in food preparation and preservation. Rice, fruits, and vegetables are staples in the diet.	Egalitarian relationships. Respect is important and caring for aging parents is integral.	Fatalistic—accept events as up to God. Health is a result of balance. Illness is the result of imbalance, that is, personal irresponsibility or irregularity.	Share medications; take medications if they have been effective for others. Stoicism. Sick individual assumes dependent role and allows family to make decisions. Readily accept Western medicine but may also use folk healers.
Jewish Americans	English is the predominant language. First-generation immigrants may speak Yiddish. Hasidic males do not touch females other than their wife. Non-Hasidic—more informal.	Live for today but plan for the future and always have respect and honor for the past. Holidays and Sabbath begin at sunset.	Religious Jews follow Kosher rules—no pork, no dairy and meat at the same meal.	Family is the core unit of society. Genders share roles for work and child rearing. Respect and honor parents.	Each person has a duty to maintain physical and mental health. Preservation of life is paramount.	Health conscious. Respect for physicians. Follow instructions to maintain health and readily seek help for problems.
Mexican Americans	Dominant language is Spanish. There are many regional dialects. Speech is often high pitched, rapid, and loud. Eye contact is considered rude. Touch is acceptable. Reveal personal information when trust is established.	Present oriented. Relaxed concept of time. Schedules and appointment times are flexible.	Diet varies according to region. Rice, beans, and tortillas are staples. Spices are used in preparation. Food is source for socialization.	Patriarchal. Machismo—men are wiser and stronger. Family takes precedence over work or any other obligation.	Fatalism—illness is God's will. Good health is equated with being free of pain. Belief in hot and cold theory of disease and evil eye.	Folk and Western medicine used—often dictated by economics. Stoicism. Physicians and nurses often seen as outsiders. Liberal use of OTC and antibiotic medications.

(continued)

Table 2-1	Cultural Phenomena Impacting Healthcare (Continued)					
Cultural Group	**Communication**	**Temporal Relations**	**Dietary Concerns**	**Family Patterns**	**Health Beliefs**	**Health Practices**
Native Americans	Dominant language varies with tribe. Many use English and native language. Some distrust of outsiders. Reveal personal information only when trust is established. Personal space requirement is greater than European Americans. Touch and eye contact vary with tribe.	Not future oriented. Time has little meaning or importance.	Corn is a staple in diet. Few fruits and vegetables. Lamb and fried chicken are frequent meat sources. Many are lactose intolerant.	Matrilineal. Grandmothers and mothers are most important. Elders are respected.	Wellness is equated with harmony with surroundings.	Medicine men are used to diagnose and treat disharmony. Variable acceptance of Western medicine.
Vietnamese Americans	Dominant language is Vietnamese. English is spoken by second generation. Personal feelings are not discussed openly with others. Eye contact is disrespectful. Touch is limited outside of the home. Silence is used to demonstrate negative emotions. Prefer more personal space than in other cultures.	Less concerned about the present and time schedules than are European Americans. Frequently late for appointments. Little attention to precise age.	Rice is a dietary staple. Fish, chicken, tofu, and green vegetables in abundance.	Patriarchal. Always includes an extended family structure. Immigrants are more egalitarian as women are increasingly employed and as they assimilate. Respect for elders.	Fatalism. Life is predetermined and illness is a punishment for wrongdoing. Good health is equated with harmony in hot and cold.	Family is the main provider of care. Prefer same-sex healthcare providers. Believe Western medicine is effective but not always accurate. As a result may over- or underuse prescribed drugs. Some use folk healers and prohibit female touching by healthcare providers—use a doll to explain and indicate problems.

Source: D'Amico, D. & Barbarito, C. (2007). *Health & physical assessment in nursing.* Upper Saddle River, NJ: Pearson Education, Inc., Table 4.1, pp. 73–76.

VI. LIFESPAN CONSIDERATIONS

A. Infants: assessment is not as difficult as long as infant feels secure
1. Have parents stay with infant to provide security
2. Place infant on examination (exam) table or permit parent to hold him or her for aspects of exam where feasible
3. Proceed with exam after infant is fed
4. Keep infant warm and warm all equipment
5. Use a soft tone of voice and make eye contact with infant
6. Auscultate heart, lungs, and abdomen when infant is asleep if possible
7. Perform all invasive steps last

B. Toddler: assessment is often difficult because of child's developmental stage and possible fear; keep in mind that restraint by device or parent/caregiver may be needed
1. Position child in parent's lap
2. Provide security and distraction
3. Children may need to be undressed one article of clothing at a time as assessment progresses
4. Provide simple instructions
5. Demonstrate procedure on a favorite toy or on child's parents
6. Offer praise for child's assistance
7. Perform all invasive steps last
8. Engage child whenever possible

C. Preschool child: assessment will be easier if the child is permitted to be independent
1. Have a parent present; a parent may hold child or child may be placed on exam table depending on child's development
2. Include child in any conversation and give simple direction
3. Remember that child may not like to undress
4. Do not offer child a choice unless there is a choice
5. Permit child to explore equipment
6. Use distraction and engage child in play where appropriate
7. Reassure child

D. School age child: assessment is generally easy because a child at this age is usually cooperative
1. Position child on exam table
2. Speak to child but remember that child may not fully understand procedure
3. Drape the children appropriately
4. The child should be in underwear even after clothing is removed and drape is placed
5. Answer the child's questions
6. Proceed with the assessment in a systematic manner

E. Adolescent: assessment is performed as it is for an adult
1. Provide privacy unless the adolescent wishes that his or her parent be present; usually the assessment is performed in private
2. Position on the exam table
3. During the exam provide education about the body as well as health teaching
4. Proceed in systematic manner
5. Apprise parents of findings after child is dressed

F. Older adult client: assessment may be difficult due to chronic health conditions
1. Have client sit on exam table until assessment requires lying; minimize position changes and assist with position changes as needed
2. Slow pace of examination as needed to accommodate client's physical condition
3. Provide for psychosocial needs as appropriate
4. Provide health teaching as appropriate

5. Answer questions and explain findings
6. Summarize findings after client is dressed; provide dressing assistance if needed

Case Study

The health center is conducting health screenings for clients who do not have health insurance. The male nurse is assigned to conduct the physical assessment on a Middle Eastern female client. The client looks anxious and states, "I do not wish to be examined."

1. What should the nurse do at this time?

2. What factors should be considered for this client?

3. What are the culture beliefs of Middle Eastern clients?

4. How should the nurse reassure the client?

5. Should the nurse encourage the client to be examined with family members present? Briefly explain your rationale.

For suggested responses, see page 308

POSTTEST

1 The nurse has just percussed a client's abdomen and wishes to document the characteristics of the sounds produced. Which descriptor would the nurse use to document the sound quality if there were normal abdominal findings?

1. Soft and dull over the right and left lower quadrants
2. Tympany over the left upper quadrant and dullness over the right upper quadrant
3. Hyperresonance over the right upper quadrant
4. Many gurgling sounds over all aspects of the abdomen

2 Upon completion of the physical examination of a client, the nurse should take which action?

1. Have another nurse confirm all findings
2. Notify the healthcare provider of all findings
3. Inform the client of the findings
4. Verify all findings with the client

3 When using the bell of the stethoscope it is essential that the nurse implement which action?

1. Have the client lie supine
2. Encourage the client to cough prior to auscultating the chest
3. Hold the stethoscope lightly against the chest
4. Verify findings with a Doppler

4 To assess the eyes of the client who is farsighted, the nurse should use which part of the ophthalmoscope?

1. Small aperture
2. Black numbers in a clockwise position
3. Red numbers in a counterclockwise position
4. Red filter aperture

5 The nurse is using the otoscope to assess the nares of a client. The nurse would select which type of speculum for use in this assessment?

1. Smallest speculum
2. Largest speculum that will fit in the client's ear
3. Shortest broadest speculum
4. Speculum that will provide a broad beam of light

6 To properly prepare the client for a physical assessment, the nurse would utilize which strategy?

1. Obtain written consent to examine the client
2. Provide comfort and privacy for the client
3. Allow the client to keep clothing on if desired
4. Have a family member present to verify findings

7 The nurse is using the skill of percussion to examine the sinuses of an adult client. Which type of percussion technique would be most appropriate for the nurse to use?

1. Direct
2. Blunt
3. Indirect
4. Light

8 The nurse is assessing the client during an employment physical examination. At what point during the examination would the nurse use bimanual palpation?

1. To palpate the chest wall
2. To examine the cardiovascular system
3. To palpate the abdomen
4. To assess the musculoskeletal system

9 A client who is mildly anxious is to undergo a physical assessment. Which of the following is the most appropriate action for the nurse to take?

1. Stay with the client at all times to provide assistance
2. Use an unhurried manner and reassure the client as necessary
3. Proceed with the exam by completing invasive aspects first
4. Ask for a consult to assess the extent of the anxiety

10 When assessing the client's skin, the nurse observes an open draining wound. What action would be most appropriate for the nurse to take at this time?

1. Notify the healthcare provider who is on call to evaluate the wound
2. Stop examining the wound, wash hands, and proceed with the remainder of the examination
3. Consult the wound care nurse for additional assessment
4. Wash hands, apply gloves, and continue assessing the wound

➤ *See pages 31–33 for Answers and Rationales.*

ANSWERS & RATIONALES

Pretest

1 **Answer: 1, 2, 4, 5** **Rationale:** Prior to performing any assessment or procedure the nurse should wash hands (option 1) or use another method of hand hygiene, such as an alcohol rub, to prevent infection. The nurse should also ensure client privacy (option 2) and make the client as comfortable as possible (option 5). The nurse should explain the procedure to the client (option 4) so the client can anticipate what is to follow, which may help the client to be more relaxed. The nurse would not need a healthcare provider's order to carry out the assessment (option 3) because physical assessment is within the scope of nursing practice.
Cognitive Level: Application **Client Need:** Health Promotion and Maintenance **Integrated Process:** Nursing Process: Planning **Content Area:** Fundamentals **Strategy:** First note that the question indicates that more than one response is correct, by the words *select all that apply*. Next, note that the wording of the question indicates the correct responses are items that the nurse would do in the situation. Read each option, one at a time, to make each selection. Consider that client preparation for any procedure should include washing hands, providing privacy, explaining what will happen during the procedure, and positioning the client. **Reference:** D'Amico, D. & Barbarito, C. (2007). *Health & physical assessment in nursing.* Upper Saddle River, NJ: Pearson Education, p. 96.

2 **Answer: 4** **Rationale:** The nurse should use an ultrasound device called a Doppler to listen for a pulse that is unable to be found by palpation. The healthcare provider (option 2) would not be notified until the assessment is complete. Additional nurses (options 1 and 3) would not

be used to verify the finding as the most effective assessment technique would be to use the Doppler.
Cognitive Level: Application **Client Need:** Health Promotion and Maintenance **Integrated Process:** Nursing Process: Implementation **Content Area:** Fundamentals **Strategy:** Note that options 1 and 3 are similar and therefore neither of them can be correct. Recall that it is important to fully assess a client prior to notifying another individual to help eliminate option 2. Alternatively, reason that the nurse should exhaust all nursing interventions that the individual nurse could perform before consulting with another healthcare team member. **Reference:** D'Amico, D. & Barbarito, C. (2007). *Health & physical assessment in nursing.* Upper Saddle River, NJ: Pearson Education, p. 103.

3 **Answer: 1** **Rationale:** The nurse would use the ulnar aspect of the hand (option 1) to detect vibrations. The pointer finger (option 2) may be used for fine tactile discrimination to determine lumps, swelling, pulsations, and texture. The palm (option 3) is not usually used in the assessment of a client. The dorsum of the hand (option 4) is used determine temperature.
Cognitive Level: Application **Client Need:** Health Promotion and Maintenance **Integrated Process:** Nursing Process: Assessment **Content Area:** Fundamentals **Strategy:** Recall the various methods used to perform palpation and then consider assessing vibration as a particular type of palpation. Eliminate option 2 first because the pointer finger is useful for tactile sensation. Next consider that the dorsum of the hand is used to determine temperature to eliminate option 4. Choose option 1 over option 3

recalling that the ulnar aspect of the hand, not the palm, is useful in assessing vibration. **Reference:** D'Amico, D. & Barbarito, C. (2007). *Health & physical assessment in nursing.* Upper Saddle River, NJ: Pearson Education, pp. 97–98.

4 Answer: 3, 4, 1, 2 Rationale: The nurse uses inspection first when assessing the client because this is the least invasive. This helps to promote trust and relaxation in the client for the parts of the examination to follow. Palpation is done next except in an abdominal assessment, in which a nurse would use auscultation prior to palpation to prevent stimulation of bowel sounds. Percussion is usually the third step of the examination process and auscultation is last. **Cognitive Level:** Application **Client Need:** Health Promotion and Maintenance **Integrated Process:** Nursing Process: Assessment **Content Area:** Fundamentals **Strategy:** Specific knowledge of the sequence of physical examination techniques is needed to answer the question. Recall that the first step is to visualize the area under examination. From there, you can use memory to place the skills in order of use. Take time to memorize this fundamental information if this question is difficult. **Reference:** D'Amico, D. & Barbarito, C. (2007). *Health & physical assessment in nursing.* Upper Saddle River, NJ: Pearson Education, p. 104.

5 Answer: 3 Rationale: The liver, located in the right upper quadrant of the abdomen, elicits dullness (option 3) during percussion because of the density of the organ. Tympany (option 1) is produced over hollow air-filled spaces, such as the stomach or the area below the margins of the liver. Resonance (option 2) is produced over lung tissue with no pathology. This sound would be percussed above the upper border of the liver, where lung tissue is found. Hyperresonance (option 4) is produced over the lung of a client with chronic obstructive pulmonary disease. **Cognitive Level:** Application **Client Need:** Health Promotion and Maintenance **Integrated Process:** Communication and Documentation **Content Area:** Adult Health: Gastrointestinal **Strategy:** Review characteristics of percussion. Recall that percussion is used to determine the size and location of an organ, to determine the density of organ, to detect masses, and to elicit pain or reflexes. Recall the various percussion notes, and conclude that dullness is the sound heard over dense organs to choose correctly. **Reference:** D'Amico, D. & Barbarito, C. (2007). *Health & physical assessment in nursing.* Upper Saddle River, NJ: Pearson Education, pp. 98–100.

6 Answer: 1, 2, 4, 5 Rationale: The nurse would palpate the skin for temperature (option 1), which should be warm. Texture (option 2) should be smooth, firm, and even. Palpation is also used to evaluate the skin for moisture (option 4) and the skin should be dry. Palpating for elasticity (option 5) is done by assessing for mobility and turgor. The skin should immediately return to the normal position and not tent. Pigmentation (option 3) is assessed through the use of inspection rather than palpation.

Cognitive Level: Application **Client Need:** Health Promotion and Maintenance **Integrated Process:** Nursing Process: Assessment **Content Area:** Adult Health: Integumentary **Strategy:** To answer this question, visualize how each assessment technique is performed. Recall that palpation indicates touch and then eliminate the single option that is assessed visually with the eyes. **Reference:** D'Amico, D. & Barbarito, C. (2007). *Health & physical assessment in nursing.* Upper Saddle River, NJ: Pearson Education, p. 202.

7 Answer: 2 Rationale: To listen to low frequency sounds, the nurse would use the bell of the stethoscope by placing it lightly on the skin. Murmurs are most often low-pitched sounds. In contrast, the diaphragm of the stethoscope is used to elicit high-pitched sounds, which may characterize some murmurs. A Doppler (option 1) is used to auscultate for peripheral pulses that are not palpable. Percussion (option 3) will provide information on body structures but will not provide information on low- or high-pitched sounds. Palpation (option 4) will not provide information on sounds, although it gives information about characteristics of the body. **Cognitive Level:** Application **Client Need:** Health Promotion and Maintenance **Integrated Process:** Nursing Process: Assessment **Content Area:** Adult Health: Cardiovascular **Strategy:** Recall that a cardiac murmur must be heard using the skill of auscultation, which helps you to eliminate options 3 and 4 first. To choose correctly between the remaining options, it is necessary to know the uses for a Doppler in contrast to uses of the bell and the diaphragm of the stethoscope. **Reference:** D'Amico, D. & Barbarito, C. (2007). *Health & physical assessment in nursing.* Upper Saddle River, NJ: Pearson Education, p. 96.

8 Answer: 3 Rationale: Deep palpation (option 3) is used to assess organs that lie deep in the abdominal cavity such as the kidney. Light palpation (option 1) is used to assess the characteristics of the skin such as temperature, pulses, and texture. Moderate palpation (option 2) is not a defined palpation technique. In hydronephrosis there would be no flank edema (option 4). **Cognitive Level:** Application **Client Need:** Health Promotion and Maintenance **Integrated Process:** Nursing Process: Assessment **Content Area:** Adult Health: Renal and Genitourinary **Strategy:** Think about the anatomy of the kidney and consider that this health problem cannot be assessed by inspection; this will help to eliminate option 4. Recall basic physical assessment techniques and use the process of elimination to choose option 3, deep palpation, which is needed to obtain information about this deeply placed organ. **Reference:** D'Amico, D. & Barbarito, C. (2007). *Health & physical assessment in nursing.* Upper Saddle River, NJ: Pearson Education, p. 98.

9 Answer: 2 Rationale: The nurse will palpate the right upper quadrant to assess the size, shape, depth, consistency, and mobility of the organ. The liver does not produce sounds that can be auscultated (option 4). Inspection of the left upper quadrant (option 1) will not provide information about the condition of the liver, because the stomach lies anteriorly in that quadrant. Percussion of the left upper quadrant (option 3) will provide information about either the spleen or stomach. **Cognitive Level:** Application **Client Need:** Health Promotion and Maintenance **Integrated Process:** Nursing Process: Assessment **Content Area:** Adult Health: Gastrointestinal **Strategy:** Think about the location and anatomy of the liver to eliminate options 1 and 3. Review the techniques of assessment to choose correctly between the remaining options. **Reference:** D'Amico, D. & Barbarito, C. (2007). *Health & physical assessment in nursing.* Upper Saddle River, NJ: Pearson Education, p. 98.

10 **Answer: 1** **Rationale:** Properly draping a client will provide warmth during the exam and help to avoid client embarrassment. While clients should seek treatment for abnormal findings (option 2), this is not part of promoting a comfortable environment. When coming in contact with body fluids during the exam, the nurse must follow standard precautions (option 3), so gloves may be worn during part of the exam. There is no need for a specific signed consent for physical assessment (option 4). **Cognitive Level:** Application **Client Need:** Health Promotion and Maintenance **Integrated Process:** Nursing Process: Implementation **Content Area:** Fundamentals **Strategy:** Think about comfort measures, which include positioning the client, providing a blanket for warmth, providing privacy, offering a pillow or raising the head of the examination table, and using standard precautions. **Reference:** D'Amico, D. & Barbarito, C. (2007). *Health & physical assessment in nursing.* Upper Saddle River, NJ: Pearson Education, p. 106.

Posttest

1 **Answer: 2** **Rationale:** Quality of percussion is described by using specific descriptors. In the left upper quadrant the stomach can yield tympany (a hollow sound), while in the right upper quadrant the liver (a dense organ) will produce dullness (option 2). Softness is not a characteristic of percussion but rather palpation (option 1). Hyperresonance is produced on percussion over air-filled organs such as the lungs (option 3). Gurgling may be heard upon auscultation of the abdomen (option 4). **Cognitive Level:** Application **Client Need:** Health Promotion and Maintenance **Integrated Process:** Communication and Documentation **Content Area:** Adult Health: Gastrointestinal **Strategy:** Specific knowledge is needed to correctly answer this question. Recall that the sounds produced by percussion include tympany (a high-pitched sound over hollow organs), resonance (a loud, low-pitched sound), hyperresonance (sound produced when an area of the body has trapped air), dullness (produced over consolidated or solid organs), and flatness (high-pitched tone produced over bone). **Reference:** D'Amico, D. & Barbarito, C. (2007). *Health & physical assessment in nursing.* Upper Saddle River, NJ: Pearson Education, p. 100.

2 **Answer: 3** **Rationale:** The client will wish to know the results of the examination and has a right to the results (option 3). Another nurse is not needed to confirm the results unless the examining nurse is unsure of the findings and would like another nurse to validate a finding (option 1). Health assessment findings need not be reported to the healthcare provider unless there is an abnormality (option 2). The client will not necessarily be able to verify findings due to a lack of healthcare knowledge (option 4). **Cognitive Level:** Application **Client Need:** Health Promotion and Maintenance **Integrated Process:** Nursing Process: Implementation **Content Area:** Fundamentals **Strategy:** Terminating a physical assessment includes providing the client with a recap of the findings and documentation of the findings. Clients usually prefer to have an update on their health. Eliminate option 1 as the nurse does not need a second opinion from another healthcare professional unless there is a questionable finding. Eliminate option 4 as the client cannot verify the findings. Unless there is a grossly abnormal finding the nurse would not notify the physician so eliminate option 3. **Reference:** D'Amico, D. & Barbarito, C. (2007). *Health & physical assessment in nursing.* Upper Saddle River, NJ: Pearson Education, p. 106.

3 **Answer: 3** **Rationale:** When using the bell of a stethoscope the nurse places the stethoscope lightly on the chest wall (option 3). If the nurse uses firm pressure on the bell of the stethoscope it will act as a diaphragm. The bell is used to detect low-pitched sounds. The client may be asked to lie in the left lateral position while performing auscultation of cardiac murmurs. Lying supine will not increase the quality of the sound in the stethoscope (option 1). Encouraging the client to cough prior to auscultating the chest will clear the airways so baseline data can be obtained (option 2). It is not possible to reproduce stethoscope sounds with a Doppler (option 4); a Doppler will detect a pulse that may not be palpated. **Cognitive Level:** Application **Client Need:** Health Promotion and Maintenance **Integrated Process:** Nursing Process: Assessment **Content Area:** Fundamentals **Strategy:** Recall that when using a stethoscope that has both a bell and a diaphragm, the bell of the stethoscope is used for auscultating low-pitched sounds, whereas the diaphragm is used for high-pitched sounds. This will enable you to correctly choose option 3. **Reference:** D'Amico, D. & Barbarito, C. (2007). *Health & physical assessment in nursing.* Upper Saddle River, NJ: Pearson Education, pp. 100–103.

4 **Answer: 2** **Rationale:** The black numbers on the ophthalmoscope are used to examine the eyes of the client who is farsighted (option 2). The small aperture is used to examine the eyes of the client whose pupils are undilated (option 1). The red numbers on the stethoscope are used to examine the eyes of the client who is nearsighted (option 3). The red aperture is used to examine the eyes of the client who may be experiencing a hemorrhage (option 4).

Cognitive Level: Analysis Client Need: Health Promotion and Maintenance Integrated Process: Nursing Process: Assessment Content Area: Adult Health: Eye, Ear, Nose, and Throat Strategy: Specific knowledge of this equipment is needed to answer the question. Recall that the large aperture is used for viewing dilated pupils, and the small aperture is used for undilated pupils. The red free filter shines green light so the optic disk can be inspected for hemorrhage. The grid is used to assess the size and location of lesions. The slit aperture permits the visualization of the elevation or depression of lesions. Reference: D'Amico, D. & Barbarito, C. (2007). *Health & physical assessment in nursing*. Upper Saddle River, NJ: Pearson Education, pp. 103–104.

5 Answer: 3 Rationale: The otoscope is used to examine nares when a nasal speculum is not available. The nurse should select the shortest broadest speculum (option 3). The smallest speculum is not selected for examination of an ear or nares as it will not permit the greatest visualization (option 1). Ear size has no bearing on nares size so it would not be pertinent to measure the speculum that would fit into the ear (option 2). The purpose of the speculum is to provide the narrow beam of light to visualize the nares (option 4).

Cognitive Level: Application Client Need: Health Promotion and Maintenance Integrated Process: Nursing Process: Implementation Content Area: Adult Health: Eye, Ear, Nose, and Throat Strategy: The otoscope is used to inspect the nose or ear. Recall that the nurse should use the broadest speculum that fits in the nose to maximize visualization of the structure. Reference: D'Amico, D. & Barbarito, C. (2007). *Health & physical assessment in nursing*. Upper Saddle River, NJ: Pearson Education, p. 104.

6 Answer: 2 Rationale: Providing privacy and comfort will make the client more comfortable during the assessment (option 2). Most facilities do not require a consent form to conduct a health assessment (option 1). The client should remove clothing and don a gown prior to being examined (option 3). Clothing may prevent adequate access to body structures or interfere with the quality of the examination. Family members should only be permitted in the examination room if the client desires their presence (option 4).

Cognitive Level: Application Client Need: Health Promotion and Maintenance Integrated Process: Nursing Process: Implementation Content Area: Fundamentals Strategy: The client preparation for physical assessment includes providing for privacy, warmth, and comfort and the use of standard precautions. Eliminate option 1 because the physical assessment procedure does not require consent. Eliminate option 3 because the clothing needs to be removed to perform an assessment. Eliminate option 4 because a family member does not verify or receive client health information unless the client approves. Reference: D'Amico, D. & Barbarito, C. (2007). *Health & physical*

assessment in nursing. Upper Saddle River, NJ: Pearson Education, p. 96.

7 Answer: 1 Rationale: The nurse would use direct percussion (option 1). The sinuses would be tapped with the fingertips of the dominant hand. Blunt percussion involves using the non-dominant hand on the body and using a closed fist to strike the non-dominant hand to assess pain and tenderness (option 2). Indirect percussion involves using a finger to strike the hand over the body surfaces to produce a sound (option 3). Light percussion is not a technique (option 4).

Cognitive Level: Application Client Need: Health Promotion and Maintenance Integrated Process: Nursing Process: Assessment Content Area: Adult Health: Eyes, Ears, Nose, and Throat Strategy: Recall that the technique of percussion involves the striking of the examiner's finger to produce sounds over various areas of the body, which is direct percussion. Percussion is used to determine the size and location of organs, to determine density, to detect masses, and to determine pain and elicit reflexes. Eliminate option 4 as there is no technique of light percussion. Eliminate options 2 and 3 as these techniques will be painful on the face. Reference: D'Amico, D. & Barbarito, C. (2007). *Health & physical assessment in nursing*. Upper Saddle River, NJ: Pearson Education, p. 98.

8 Answer: 3 Rationale: The bimanual palpation technique requires the use of both hands to encircle the part of the body to be examined and is used for palpating organs in the abdomen (option 3). The chest wall is not palpated (option 1). Techniques used to examine the chest wall and cardiovascular system include inspection, percussion, and auscultation (option 2). The musculoskeletal system is inspected and lightly palpated but moderate or bimanual palpation is not required as no structures lie deep within the body cavity (option 4).

Cognitive Level: Application Client Need: Health Promotion and Maintenance Integrated Process: Nursing Process: Assessment Content Area: Fundamentals Strategy: Recall that the technique of palpation includes using the fingertips for tactile discrimination. The grasping technique is used to determine the shape of organs, the back of hand is used to discern temperature, and the base of the fingertip is used to detect vibration. The chest wall and musculoskeletal system are not generally palpated. In the abdomen this technique of assessment is used last. The only answer in which a two-handed technique could be utilized is option 3. Reference: D'Amico, D. & Barbarito, C. (2007). *Health & physical assessment in nursing*. Upper Saddle River, NJ: Pearson Education, pp. 95, 96, 100–103.

9 Answer: 2 Rationale: The nurse must display a confident, unhurried attitude and provide reassurance to the client to decrease anxiety (option 2). The nurse should not remain with the client while the client is

dressing or undressing (option 1). Invasive aspects of the physical examination should be deferred until the end to help the client relax and decrease anxiety (option 3). A healthcare provider would not be consulted as anxiety prior to an examination is normal (option 4).
Cognitive Level: Application **Client Need:** Psychosocial Integrity **Integrated Process:** Caring **Content Area:** Fundamentals **Strategy:** Recall that psychosocial needs are addressed with physical needs. To decrease anxiety the nurse should introduce him- or herself, provide privacy, explain all procedures, and proceed in an unhurried manner. **Reference:** D'Amico, D. & Barbarito, C. (2007). *Health & physical assessment in nursing.* Upper Saddle River, NJ: Pearson Education, p. 96.

10 **Answer: 4** **Rationale:** The nurse should employ standard precautions, utilize gloves, and continue the examination (option 4). The physician should not be notified

until all assessment data is gathered so complete information can be related (option 1). The nurse should continue assessing the wound to proceed in a systematic organized manner (option 2). The nurse would not consult the wound care nurse until the initial assessment of the wound is completed (option 3).
Cognitive Level: Analysis **Client Need:** Safe Effective Care Environment: Safety and Infection Control **Integrated Process:** Nursing Process: Implementation **Content Area:** Adult Health: Integumentary **Strategy:** It is essential to prevent the spread of infection through the use of standard precautions. Standard precautions include the use of gloves with every client contact and goggles and gowns when there is danger of coming in contact with blood and body fluids. Recognize that option 4 is the only answer that protects the nurse and the client.
Reference: D'Amico, D. & Barbarito, C. (2007). *Health & physical assessment in nursing.* Upper Saddle River, NJ: Pearson Education, p. 97.

References

Bickley, L. (2010). *Bates guide to physical examination and history taking* (10th ed.). Philadelphia: Lippincott Williams & Wilkins.

D'Amico, D. & Barbarito, C. (2007). *Health & physical assessment in nursing.*

Upper Saddle River, NJ: Pearson Education, Inc.

Jarvis, C. (2008). *Physical examination and health assessment* (5th ed.). St. Louis, MO: Elsevier Saunders.

Zator Estes, M. (2009). *Health assessment and physical examination* (4th ed.). Clifton Park, NY: Delmar Cengage Learning.

ANSWERS & RATIONALES

3 Psychosocial Assessment

Chapter Outline

Overview of Psychosocial Assessment

Conducting a Psychosocial Assessment

Expected Findings

Unexpected Findings

Lifespan Considerations

Documentation

NCLEX-RN® Test Prep

Visit the Companion Website for this book at www.pearsonhighered.com/hogan to access additional practice opportunities and more.

Objectives

➤ Describe factors that affect mental health that are part of psychosocial assessment.

➤ Discuss the various parts of a psychosocial assessment.

➤ Explain how culture is a part of the psychosocial assessment.

➤ Review focused questions to ask during a psychosocial history.

➤ Differentiate normal from abnormal findings obtained during psychosocial assessment.

Review at a Glance

affect outward expression of emotions such as joy, sorrow, anger

anergia lack of energy

anhedonia loss of pleasure; loss of interest in pleasurable activities previously enjoyed

anxiety state of apprehension, dread, uneasiness, or uncertainty generated by a real or perceived threat whose actual source is unidentifiable

body image person's internal image of external physical self

coping mechanisms ways of adjusting to external stressors without changing one's goals or life direction

culture pattern of learned behavior based on values, beliefs, and perceptions of the world taught and shared by members of a group or society

depression severe feeling of sadness, lack of motivation, changes in sleep patterns and appetite, and wanting to withdraw or isolate from others

mental health ability to see oneself as others do and to fit into culture and society where one lives

mental status examination (MSE) tool used to assess ability to think, reason, cope with feelings and stressors, and behave in a socially and culturally acceptable manner

psychosis a disorderly mental state in which a client has difficulty distinguishing reality from his or her own internal perceptions

self-concept feelings and understanding of one's own status as a person

self-esteem feelings of self-respect or self-worth

spirituality belief that there is someone or something in the world more powerful and able to guide individuals

substance abuse purposeful use for at least one month of a drug that results in adverse effects to self or others

suicide the intentional and voluntary taking of one's life

PRETEST

1 The triage nurse in the emergency department (ED) is caring for a 59-year-old male who has a broken leg. The client demands to be taken to the x-ray department immediately because of the stress of the injury on his heart condition. What would be the nurse's first action to care for this client's immediate needs?

1. Bring the client to the x-ray department immediately
2. Begin to establish a therapeutic relationship with the client
3. Sit with the client; maintain good eye contact; and speak in a calm, even voice
4. Begin asking the client what happened and what he was doing when he injured his leg

2 The medical-surgical unit nurse is doing an intake interview with a male client scheduled for left leg amputation the next morning. The client says he has taken lithium (Eskalith) for four years but stopped two days ago because he ran out and could not afford to buy more. The client states he knew he would be okay for a few days until he got to the hospital. What question would the nurse ask next?

1. "Who prescribes your medication and when was your last dose?"
2. "Who prescribes your medication and how often does your prescription indicate you should take it?"
3. "Can you tell me a little about how you began taking lithium?"
4. "Have you had any symptoms of your disorder since you have not been taking your medication?"

3 The nurse has conducted a Folstein Mini Mental Status Exam on a client. After noting that the client had a perfect score, what number would the nurse document on the medical record as the score for this assessment? Provide a numerical response.

4 Once the nurse has established that the client is hearing other voices while the nurse is talking with him or her, the nurse would use which communication strategy?

1. Tell the client that the voices are not real and should be ignored.
2. Indicate that this happens sometimes when clients are stressed.
3. Let the client know that the nurse believes the client is hearing voices, but that the nurse does not hear them.
4. Tell the client the nurse will notify the physician about the client hearing voices.

5 The client reports being hospitalized two weeks ago in another state but for something the client is "not sure should be discussed right now." Which therapeutic communication skill would be most beneficial for the nurse to use at this time?

1. Reframing
2. Keeping in the here and now
3. Use of silence
4. Refocusing

6 The client is standing next to the bed with eyes closed, breathing evenly, with hands clasped, and humming almost inaudibly. When the nurse enters the room the client opens the eyes slowly and says, "I was just taking a moment for myself. This is very stressful but I have a way to work through it now." The nurse believes that the client was involved in which of the following?

1. Prayer
2. Reiki
3. Meditation
4. Yoga

7 When asked to describe himself the client states, "I am fat, too short, and ugly, but I dress well and have good posture, although that does not mean anything about me. My mother made me practice walking and taught me how to buy the right clothes." The nurse concludes that the client has which of the following?

1. High self-esteem
2. Low self-esteem
3. High self-concept
4. Low self-concept

8 The nursing assistant (NA) tells the nurse about a client who "always stands too close to me when I talk with him. I am feeling very uncomfortable. I am going to tell him one more time to back off or I will have to call someone from security." The nurse should do which of the following?

1. Explain this may be part of the client's cultural norms and have the NA talk with the client about concerns.
2. Tell the client that he cannot stand close to the NA.
3. Tell the NA to read some articles about the client's culture to avoid calling security.
4. Accompany the NA to the client's room to talk about culture and the NA's needs.

9 The nurse has just finished talking with a client about depression and anxiety. The client says, "I understand that having these diseases is something I got because of my mother's family." The nurse recognizes that the client is referring to which of the following?

1. Physical illness
2. Genetic predisposition
3. Family illness
4. Family partiality

10 The nurse in an urban neighborhood health clinic is interviewing a 16-year-old client who reports "It's hard to deal with life. No one cares." When asked who the client usually talks with when feeling "down" the client answers, "There is no one." Which question should the nurse ask next?

1. "Do you or anyone you live with own a gun?"
2. "Whom do you live with?"
3. "Are you having thoughts about hurting yourself?"
4. "Have you ever cut yourself or do you know of anyone in your family who cuts to relieve pain?"

➤ *See pages 51–53 for Answers and Rationales.*

I. OVERVIEW OF PSYCHOSOCIAL ASSESSMENT

A. **Psychosocial assessment or intake interview is part of a client's admission to a psychiatric inpatient unit, or general hospital, rehabilitation center, extended-care facility, healthcare clinic, and home setting; the assessment should:**

1. Focus on the effects of an illness on the client's and family's psychological, emotional, and spiritual needs

2. Begin the process of identifying key psychological factors that contribute to the client's **mental health** (an ability to see oneself as others do and to fit into culture and society where one lives) and begin formulating pertinent nursing diagnoses

3. Provide data about client's body language, mood, affect, attitude, and changes in behavior

4. Provide results of a **mental status examination (MSE)** (assesses an individual's ability to think, reason, cope with feelings and stressors, and behave in a socially and culturally acceptable manner); components of the MSE are usually integrated throughout the health interview; however, they consist of a specific set of assessments, as outlined in Box 3-1

5. The MSE can be done using the Folstein Mini Mental Status Exam tool; this tool consists of 11 items that focus on cognitive functioning, not mood or thought processes; the maximum score on this tool is 30, while the average score is 27; scores between 24 and 30 indicate no cognitive impairment, scores between 18 and 23 indicate mild cognitive impairment, scores between 8 and 17 indicate moderate cognitive impairment, and scores from 0 to 7 indicate severe cognitive impairment

B. **Internal and external key factors, which are utilized to formulate nursing diagnoses and an individualized nursing care plan**

1. Internal factors affecting psychosocial health

a. Genetics

1) Influences physical and psychosocial health throughout one's lifetime; i.e., children of parents with alcoholism, hypoglycemia, or other health disorders are genetically predisposed to those disorders

2) Genetic factors are dependent upon inherited ability and are enhanced or diminished in response to environmental and education factors

b. Ability to cope with stress

1) Individuals considered psychologically and physically healthy are able to cope with life events and make necessary adaptations in times of stress
2) Individuals may demonstrate effects of stress with physical symptoms (back pain, neck pain, chest pain, difficulty breathing, dry mouth, nausea, palpitations, hypertension, and weight loss/gain)
3) Some individuals use destructive **coping mechanisms** (ways of adjusting to external stressors without changing one's goals or life direction) during periods of stress, such as use of alcohol, nicotine, or sleep aids

---

Box 3-1

Components of Mental Status Examination

Appearance

Posture (should be erect with relaxed position)

Body movements (should be voluntary, coordinated, deliberate, smooth, and even)

Dress (should be appropriate for age, gender, social group, season, and setting)

Grooming and hygiene (should be clean and well-groomed; note that dress may also reflect economic status and fashion trends)

Behavior

Level of consciousness (should be awake, alert, aware of and appropriately responding to internal and external stimuli)

Facial expression (should be appropriate to situation with eye contact according to cultural norm)

Speech (laryngeal sounds should be effortless and client engages in conversation appropriately, with steady pace and clear articulation of words, and effortless word choice that is appropriate to educational level)

Mood and affect (should be appropriate to place and condition, and should change appropriately with change in topic of conversation; judged also by answers to specific questions about feelings)

Cognitive Function (Cognition)

Orientation (should be correct as to time [day of week, date, year, season], place [present location, city, state, and where client lives], and person [own name and age, type of worker that examiner is]

Attention span (should be able to concentrate and complete a thought without distraction)

Recent memory (should be able to recall time arrived at agency or 24-hour diet recall in context of health history interview)

Remote memory (should be able to verify past health, birthday, and historic events that are relevant to client)

New learning (should be able to repeat four words stated by examiner at 5, 10, and 30 minutes after examiner stated them if under age 60 years)

Higher intellectual function (assessed during context of interview; should be able to exhibit problem-solving and reasoning abilities)

Judgment (assessed during context of interview; should be realistic about personal healthcare, compliance with prescribed health regimen, general goals for future)

Thought Processes and Perceptions

Thought processes (should be logical, coherent, relevant, and goal-directed)

Thought content (should be consistent and logical)

Perceptions (should be aware of reality and congruent with examiner's perceptions)

Suicidal thoughts (should be absent; assess risk for suicide when client expresses sadness, grief, despair, or hopelessness)

      4) Positive coping strategies include talking openly about feelings with someone trusted; maintaining a positive outlook utilizing relaxation techniques such as deep breathing, guided imagery, yoga, and prayer; willfully concentrating on a positive daily regime; putting healthy eating habits into place; regular exercise; and getting sufficient rest and sleep

2. External factors affecting psychosocial health

   a. Family: core unit where individuals learn about love, caring, belonging, coping skills, social interactions, life changes, and dealing with stress; family

   b. **Culture**: complex system of learned behaviors including knowledge, beliefs, morals, and customs used as part of life

      1) Culture affects many factors related to health such as family dynamics, customs, diet, exercise, communication, membership in social organizations, and how time is perceived and utilized by the client

      2) Health beliefs and patterns to inquire about include culture-related anatomical characteristics, physiological differences or deficiencies, and hereditary considerations that can place clients at risk for certain diseases or illnesses

   c. Geography: area where an individual is raised and lives

      1) Can greatly influence how the individual lives now, habits that have been formed, and values and beliefs that are a part of life patterns

      2) Important geographic elements include how individuals live and move about, and what kind of healthcare is available to them

      3) In the United States today, urban neighborhoods tend to have individuals from many cultures and backgrounds living in close proximity (with possible crowding, congestion, and higher crime rates), while in rural areas, individuals may have fewer resources available and experience more isolation

   d. Safety is an important factor to psychosocial health because it can influence social development, emotional well-being, and stability

   e. Economic status affects individual's values and attitudes; it can help shape values and role expectations related to marriage, gender roles, family roles, sex, parenting, education, housing, leisure activities, clothing, occupation, and religious practices

   f. Other factors affecting psychosocial health

      1) **Self-concept** (belief and perception one has about self) can be positive or negative and can change over time; if positive, one may develop and maintain positive relationships and prevent mental illness; one may also be better able to make necessary changes to self-image and be better adjusted to healthy eating, sleeping, and exercising habits

      2) **Self-esteem** (self-respect/self-worth felt by a person)

      3) **Body image** (way a person sees his or her physical self); can be either positive or negative

      4) Role development (ability to function in society); assumed roles include parent–child, student–teacher, employee–employer, and sibling–sibling; we learn role expectations by socialization

      5) Relationships: essential part of life for most individuals; help establish ability to trust another

      6) **Spirituality** (belief that there is someone or something in the world more powerful and able to guide individuals); a source of internal strength and conviction about very reason for life that is based in **culture**, personal beliefs, mores, and lifestyle

II. CONDUCTING A PSYCHOSOCIAL ASSESSMENT

A. Medical record information and intake interview

1. Medical record data provide significant information such as brain trauma, brain tumors, electrolyte imbalance, multiple sclerosis, psychiatric history, or alcohol and other drug history or treatment

2. Intake interview data identify significant concerns, such as history of psychological, psychiatric, or developmental issues that may impact current reason to seek healthcare; major client stressors and how the client coped with them; and any treatment and outcome issues that are currently relevant to the present

B. When to conduct in-depth psychosocial assessment

1. If significant topics identified previously warrant further inquiry, such as unusual or bizarre behavior, unusually high anxiety levels, or any past depressed affect

2. When the client receives a poor prognosis or poor surgical outcome or when the client is hospitalized longer than expected, if unusual or bizarre behavior becomes an issue

3. For some clients, a primary healthcare problem is a psychosocial or psychiatric issue, such as **depression** (severe feeling of sadness, lack of motivation, changes in sleep patterns and appetite, and wanting to withdraw or isolate from others), **psychosis** (a disorderly mental state in which a client has difficulty distinguishing reality from his or her own internal perceptions), **anxiety** (state of apprehension, dread, uneasiness, or uncertainty), **substance abuse** (the purposeful use, for at least one month, of a drug that results in adverse effects to one's self or others), or another psychiatric disorder; the initial interview should utilize the fewest questions needed to gather accurate and detailed data about psychosocial aspects of the client's life and should include a focus interview directed toward the current problem for which the client is being treated

C. When there is a history of psychosocial issues/concerns, ask questions such as the following:

1. "How are you feeling right now about being here? Have you ever felt this way before, especially when you were ill or being treated for an illness or injury?"

2. "Were you ever treated for a psychological or psychiatric problem in the past?"; if so, ask the following questions:
   a. "Where were you treated (inpatient or outpatient treatment)?"
   b. "Do you feel the treatment was helpful?" If yes, "How did the treatment help you deal with problems differently?"

3. "Do you or did you ever use alcohol? Do you or did you ever use drugs?"
   a. "In the course of one week, what do you drink and how many drinks containing alcohol do you have?"
   b. "Does this help you decrease your stress?"
   c. "What about food—do you feel you eat more food when you are stressed?"
   d. "What kind of food gives you 'comfort' or 'good feelings'?"
   e. "Have you ever received treatment for an addiction to food, alcohol, or drugs (legal or illegal)?"; if yes:
      1) "When were you in treatment and for how long?"
      2) "How successful has treatment been for you?" (these questions can help establish past history of addiction, treatment, and the use of maladaptive coping skills)

4. "How do you currently cope with stress and anxiety? How does this work for you?"

D. History of physiological health problems (psychological, cognitive, perceptual, or affective problems may be related to physical signs and symptoms)

1. "Can you provide details about any chronic illness you have, such as asthma, arthritis, heart problems, headaches, stomach or bowel problems, skin rashes, or glandular problems?"; if so, ask the following:
   a. "How has your life changed since you were diagnosed (physically, mentally, and emotionally)?"

    b. "Do you believe this illness affects the way you feel or think?"

    c. "How does it affect you physically?"

E. Assessment of self-concept (difficult to assess during intake interview; additionally, clients need a baseline understanding of their self-concept and established trust with the interviewer to talk openly about themselves)

  1. Ask the following few questions during the intake assessment or focus assessment to establish a baseline understanding of the client's self-concept and ideas about how he or she is viewed by others:

    a. "If you were at a social gathering with a friend and the friend wanted to introduce you to another person at the party, what would you want that friend to say about you to the stranger?"

    b. "What would you say are your best characteristics?"

    c. "Are there any traits that you have that you would like to change?"

  2. "How much time do you like to spend alone? What do you like to do for fun, hobbies? How much time each week do you spend on hobbies or having fun?"

  3. "Since you were diagnosed with this illness, do you feel different about yourself, how you look, what you are able to do, or how you live each day? If so, how?"

  4. "Is there a significant other in your life right now?" (relationships with significant individuals provide information about sexual preferences, intimate relationships, and how well the client is able to relate to another in a significant way)

F. Assessment of family history (how the client's family functions can provide data about the client's present status, ability to cope with stress and adapt to change, traits based on heredity or genetic features, and baseline data about present illness and response to it)

  1. "If you look at your family tree, parents and their nuclear family, and your grandparents and their siblings and parents, are there members that you know of who suffered from...

    a. alcohol or drug abuse?"

    b. psychiatric illness such as schizophrenia, depression, bipolar disorder, or anxiety?"

    c. "Are there any other disorders that you remember your family talking about that may affect you?"

  2. "What is your birth order in your family? Are the siblings you grew up with all from the same set of parents?"

  3. "Please describe what it was like in your household growing up."

    a. "How many people lived in your home? Tell me a little about them."

    b. "Would you describe your household as functional, dysfunctional, chaotic but functional, or other? Would you give me a couple of examples?"

    c. "How were family conflicts worked out between adults/parents/caretakers? Between caretakers and children? Between siblings?"

  4. "In the family you live with now, what are your primary responsibilities? What role(s) do you have in the family (father/mother, sister/brother, daughter/son, work outside the home/stay at home, etc.)?"

  5. "When you were growing up, did you ever have a major loss (parent, grandparent, sibling, close family member)? Do you remember who helped you and how you worked through the loss?"

G. Assessment of roles and relationships (outside of family dynamics—friends, neighbors, and co-workers; individual's ability to form close relationships is important indication of his or her ability to form close bonds with others)

  1. "How long have you lived in your present home, worked in your present position?"

  2. "How long have you known some of your close friends?"

  3. "How much time or how often do you spend time with close friends? What do you usually do together and how often?"

Practice to Pass

During an initial psychosocial assessment on a busy psychiatric inpatient unit, a client asks the nurse, "Why are you asking me so many questions about my mother, father, siblings, and grandparents?" What would be the most appropriate explanation by the nurse?

4. "Describe the relationship you have with neighbors."
5. "Do you belong to any organizations, social groups or clubs (church group, golf league, or service organizations, etc.)?" (indicates that the client spends time giving back to the community or spends time with other acquaintances and friends and is able to form relationships with others)

H. Assessment of culture (data yield possible information about the client's norms, mores, beliefs, social customs, responses to illness or injury, and abilities to participate in self-care, and allows the nurse to include the client's cultural beliefs and norms in the plan of care; see also Table 3-1 for categories to include when conducting a cultural assessment)

1. "What is your primary language? Do you speak any other languages?"
2. "Is there any significance to you about how close or far apart people should be when they are talking?"
3. "Can you tell me a little about what is acceptable and not acceptable to you concerning eye contact? Touching? Display of feelings to a healthcare provider? Facial expressions used during conversation? The use of silence?"
4. "Are there any other customs that you would share with me to make it easier for me to understand what is important to you?"
5. "Let's talk a little about *time*. Are you usually on time for appointments, school, work, or social gatherings? Is being on time important to you?"
6. "What foods are important in your culture? How often are they a part of your meals?"
   a. "Do you have some favorite foods?"
   b. "Are there any foods that you do not like?"
   c. "Are there foods that you do not eat because of religious beliefs?"
   d. "Do you have other special considerations about food that are related to religious beliefs (fasting, rituals, holiday foods, etc.)?"
7. "What do you do when you are not feeling well?"
   a. "Do you ever use herbs or other non-traditional remedies for medicinal purposes?"
   b. "How do you feel about taking medications prescribed by a physician or nurse practitioner?"
   c. "Where do you go for your healthcare needs (physician, nurse practitioner, hospital, clinic, shaman, older members of family, etc.)?"
   d. "If you are given prescriptions or medicine, do you follow the instructions yourself or does someone else care for you when you are ill?"

I. Assessment of ability to cope with stressors (a learned ability in childhood, but methods usually change over time depending on age, culture, level of cognitive ability, adaptability, and severity of stressors)

1. "What are major sources of stress in your life right now?"
   a. "How are you coping with them?"
   b. "When you feel upset, what do you usually do to cope? Who do you usually call on to help?"
   c. "Are there any comfort measures that make it easier to cope with stress?"
2. "How are you coping with your present illness?"
   a. "Have you had difficulty adjusting your daily activities to adapt to the changes you needed to make because of the illness?"
   b. "How has this illness affected relationships in your life?"
   c. "How do you feel about the life changes you have had to make?"
   d. "Are you taking any medications, smoking, using alcohol, or using illegal drugs because of the stress you are under now? If yes, can you describe how much, how often, and how the drugs/alcohol affect your daily life?"

!

Practice to Pass

What is the purpose when the nurse asks the client about where he or she lives and with whom he or she lives?

!

Practice to Pass

Identify the major components of the individual client's culture and why these components are included in a psychosocial assessment.

Table 3-1		
Guidelines for Cultural Assessment	**Ethnicity**	Does the client identify with a particular ethnic/racial/cultural group? Where was the client born? How long has the client lived in this country?
	Communication	What language is spoken? Can the client communicate in English? If yes, both spoken and written? Does the client speak for self or defer to another? What nonverbal communication behaviors are observed (e.g., touching, eye contact)? What significance do these behaviors have for the nurse—client interaction?
	Space	Observe the client's proximity to other people and objects within the environment. How does the client react to the nurse's movement toward the client? Assess the client's physical environment (especially important in home health nursing, community nursing, and long-term care nursing). What cultural objects within the environment have importance for health promotion/health maintenance?
	Social Organization	What are the client's roles? Is the client the primary decision maker for healthcare behaviors? Must the client consult another to make health decisions? If yes, who? What other family members are important to the client's decision making? Are there cultural or religious leaders who are important in the client's health decision making? Is there a religious affiliation linked with cultural affiliation (e.g., Jewish, Latino, Catholic)?
	Time	What is the client's time orientation: past, present, or future? What is the significance of time for the client? Does the client talk about time in specifics, such as dates or times, or in generalities, such as "a long time" or "a short time"?
	Environmental Control	How is health defined by the culture? What does the client believe to be the cause of the illness or health concern? Has the client used the services of cultural healers? What healing practices has the client used? Have folk healing behaviors been used? Is the client wearing or carrying any amulets or artifacts that are believed to have healing properties?
	Biological Variations	Are there normal variations in anatomical characteristics (e.g., body structure or size, skin color, facial characteristics)? What are the dietary preferences of the client? Are the dietary preferences related to the client's ethnicity? Is the client at risk for nutritional deficiencies because of ethnicity (e.g., pernicious anemia, lactose intolerance)? Are there variations in physiological functioning related to the client's ethnicity or race (e.g., drug metabolism, alcohol metabolism)? Are there illnesses or diseases that the client is at risk for because of ethnicity or race (e.g., hypertension, diabetes mellitus, sickle-cell anemia)?

Source: Kozier, B., Erb, G., Blais, K., Wilkinson, J. M.. (1998). *Fundamentals of nursing: Concepts, process, and practice*, (5th ed.). Pearson Education, Inc. Cited in D'Amico, D. & Barbarito, C. (2007). *Health & physical assessment in nursing.* Upper Saddle River, NJ: Pearson Education, Inc., p. 78, Table 4.2.

3. "Have you had any periods of sadness or crying spells recently?"
    a. "Have you experienced changes in your appetite recently? Any difficulty with fatigue or problems sleeping?"
    b. "What is your current weight? Have you gained or lost weight recently? If so, how much?"
    c. "Has your interest in sexual activity changed recently?"
    d. "Do you ever feel hopeless, irritable, indecisive, or confused?"
    e. "Do you have times when your heart pounds or you have trouble concentrating?"
    f. "Have you had any thoughts about taking your life or hurting yourself? If so, have you thought of how you would hurt yourself or end your life? Please elaborate."

J. **Assessment of senses and cognition (data obtained by asking in a non-threatening manner about hallucinations [perceiving stimuli that are not present], delusions [false beliefs], or other cognitive impairment)**

!

Practice to Pass

The client is admitted to an inpatient medical unit for exacerbation of chronic obstructive pulmonary disease. Which aspect of a psychosocial assessment would prevent the nurse from beginning the admission process with the client?

1. "Please tell me your first, middle, and last name; how old you are; and the city and state in which you were born."
    a. "Please tell me where you are right now and how you got to be here."
    b. "What day of the week is it? What is today's date?" (these questions test the client's orientation to person, time, and place)

2. "Now I would like to ask you a series of questions to test your senses and how you think and feel about things. Are you ready?"
    a. "Do you have any trouble deciding things, like what to do or what not to do? Can you give me some examples of how you make decisions such as when to eat lunch or go to the store?" (these questions give information about process of decision making)
    b. "Please count backward subtracting 7 each time, starting with 100." (tests cognitive functioning)
    c. "If I say, 'A rolling stone gathers no moss,' what does that mean to you?" (tests abstract/concrete thinking ability)
    d. "Do you ever have a problem with thinking or just sitting quietly and reading the paper or watching the news on TV? What was one news item you remember from the last time you watched the news?" (helps determine the client's ability to think and process information; clients with bipolar, psychotic, or anxiety disorder may or may not (because of racing thoughts) be able to think/reason; if client can remember news items from one day ago, this indicates intact short term memory)
    g. "Who was the 16th president of the United States?" (example of a test for long-term memory)
    h. "Have you ever heard voices inside your head that no one else hears?"
        1) "What did the voices say?"
        2) "Do the voices tell you to do things to yourself or to others?" (address psychosis, delusions or hallucinations, and client safety; command hallucinations benign or telling client to hurt self or others)
    i. "Did you ever misunderstand or think an object is something it is not, like seeing a tree and thinking you're looking at a bear? Or hear a bell and think someone is singing, or smell something and find out it is not what you thought it was? If yes, please describe what you saw, heard, smelled, or felt that was not what it seemed."

K. **Assessment of spirituality and belief systems (may influence the client's health and decisions about health and healing; see the following suggested questions)**

1. "Are there health- or nutrition-related guidelines that you follow as part of your beliefs?"

2. "In your present experience with healthcare, have you had any ethical or moral difficulties from the treatment you are being offered here so far? If yes, please explain. If there are difficulties now or while here, how do you plan to address them with those providing care?"

3. "Do you have 'faith' or 'spiritual beliefs' that are a part of your life?"
   a. "How will they help now with this illness?"
   b. "Do you use a form of prayer or meditation? Please elaborate."
   c. "As you think about your present illness do you feel angry with God, your higher power, or your religious healers because you have this illness? Please explain."
   d. "Do you think you have this illness as a punishment for some past deeds?"

L. **Physical cues about psychosocial status (provides valuable cues and data)**
   1. Observe client's posture, grooming, speech pattern, eye contact and verbalization method, rate and clarity; rapid or loud, pressured or high-pitched speech may indicate anxiety, fear, or presence of hallucinations
   2. If client is experiencing hallucinations, he or she may talk or gesture while nurse does not witness anyone except client; if this occurs, note content of client's speech so if client is hearing command hallucinations that would put someone in danger, nurse can assess need for intervention
   3. Assess clients who are disheveled, dirty, and/or have strong body odor for skin or nutritional disorders; disheveled or unkempt appearance may also indicate depression or low self-esteem; body posture may also indicate fear or anxiety; eye contact should be direct, if appropriate for ethnic group
   4. Note client's movements, which should be fluid and relaxed; tics or restlessness could indicate anxiety, high stress, or apprehension
   5. Observe client's facial expressions, which should be appropriate for conversation and setting; note any rapid movement or quick changes in mood because this could also indicate a mood disorder
   6. Note client's dress, which should be appropriate for time of year, event, and age

M. **Miscellaneous psychosocial assessments: some very useful level-of-wellness assessment tools, social skills tests, and other quality-of-life scales can be found online (see Box 3-2)**

Practice to Pass

Which physical cues are most relevant for the nurse to utilize to determine a client's psychosocial status?

III. EXPECTED FINDINGS

A. **Health history, current level of wellness, and treatment and history of any chronic conditions**
   1. Client is able to relate history of health and give information about how he or she copes with anxiety, pain, and illness/injury with minimum difficulty
   2. Client with little or no history of severe illness is able to care for self, follow treatment recommendations, and understand client teaching for present medical problem, depending on the presenting illness/injury
   3. Client with healthy self-concept is able to provide data needed to formulate plan of care based on his or her physical, psychological, and emotional needs
   4. Psychosocial focus interview is usually only done on an as-needed basis, but might be done during the admission interview to look at past behavior and coping skills to prepare for any adverse incidents that may arise during the client's care

Box 3-2	This is a sample list of reputable websites for psychosocial assessment:
Online Links to Tools for Psychosocial Assessment	Centers for Disease Control and Prevention: www.cdc.gov/mentalhealth/resources.htm
	Columbia University TeenScreen Program: www.teenscreen.org
	U.S. Department of Health & Human Services: www.healthfinder.gov/HealthTools/

5. If the client is able to accept a chronic illness diagnosis and changes needed to adjust to that illness, the client describes him- or herself as being aware of changes that are happening and describe how he or she is adjusting to changes in body image and self-concept

B. **Family history and roles and relationships**
1. Client who describes uneventful healthcare history is likely to demonstrate positive attitude, **affect**, (the outward expression of emotions) and coping skills; this client can generally be expected to cope with illness and injuries emotionally, physically, and psychologically
2. Client's nuclear family and amount of structure and care can help the nurse establish the client's ability to cope and change now based on how he or she was taught and environment where he or she grew up, whether a loving, trusting, chaotic, or dysfunctional environment
3. If client lost a significant individual early in his or her development and was given necessary help to grieve the loss, client will be able to talk about the loss without undue distress

C. **Culture**
1. Cultural topics including ethnicity, communication, space, social organization, time, environmental control, and biological variations; refer again to Table 3-1
2. Any important cultural factors that client identifies should be included in plan of care to help client respond in a positive way to illness/injury

D. **Coping with stressors**
1. If client has a physical or psychiatric illness, ability to adjust and to reach out for help as a past pattern of behavior indicates healthy coping
2. If client is diagnosed with a fatal or chronic illness, expected responses include ability to acknowledge emotional response, grieve loss, and vent negative feelings and adjust to life change

E. **Senses and cognition (mental status exam)**
1. Client is oriented to time, place, and person
2. Client is able to think and process information
3. Client can remember a news item from one day ago to indicate intact short-term memory
4. Client can answer common knowledge questions, such as a previous president of United States, etc. to indicate intact long-term memory
5. Client has upright posture and ability to remain focused during interview

F. **Spirituality and belief systems**
1. Client can identify personal belief systems
2. Client expresses satisfaction with belief systems

IV. UNEXPECTED FINDINGS

A. **Health history, current level of wellness and treatment, and chronic conditions**
1. Past relevant medical or psychosocial findings include such problems as brain tumors, brain trauma, electrolyte imbalance, multiple sclerosis, or psychiatric or alcohol and other drug history
2. If past history findings give information about current status, it will help establish client's ability to cope with stressors, past patterns of behavior related to treatment, and compliance with prescribed care

B. **Self-concept**
1. Poor self-concept and self-image may be accompanied by reduced coping abilities as well as increased anxiety level, depression, and reality testing
2. This information helps determine if client is able to participate in formulating a plan of care

C. Family history and roles and relationships

1. If client is from a family where alcohol and drugs were abused by many family members, this can indicate genetic predisposition; this can add to support if family is in recovery or it can be detrimental if client's family members are actively drinking or abusing drugs; client's coping skills may not be optimal because effective coping was not learned in past

2. Diagnosis of schizophrenia or other psychiatric disorders in a client with a positive family history can also be devastating and indicates that plan of care should include developmental skills as well as treatment needs

3. Most clients brought up in a family where there was chaos and dysfunction usually have difficulty coping with illness/injuries

   a. Client's birth order becomes important when assessing present coping abilities; he or she was probably not taught the skills of becoming an adult from parents but may have learned to "take care of him- or herself" from older siblings who themselves were "surviving" rather than living a positive, productive life

   b. Dysfunctional family environments during youth can also negatively impact how an individual will view and cope with losses in life, including loss of health

4. Inadequate relationships with others can lead to decreased support available to the client during times of illness

5. Sexually active clients may have a difficult time with changes in lifestyle or separation from the partner while hospitalized, or the partner may have difficulty with changes to his or her life as well

D. Culture

1. If a client being treated in a healthcare facility has a cultural norm to seek care only from a healer specific to his or her culture, the client could experience distress or demonstrate negative behaviors because of fear, shame, confusion, or devastation

2. Client could also experience distress if healthcare environment does not attempt to incorporate cultural norms regarding food or other basic needs

E. Coping with stressors

1. Client presenting with psychosis would demonstrate withdrawal and a change in affect and thought processes, and possibly hallucinations or delusions

2. Client presenting with depression will demonstrate changes in mood, eating and sleeping patterns, and other signs of depression such as **anergia** (lack of energy) and **anhedonia** (inability to experience pleasure)

3. If alcohol and drugs were used excessively in the past, it can indicate past maladaptive coping behaviors or dysfunction and could be a major safety issue for the client; this should be included in the plan of care

4. If client has past psychiatric diagnoses and treatment, nurse can follow up with a focus interview about pattern of treatment and recovery since initial diagnosis

   a. If client has followed through with treatment and medication and is still compliant, nurse indicates this on plan of care

   b. If client is not taking medications or following plan of care and is showing signs and symptoms of psychiatric diagnosis, nurse collaborates the healthcare team to ensure client receives appropriate care and follow-up services, including monitoring for risk of self-harm or **suicide** (intentional and voluntary taking of one's life) as indicated

5. Client who has a chronic illness and is not able to cope with the illness may refuse treatment or may not be motivated to participate in self-care

6. If diagnosed with a chronic or fatal disorder, maladaptive coping could lead to depression, anxiety, and possible suicidal ideations

F. Senses and cognition (mental status exam)

1. Hallucinations, delusions, or other cognitive impairments are unexpected findings that are described and documented; when client experiences auditory hallucinations (hears

voices), nurse must also determine client's safety—command hallucinations can be a danger if client determines that voice(s) must be obeyed

! 2. Impaired judgments, insufficient capacity for abstract thinking, and/or impaired short-term and long-term memory are unexpected findings and require further follow up and documentation

G. **Spirituality and belief systems: client could experience distress if healthcare environment does not provide opportunity to incorporate spiritual beliefs during care**

H. **Miscellaneous findings**

1. Clients who are disheveled, have poor posture, grooming, speech patterns, and poor eye contact need further assessment for signs and symptoms of thought, mood, or other disorders

2. Clients with rapid, loud or pressured, or high-pitched speech may be experiencing anxiety

3. If client is talking while no one is present nearby, a focus assessment for hallucinations is indicated

4. If client demonstrates tics (involuntary muscle movements or twitches) or restlessness, it could indicate anxiety, high stress, or fear

V. LIFESPAN CONSIDERATIONS

A. **Psychosocial development occurs across the lifespan**

B. **Eric Erikson's theory of psychosocial development outlines developmental stages from infancy through older adulthood, each with inherent tasks that are unique to that stage**

1. The course of development is determined by the interaction of the body (genetics or biology), mind (psychological), and cultural (ethos) influences

2. Personality traits are learned, based on challenges and support individuals receive while growing up

! C. **Erikson's stages (see Table 3-2)**

1. Stage 1 - Infancy: birth to 18 months; trust vs. mistrust

a. Infant establishes a sense of trust, especially with a primary caregiver through continuous visual contact and touch; if infant experiences repeated frustration and deprivation of contact and touch, mistrust will develop

Table 3-2	Stage	Timeframe	Ego Development Outcome	Basic Strength
Summary of Erickson's Stages of Psychosocial Development	**Stage 1: Infancy**	Birth to 18 Months	Trust vs. Mistrust	Drive and hope
	Stage 2: Early Childhood	18 months to 3 years	Autonomy vs. Shame	Self-control, courage, and will
	Stage 3: Preschool	Age 3 to 5 years	Initiative vs. Guilt	Purpose
	Stage 4: School Age	Age 6 to 12 Years	Industry vs. Inferiority	Method and competence
	Stage 5: Adolescence	Age 12 to 18 Years	Identity vs. Role Confusion	Devotion and fidelity
	Stage 6: Young Adulthood:	Age 18 to 35 Years	Intimacy and Solidarity vs. Isolation	Affiliation and love
	Stage 7: Middle Adulthood:	Age 35 to 55 or 65 Years	Generativity vs. Self-absorption or Stagnation	Production and care
	Stage 8: Late Adulthood	Age 55 or 65 to Death	Integrity vs. Despair	Wisdom

   b. While learning to trust caregiver, infant also learns to trust the world; if infant is frustrated and receives little or inconsistent touch or visual contact, then infant learns deep-seated feelings of worthlessness and mistrust

2. Stage 2 - Early Childhood: 18 months to 3 years; autonomy vs. shame
   a. Learn to master skills of walking, talking, feeding self, and fine motor skills
   b. Master toilet training and build self-esteem while developing control over body functions
   c. Begin to learn right from wrong and use more autonomy (such as using word "no") as will develops
   d. Those not developing autonomy are learning shame and doubt; a child who is ashamed about toilet training or learning other skills at this level may experience low self-esteem as well

3. Stage 3 - Preschool Age 3 to 5 years; initiative vs. guilt
   a. Try to explore world and imitate adults environment by acting out roles experienced in life
   b. They also begin to ask "why?"
   c. Those who receive encouragement and reassurance learn direction, purpose, self-sufficiency, and self-assertion—they develop initiative
   d. Those who are punished, ridiculed, or otherwise prevented from developing initiative develop guilt

4. Stage 4 - School Age: 6 to 12 years; industry vs. inferiority
   a. Develop new skills and knowledge
   b. If children master skills that promote a sense of worth, such as school work, sports, arts, and social interaction, they receive recognition and approval and develop a sense of industry, confidence, and competence
   c. Excessive criticism of areas where child fails to excel can lead to a sense of inferiority
   d. Peer group acceptance becomes more important and children learn to cooperate with others
   e. Major relationships include people in school and neighborhood; in last part of stage (10–12 years) they begin to question and possibly reject parental ideas and values, but family still has most influence on decisions and behavior

5. Stage 5 - Adolescence: 12 to 18 years; identity vs. role confusion
   a. Beginning in this stage, development depends on what person now does for him- or herself
   b. In this stage person is neither child nor adult and life becomes more complex as person strives to find his or her identity
   c. As person struggles with moral decisions and social interactions, tasks the individual chooses can lead to either identity (if successful) or role confusion (if unsuccessful)
   d. Important relationships are acquaintances and members of a wider society; family becomes decreasingly important and peers become more important
   e. "Causes" also become important while developing a life philosophy and trying to think altruistically rather than realistically

6. Stage 6 - Young Adulthood: 18 to 35 years; intimacy and solidarity vs. isolation
   a. Begin to look for intimacy with another for a permanent relationship; this requires ability to establish mutual trust, cooperate with another, share goals and feelings, and accept others
   b. If successful during this stage, will usually experience intimacy; if not, a sense of distancing from others can result
   c. Most important relationships are with a few close friends, spouse, and children; if not successful, person's world can become more and more narrow until person tries to feel superior to others in order to protect him- or herself

7. Stage 7 - Middle Adulthood: 35 to 55 or 65; generativity vs. self-absorption or stagnation
    a. Significant tasks include concern for establishing and guiding next generation (including home, work, social, and other areas of life)
    b. Individual strives for productivity (what Erikson calls *generativity*)
    c. Most individuals fear inactivity, which could lead to stagnation
8. Stage 8 - Late Adulthood: 55 or 65 to death; integrity vs. despair
    a. Many look back on their lives with happiness and contentment, feeling as though they have accomplished a great deal in earlier years
    b. If they are fulfilled they have a sense of integrity and wisdom gained from life experiences
    c. If they are not fulfilled, they can have a sense of despair if they perceive themselves as failures; they may fear death and need to find a sense of accomplishment
    d. Significant relationship is with all others in their world and those who are most like themselves

VI. DOCUMENTATION (SEE TABLE 3-3 FOR SAMPLE FORM)

A. **Main reason client seeks care**
B. **History of psychosocial issues/concerns**
C. **History of physiological health problems**
D. **Important self-concept and self-esteem issues**
E. **Relevant family issues and relationships**
F. **Cultural factors relevant to healthcare needs**
G. **Current and past coping skills and effectiveness**
H. **Mental Status Examination (MSE)**
    1. Assessment of senses and cognition
    2. Spirituality and beliefs system factors
    3. Physical cues about psychosocial status

Table 3-3	Components of the Psychosocial Assessment	
Sample Psychosocial Assessment Documentation Tool	Medical record available/examined: Yes No	Date, time. and place of interview:
	Significant data obtained: Yes No	Reason for seeking care today:
	If yes, make notes on reverse side.	
	History of psychosocial issues/concerns	History of physiological health problems
	Family history related to psychosocial health	
	Assessment of self-concept	Assessment of roles and relationships
	Assessment of culture (using guidelines for cultural assessment)	
	Assessment of the ability to cope with stressors	
	Assessment of senses and cognition	
	Attitude/behavior:	Memory
	Mood/affect:	Concentration:
	Orientation:	Attention:
	Speech (rate, tone, etc.):	Thought Processes:
		Suicide/Homicide/Plan:
	Assessment of spirituality and beliefs	Physical cues r/t psychosocial status

Case Study

A 54-year-old male client comes to the day-surgery suite for a biopsy and surgical excision of a squamous cell carcinoma lesion near his left eye. The client's vital signs are BP 156/94, T 98.2, P 86, R 32. The client states having no allergies and having not eaten since 7 p.m. the previous evening.

The client is accompanied by his wife, who says she is concerned because her husband acted strangely most of the previous night and again this morning. She says that he has not had any alcohol or other substances, but he talks to himself and gets mad and talks loudly. "When I ask what he is saying, he just says he was not talking to me, but there is no one else in the room."

The client is currently sitting on the stretcher, talking very softly and gesturing with his hands as though involved in a conversation. There is no one near the client at this time, as the nurse and the client's wife are in the hallway outside the room.

1. What should the nurse ask to verify the history of alcohol intake?

2. How will the nurse proceed to care for this client?

3. What is the major nursing diagnosis for this client?

4. Which diagnostic tests should be performed on this client?

5. Should the client's preparation for surgery be continued so that he can be in the operating room in ½ hour?

For suggested responses, see page 308

POSTTEST

1 The nurse conducting a psychosocial assessment asks the client to talk about whom he lives with. The client looks at the floor, answers the questions, and then continues to look down without eye contact. The nurse should take which action next?

1. Ask the client why he will not communicate.
2. Stand up and say that he or she will be back when the client is ready to communicate.
3. Quietly sit with the client until he is ready to communicate verbally and non-verbally.
4. Ask if there is a reason that the client is looking down at the floor.

2 The nurse is going to conduct a psychosocial assessment on a client. Arrange in order the sequence for completing the sections of the psychosocial assessment. All options must be used.

1. Senses and cognition
2. History of physiological health status
3. Ability to cope with stressors
4. Spirituality and beliefs
5. Role and relationships

3 While preparing a client for discharge from the inpatient unit, the nurse describes how the client can maintain a healthy eating pattern, daily exercise, and adequate sleep and rest. The nurse later explains to a mental health assistant that this teaching is related to which concept?

1. Healthy self-concept
2. External factors of healthy living
3. Physical fitness
4. Cognitive wellness

4 The new nurse orientee asks the preceptor about conducting a psychosocial assessment examination with a client. The preceptor suggests beginning the assessment using which approach?

1. Looking at the client's medical record
2. Sitting with the client for 15 minutes to get acquainted
3. Asking the physician for information pertinent to nursing
4. Asking peers on the unit if anyone has ever taken care of this client before

5 The nurse conducts a psychosocial intake assessment for a client brought to the emergency department by her mother who found the client barely conscious and is afraid she took "some drugs or something." The client says, "I just want to sleep right now." What would be the most important question at this time?

1. Ask the mother about the client's recent state of mind
2. Ask the client about her last visit to a healthcare facility or practitioner
3. Ask the mother about the client's history of alcohol/drug use
4. Ask the client about regular use of alcohol and/or drugs

6 A 58-year-old male client is hospitalized on the inpatient medical surgical nursing unit for pneumonia. The client has a history of schizophrenia, which is being treated with medication and psychiatric care as needed. The nurse would use which method to obtain information for the psychosocial assessment?

1. Ask the client directly
2. Wait to conduct the assessment until a family member comes to visit the client
3. Find medical records to get information about the diagnosis rather than talking to the client
4. Ask an immediate family member about the client's history of schizophrenia

7 The nurse is conducting a psychosocial interview with a female client and asks who she looks to, relates with, and how she interacts with others. The nurse would document the client's answers under which category of the psychosocial assessment?

1. Self-examination
2. Self-concept
3. Self-esteem
4. Self-image

8 The nurse is conducting a psychosocial intake interview with a 7-year-old female client hospitalized several times this year for unstable asthma. The nurse asks how the client is doing right now, being hospitalized again. The client states, "I use my deep breathing exercises and it helps me feel better." The nurse concludes that the client has most likely learned her coping skills from source?

1. A social worker in the outpatient department where she visits her physician
2. Her grandparents, who take care of her when her mother has to work
3. Significant individuals in her life
4. The nurses who take care of her on the unit where she is usually hospitalized

9 The nurse would document which of the following as physical observations during the psychosocial assessment of a client?

1. Self-image
2. Self-concept
3. Body language
4. Ability to cope with stress

10 The nurse gathering psychosocial assessment data from a 9-year-old client learns that the client is withdrawing from peers at school and feels incompetent as a member of the swim team. The nurse concludes the client is in which stage of development according to Erikson?

1. Autonomy vs. Shame
2. Initiative vs. Guilt
3. Industry vs. Inferiority
4. Integrity vs. Despair

➤ *See pages 53–55 for Answers and Rationales.*

ANSWERS & RATIONALES

Pretest

1 **Answer: 3** **Rationale:** Option 1 would not help the client to calm down; if anything it would only escalate his mood and behavior because it would not lower his stress level. Option 2 is what the nurse does to begin to assess the client's needs, but first the nurse must use option 3 and sit with him, maintain good eye contact, and help him to begin to focus and break the cycle of high emotions that he is displaying. Option 4 would only add to his already high stress level.
Cognitive Level: Application **Client Need:** Psychosocial Integrity **Integrated Process:** Communication and Documentation **Content Area:** Mental Health **Strategy:** Bringing the

client to the x-ray department will not help his feeling of fear. Before physical care can begin, the nurse must help the client to reduce his stress. The best approach is to use "therapeutic use of self" to help him focus on the present and reassure him by centering him on the immediate need to reduce his stress. **Reference:** D'Amico, D. & Barbarito, C. (2007). *Health & physical assessment in nursing.* Upper Saddle River, NJ: Pearson Education, Inc., p. 85.

2 **Answer: 1** **Rationale:** First the nurse needs to establish the last dose and who prescribed the lithium so the prescribing physician and the surgeon can be notified (option 1). How often the client was taking the medication is not as important as the last dose taken (option 2). The history of how the client began taking lithium is not a first priority (option 3) nor are the objective symptoms which the client may or may not be sure of (option 4). **Cognitive Level:** Application **Client Need:** Psychosocial Integrity **Integrated Process:** Communication and Documentation **Content Area:** Mental Health **Strategy:** Maintaining safety during hospitalization is an important consideration, especially after noting there is no history of the client's lithium use, behavior when not taking lithium, or knowledge if the prescribing physician or surgeon is aware that the client has stopped the lithium. Eliminate option 3 first since it involves more remote client history and option 4 because the time span has only been 2 days. Choose option 1 over option 2 because although both options ask about the prescriber, option 2 addresses dosage frequency while option 1 determines the time that has elapsed since the client has taken any medication. **Reference:** D'Amico, D. & Barbarito, C. (2007). *Health & physical assessment in nursing.* Upper Saddle River, NJ: Pearson Education, Inc., p. 89.

3 **Answer: 30** **Rationale:** The Folstein Mini Mental Status Exam is a test that has 11 items with a maximum score of 30. The test measures cognitive functioning exclusively and does not cover mood or thought processes. It includes items such as orientation, memory, attention and calculation, naming, repetition, writing, and drawing. **Cognitive Level:** Application **Client Need:** Psychosocial Integrity **Integrated Process:** Nursing Process: Assessment **Content Area:** Mental Health **Strategy:** Specific knowledge is needed to answer this question. Recall that the score can range from 0 to 30, with 30 being a perfect score. **Reference:** Jarvis, C. (2008). *Physical examination and health assessment* (5th ed.). St. Louis, MO: Saunders, pp. 103–104.

4 **Answer: 3** **Rationale:** Option 1 discounts the client's feelings and beliefs. Options 2 and 4 are not being honest with the client, which is cruel and unethical, as well as dishonest. The statement in option 3 supports the client, but also reinforces reality. **Cognitive Level:** Application **Client Need:** Psychosocial Integrity **Integrated Process:** Nursing Process: Implementation **Content Area:** Mental Health **Strategy:** It is important not to lie to a client or to discount the

client's feelings. The only correct response available is to let the client know that the nurse understands he or she is hearing voices but that the nurse does not hear those voices. This response affirms the client's reality but does not validate those perceptions. **Reference:** D'Amico, D. & Barbarito, C. (2007). *Health & physical assessment in nursing.* Upper Saddle River, NJ: Pearson Education, Inc., p. 91.

5 **Answer: 3** **Rationale:** Reframing is not necessary with the client's statement (option 1). It is an awkward moment but the client is very clear about being reluctant to talk about the last hospitalization. The client is in the here and now and does not need to be refocused (options 2 and 4). The only correct option therefore is to use silence and allow the client time to say more (option 3). If not, then the nurse should move on and come back to the topic later in the interview. **Cognitive Level:** Application **Client Need:** Psychosocial Integrity **Integrated Process:** Communication and Documentation **Content Area:** Mental Health **Strategy:** Using silence gives the client time to decide whether to choose to share the information about the last hospitalization or not. The client does not need to be coaxed or encouraged at this time and should be allowed to be autonomous. **Reference:** D'Amico, D. & Barbarito, C. (2007). *Health & physical assessment in nursing.* Upper Saddle River, NJ: Pearson Education, Inc., p. 91.

6 **Answer: 3** **Rationale:** The client was humming very softly and standing with eyes closed, breathing evenly. This is a form of meditation, a way for the client to become calm and reduce stress by using breathing and body alignment (option 3). Reiki involves more than the client alone (option 2), while prayer is usually silent or spoken rather than hummed (option 1). Yoga involves body movement, while this client is not moving (option 4). **Cognitive Level:** Comprehension **Client Need:** Psychosocial Integrity **Integrated Process:** Nursing Process: Assessment **Content Area:** Mental Health **Strategy:** Recall that closing the eyes, concentrating on internal peaceful thoughts, putting the body in a comfortable relaxed position, and having control of breathing is known as meditation. Consider that it is very helpful if overwhelmed or very anxious. **Reference:** D'Amico, D. & Barbarito, C. (2007). *Health & physical assessment in nursing.* Upper Saddle River, NJ: Pearson Education, Inc., p. 91.

7 **Answer: 4** **Rationale:** A client with high self-esteem (option 1) would have positive feelings about self while one with low self-esteem (option 2) would have negative feelings about self. A high self-concept is a positive "image of self" rather than "feelings about self" (option 3). The client would be realistic but kind to himself rather than negative toward his appearance and behavior. Therefore, this client is projecting a low self-concept (option 4). **Cognitive Level:** Analysis **Client Need:** Psychosocial Integrity **Integrated Process:** Nursing Process: Assessment **Content Area:** Mental Health **Strategy:** To choose correctly recall that *self-concept* is the ideas or image of self in the mind while *self-esteem* is the feelings and thoughts one has about self. **Reference:** D'Amico, D. & Barbarito, C. (2007). *Health & physical assessment in nursing.* Upper Saddle River, NJ: Pearson Education, Inc., p. 88.

8 **Answer: 1** **Rationale:** For the NA to understand the client's cultural norm related to space, the nurse would explain the norms related to his culture (option 1). The nurse should then allow the NA to talk with the client. Option 2 is incorrect because the nurse does not need to interfere in the NA's relationship with the client. Option 3 is irresponsible on the nurse's part; the NA can acquire knowledge to work on communication skills with the client. The nurse does not need to intercede between the NA and the client unless there is a valid purpose (option 4).
Cognitive Level: Application **Client Need:** Psychosocial Integrity **Integrated Process:** Nursing Process: Implementation **Content Area:** Mental Health **Strategy:** Recognize that the actual client in this situation is the NA who needs to understand the culture and norms of the client to then make better decisions about how to work with a particular client while being considerate of culture and norms. **Reference:** D'Amico, D. & Barbarito, C. (2007). *Health & physical assessment in nursing.* Upper Saddle River, NJ: Pearson Education, Inc., p. 77.

9 **Answer: 2** **Rationale:** The correct terminology is genetic predisposition (option 2). These illnesses are not physical; therefore, option 1 is incorrect. Options 3 and 4 are not true: Not every person in the family will have these illnesses, nor is *family partiality* a nursing term. The nurse needs to verify that the client understands the terminology being used.
Cognitive Level: Comprehension **Client Need:** Psychosocial Integrity **Integrated Process:** Teaching and Learning **Content Area:** Mental Health **Strategy:** To answer this question correctly, utilize knowledge of medical terminology. Recall that knowledge of genetic predisposition can help clients to look for signs and symptoms of those illnesses to which they are predisposed. **Reference:** D'Amico, D. & Barbarito, C. (2007). *Health & physical assessment in nursing.* Upper Saddle River, NJ: Pearson Education, Inc., p. 81.

10 **Answer: 3** **Rationale:** The symptoms suggest that the client might be thinking about self-harm, which explains being at the clinic seeking help. It is important to establish the safety level quickly so that this can be addressed first. The other options are important to intake assessment but not as important as option 3.
Cognitive Level: Application **Client Need:** Psychosocial Integrity **Integrated Process:** Nursing Process: Planning **Content Area:** Mental Health **Strategy:** Consider that when working with a client who has mental health issues, safety needs come first. To verify that the client is safe, the nurse must be sure there is no thought of self-harm at this time, using a direct question such as in option 3. **Reference:** D'Amico, D. & Barbarito, C. (2007). *Health & physical assessment in*

nursing. Upper Saddle River, NJ: Pearson Education, Inc., p. 89.

Posttest

1 **Answer: 4** **Rationale:** The client is looking down and does not make eye contact. The most reasonable answer for this behavior would be the client's cultural beliefs/customs. By asking the question in option 4, it gives the client an opportunity to respond. Asking the client why he is not communicating (option 1) could put the client on the defensive. Getting up and leaving the client (option 2) would give the client the message that the nurse is angry, and option 3 is inappropriate because this would only make the nurse and the client non-communicative and uncomfortable.
Cognitive Level: Application **Client Need:** Psychosocial Integrity **Integrated Process:** Communication and Documentation **Content Area:** Mental Health **Strategy:** Recall that eye contact is influenced by a client's culture. Next consider that asking the client directly is the most respectful and direct method for inquiring about his behavior and cultural norms. **Reference:** D'Amico, D. & Barbarito, C. (2007). *Health & physical assessment in nursing.* Upper Saddle River, NJ: Pearson Education, Inc., p. 76.

2 **Answer: 2, 5, 3, 1, 4** **Rationale:** The sequence of the psychosocial assessment is as follows: review of medical record and intake information, history of psychosocial concerns, history of physiological alterations or diseases (option 2), self-concept, family history, other roles and relationships (option 5), stress and coping (option 3), senses and cognition (option 1), spirituality and belief systems (option 4).
Cognitive Level: Application **Client Need:** Psychosocial Integrity **Integrated Process:** Nursing Process: Assessment **Content Area:** Mental Health **Strategy:** Familiarity with the process and sequence for conducting a psychosocial assessment is needed to answer the question. Consider that physiological data is reviewed before the psychosocial components to help make the correct initial choice. **Reference:** D'Amico, D. & Barbarito, C. (2007). *Health & physical assessment in nursing.* Upper Saddle River, NJ: Pearson Education, Inc., p. 81.

3 **Answer: 3** **Rationale:** In order to maintain physical fitness an individual needs to maintain healthy eating and sleeping patterns (option 3). Daily exercise is also a major part of the client's physical fitness that will enhance healing and recovery. The other options are not correct because they are not physiologically based.
Cognitive Level: Application **Client Need:** Psychosocial Integrity **Integrated Process:** Nursing Process: Implementation **Content Area:** Mental Health **Strategy:** Recall that for an individual to maintain psychosocial health, physical fitness must be included as part of a healthy lifestyle. Diet, exercise, and rest/sleep patterns of living make a major difference for a client who is striving to maintain health and well-being.

ANSWERS & RATIONALES

Reference: D'Amico, D. & Barbarito, C. (2007). *Health & physical assessment in nursing.* Upper Saddle River, NJ: Pearson Education, Inc., p. 82.

4 **Answer: 1** **Rationale:** This client may have had a past history of emotional or psychiatric problems that could contribute to the student's knowledge and help conduct the psychosocial assessment with insight and pertinent information about this particular client (option 1). Option 2 will help the student become acquainted with the client socially but it is not the first step to gather data about the client. Option 3 will not give the student information related to nursing. The physician will concentrate on the medical aspect of the client's care. Option 4 is not the best approach to establish a baseline of pertinent factual data for the psychosocial assessment. **Cognitive Level:** Application **Client Need:** Psychosocial Integrity **Integrated Process:** Nursing Process: Planning **Content Area:** Mental Health **Strategy:** As the student learns to conduct physical and psychosocial assessments with clients, the nurse will help the student take the most important steps first, second, etc. to gather client data in order to have accurate and helpful psychosocial assessment data. Choose option 1 after considering that medical record data can help the student determine where to begin the assessment and identify any areas of heightened concern that should be addressed first. **Reference:** D'Amico, D. & Barbarito, C. (2007). *Health & physical assessment in nursing.* Upper Saddle River, NJ: Pearson Education, Inc., p. 86.

5 **Answer: 3** **Rationale:** Option 3 will give the nurse a beginning history of the client's alcohol/drug use. This can be valuable for the intake assessment for both the physical and the psychosocial part of the intake assessment. Option 1 will not help the nurse assess the reason that the client is in the current condition. Option 2 is not the first question that the nurse should ask of the mother. Option 4 is probably not going to help get accurate information about the client's present condition. The client does not want to answer questions and will probably deny any use of substances at this time. The nurse needs to assess the client's state of health. The mother would be most likely to give accurate information. The client's rights are not being violated by the nurse asking questions of the parent. **Cognitive Level:** Application **Client Need:** Psychosocial Integrity **Integrated Process:** Nursing Process: Assessment **Content Area:** Mental Health **Strategy:** Determine first that the present psychosocial assessment should be done quickly to gain information about the client's state of health and safety level. Asking the mother about the client's history of drug use does not violate the client's rights but helps to establish the client's psychosocial well-being. The nurse will question the client later but in order to begin the assessment the nurse chooses to question the more reliable person at this time, who is the mother. **Reference:** D'Amico, D. & Barbarito, C.

(2007). *Health & physical assessment in nursing.* Upper Saddle River, NJ: Pearson Education, Inc., p. 86.

6 **Answer: 1** **Rationale:** The client is hospitalized for pneumonia. The psychosocial history should be conducted with the client as much as possible (option 1). Information from a medical record should be included in the assessment but the nurse should conduct the assessment with the client. There is no indication here that the client cannot personally answer questions, which is why options 2 and 4 are incorrect. Option 3 is partly accurate; the nurse should get information from a medical record but should still conduct the intake assessment with the client. **Cognitive Level:** Application **Client Need:** Psychosocial Integrity **Integrated Process:** Communication and Documentation **Content Area:** Mental Health **Strategy:** Consider that the nurse needs to conduct the psychosocial assessment and the best source of information should be the client. In this case, there is no indication that the client cannot be interviewed about the history of schizophrenia. If there is a medical record that the nurse can refer to, begin establishing a baseline there, but the interview should begin with the client, not with family members. **Reference:** D'Amico, D. & Barbarito, C. (2007). *Health & physical assessment in nursing.* Upper Saddle River, NJ: Pearson Education, Inc., p. 78.

7 **Answer: 2** **Rationale:** Option 2 is a combination of how the client feels he or she looks and his or her beliefs about self, which is the description given in the question. Option 1 is the client's examination of self, which is not described in this question. Options 3 and 4 are self-esteem and self-image, which are parts of one's self-concept. **Cognitive Level:** Analysis **Client Need:** Psychosocial Integrity **Integrated Process:** Nursing Process: Analysis **Content Area:** Mental Health **Strategy:** Recall the definitions of the components of the psychosocial interview. This includes all but option 1. Remember that self-examination is not usually associated with a psychosocial assessment but rather with a physical assessment such as breast "self-exam." The other 2 options (3 and 4) are a definition of the correct answer, option 2. **Reference:** D'Amico, D. & Barbarito, C. (2007). *Health & physical assessment in nursing.* Upper Saddle River, NJ: Pearson Education, Inc., p. 83.

8 **Answer: 3** **Rationale:** Option 1 is incorrect because there is no indication of this in the question and usually children learn from significant individuals in their life (option 3). A child will model those individuals as he or she grows and develops. The question does not indicate that the child spends a significant amount of time with the grandparents (option 2), and option 4 is also vague and is not presented as a significant person in the child's life. Therefore, the correct answer is option 3. **Cognitive Level:** Analysis **Client Need:** Psychosocial Integrity **Integrated Process:** Nursing Process: Analysis

Content Area: Mental Health **Strategy:** Recall that coping mechanisms that a child learns are usually learned from significant people in the child's life. To determine from where a child learns coping, recall the principles of development. **Reference:** D'Amico, D. & Barbarito, C. (2007). *Health & physical assessment in nursing.* Upper Saddle River, NJ: Pearson Education, Inc., p. 85.

9 **Answer: 3** **Rationale:** Body language is the only physical observation. Self-image and self-concept (options 1 and 2) are internal psychosocial factors. Ability to cope with stress (option 4) is not usually considered a physical observation.

Cognitive Level: Analysis **Client Need:** Psychosocial Integrity **Integrated Process:** Communication and Documentation **Content Area:** Mental Health **Strategy:** Consider that a physical indicator is one that is observable by the nurse. With this in mind, you would eliminate each of the incorrect options, as only option 3, body language, is observable by the nurse.

Reference: D'Amico, D. & Barbarito, C. (2007). *Health & physical assessment in nursing.* Upper Saddle River, NJ: Pearson Education, Inc., p. 92.

10 **Answer: 3** **Rationale:** Given the information in the question, the correct answer can be established by knowing the tasks for the stages of development and applying them to the client described. Option 3 is the correct answer because of the age of the client, which falls in the school-age stage. Option 1 refers to early childhood, option 2 refers to preschoolers, and option 4 refers to older adults.

Cognitive Level: Analysis **Client Need:** Psychosocial Integrity **Integrated Process:** Nursing Process: Analysis **Content Area:** Mental Health **Strategy:** As indicated, knowing the levels of development and some of the tasks for the levels is essential. The age of the child and the tasks are only relevant to the industry versus inferiority level of development. **Reference:** D'Amico, D. & Barbarito, C. (2007). *Health & physical assessment in nursing.* Upper Saddle River, NJ: Pearson Education, Inc., p. 49.

References

D'Amico, D. & Barbarito, C. (2007). *Health & physical assessment in nursing.* Upper Saddle River, NJ: Pearson Education, Inc.

Fontaine, K. (2009). *Mental health nursing* (6th ed.). Upper Saddle River, NJ: Pearson Education, Inc.

Gorman, L. M. & Sultan, D. F. (2008). *Psychosocial nursing: For general patient care* (3rd ed.). Philadelphia, PA: F.A. Davis.

Hermanns, M. S. & Russell-Broaddus, C. A. (2006). "But I'm not a psych nurse!" *RNWeb.* Retrieved October 24, 2008, from http://rn.modernmedicine.com/rnweb/content/printContentPopup.jsp?id=388220

4 Nutritional Assessment

Chapter Outline

Overview of Nutritional Status
General Health History Related to Nutrition
Present Health History Related to Nutrition

Equipment, Preparation, and Positioning
Nutritional Assessment
Expected Findings

Unexpected Findings
Lifespan Considerations
Documentation

NCLEX-RN® Test Prep

Visit the Companion Website for this book at www.pearsonhighered.com/hogan to access additional practice opportunities and more.

Objectives

➤ Describe factors that affect nutritional health.
➤ Describe the nutritional focus areas from Healthy People 2010.
➤ Identify the components of a diet history.
➤ Explain the techniques and tools used to gather data during a diet history.
➤ Describe how nutritional assessment techniques are customized to specific age groups across the lifespan.
➤ Differentiate between normal and abnormal findings obtained during a nutritional assessment.
➤ Differentiate between normal and abnormal laboratory test results measured as part of a nutritional assessment.
➤ Describe important information to document regarding a client's nutritional status.

Review at a Glance

anthropometric measurements collection of specific data related to physical characteristics of the body

bioelectrical impedance analysis a non-invasive tool using electroconduction through water, muscle, and fat to determine body composition

body mass index (BMI) a measurement that correlates indirectly to amount of body fat; calculated by dividing weight (kg) by height (meters)²

calf circumference a measurement obtained at maximum width of calf

diet recall a nutritional assessment in which a client verbally recalls all food, beverages, and nutritional supplements

or products ingested over a 24-hour period; also called a 24-hour recall

height total body length from heels to top of head

malnutrition a state of under- or over-nutrition with adverse metabolic consequences to body

mid-arm circumference a measurement obtained by measuring around mid-arm at tricep skinfold

nutritional health physical result of balance between nutritional intake and requirements

overweight a BMI of greater than 25 without comorbid conditions; increased

weight and fat stores in excess of normal expected body mass index

skinfold measurements use of calipers to determine thickness of skinfolds and underlying subcutaneous (SubQ) tissue; can estimate SubQ fat stores at up to eight different locations on body

underweight a BMI of less than 18.5 with associated health consequences; a weight less than expected based on body fat, height, age, and activity

weight product of force of gravity multiplied by body mass; term is used commonly as one indicator of health

PRETEST

1 The nurse is obtaining a 24-hour diet recall from a client who is losing approximately 1 to 1.5 pounds per week. What are the most appropriate questions for the nurse to ask this client about the diet consumed? Select all that apply.

1. "When was the first time you ate yesterday?"
2. "How much water did you drink yesterday?"
3. "What nutritional supplements did you take yesterday?"
4. "What did you have for breakfast?"
5. "What was the first thing you ate yesterday?"

2 During the last three months, the client's weight has decreased from 150 pounds to 120 pounds. The nurse who is assessing the client's nutritional status calculates the weight loss percentage to be ___%. Provide a numeric answer.

3 The nurse is performing anthropometric measurements on a client as part of a nutritional assessment. Which method would be most appropriate to use in calculating the risk of cardiovascular disease?

1. Weight
2. Body mass index
3. Waist circumference
4. Skinfold measurements

4 Which of the following techniques would the nurse use to perform a tricep skinfold measurement?

1. Use thumb and forefinger to grasp subcutaneous (subQ) fat and skin layers on the anterior aspect of the upper arm and then apply skinfold calipers
2. Use thumb and forefinger to grasp subQ fat and muscle in the upper third of the arm and then apply skinfold calipers
3. Use thumb and forefinger to grasp subQ fat and muscle on the bottom lateral aspect of the arm and then apply skinfold calipers
4. Use thumb and forefinger to grasp subQ fat and skin layers at the midpoint of the back of the arm and then apply skinfold calipers

5 The client has been slowly losing weight for the past several months. The client states, "I have always been of normal weight up until now." The nurse determines that it is essential to gather information about which of the following?

1. Poor dentition, and swallowing and chewing difficulties
2. Poor dentition, swallowing and chewing difficulties, and functional and physical decline
3. Past medical history and medication history over the last 12 months
4. Skinfold measurements, diet recall, and past medical history

6 The nurse is conducting a nutrition education program for the parents of school-age children. The nurse should instruct the parents that children at this developmental age are likely to be more at risk for which common nutritional concern?

1. Undernutrition due to high energy levels
2. Nutrition deficiencies due to fad dieting
3. Undernutrition due to lack of fortified food
4. Overnutrition due to frequent take-out meals

7 The nurse is performing a nutritional and physical assessment on an adult client. The nurse documents that the client has yellow subcutaneous fat deposits around the eyes. The nurse should expect which laboratory test to be ordered?

1. Albumin level
2. Iron level
3. Complete blood count
4. Cholesterol level

8 The parent of a child asks the nurse, "Why is my child's mouth bleeding?" The nurse examines the child's mouth and finds that the gums are spongy and bleeding is present. What is the nurse's best response to the parent?

1. "The bleeding is to due to the child's nervous habit of biting the inside of the mouth."
2. "It is a condition called stomatitis."
3. "Spongy, bleeding gums can occur with a vitamin C deficiency."
4. "It is probably due to a protein deficiency."

9 The client asks the nurse, "What is macrocytic anemia?" What is the nurse's best response?

1. "Anemia due to low hemoglobin."
2. "A deficiency that may be due to low folic acid or vitamin B_{12} levels."
3. "A form of malnutrition."
4. "Too few white blood cells."

10 The nurse is teaching the adult client about MyPyramid. The nurse can evaluate that the client understands the teaching when the client states that MyPyramid does which of the following?

1. Aids in group teaching
2. Reflects an individualized approach to nutrition
3. Encourages a low intake of carbohydrates
4. Indicates two servings of grains are needed daily

➤ *See pages 69–70 for Answers and Rationales.*

I. OVERVIEW OF NUTRITIONAL STATUS

A. Nutritional status: balance of nutritional intake and nutritional requirements needed for energy and to maintain health
   1. Factors influencing nutrition
      a. Physical: undernutrition, overnutrition, medication use, disease conditions
      b. Psychosocial: depression, lack of knowledge of proper nutrition
      c. Cultural: lifestyle choice—avoiding or eating certain foods
      d. Economic: poverty, inability to obtain food
B. Adequate nutrition: a state of consuming appropriate amounts and types of nutrients to sustain the body's metabolic needs
C. Inadequate nutrition (malnutrition)
   1. Overnutrition: a state in which client consumes more calories than needed; may influence development of diseases such as diabetes mellitus type 2, cardiovascular disease, cancer, and musculoskeletal disease
   2. Undernutrition: a state in which client has inadequate intake of nutrients to meet body's needs; increases risk of infection, poor wound healing, inadequate physical and mental development in children, disease, and possibly death
   3. See Box 4-1 for examples of risk factors for undernutrition or overnutrition

Box 4-1	
Risk Factors for Poor Nutritional Health	**Undernutrition** • Chronic disease, acute illness, or injury • Multiple medications • Food insecurity—lack of free access to adequate and safe food • Restrictive eating due to chronic dieting, disordered eating, faddism, or food beliefs • Alcohol abuse (proper nutrient intake) • Depression, bereavement, loneliness, social isolation • Poor dental health • Decreased knowledge or skills about food preparation and recommendations • Extreme age—premature infants or adults over 80 years of age **Overnutrition** • Excess intake of fat, sugar, calories, or nutrients • Alcohol abuse (excess calories from sugar in alcohol) • Sedentary lifestyle • Decreased knowledge or skills about food preparation and recommendations

Source: D'Amico, D. & Barbarito, C. (2007). *Health & physical assessment in nursing.* Upper Saddle River, NJ: Pearson Education, Inc., p. 137, Box 9.1.

II. GENERAL HEALTH HISTORY RELATED TO NUTRITION

A. Identifies risks to *nutritional health* (physical result of balance between nutritional intake and nutritional requirements)

B. Evaluates clues to nutritional problems utilizing age to determine nutritional requirements

C. Components of health history useful in evaluating nutritional health

1. Religious and cultural beliefs may influence dietary preferences; ask the client the following:

    a. "Do you have any religious beliefs that may influence your dietary practices? If so, what?"

    b. "Do you have any cultural practices that may influence your dietary practices? If so, what?"

2. Socioeconomic status may influence ability to eat a healthy diet; with inadequate income many people, especially children, are at risk for poor nutrition; ask client the following:

    a. "Is your income adequate to meet food needs?"

    b. "Do you have adequate access to a grocery store?"

3. Assess client for changes in health status; illness, change in mental status, and medications may influence nutritional intake; ask client the following:

    a. "Have your eating habits and appetite changed recently?"

    b. "Do you attempt to maintain your **weight** with good nutrition? How?"

4. Evaluate changes in weight and causes for these changes, which may provide information about **malnutrition** (inadequate or excessive intake of calories, protein and other nutrients) and hydration status; ask the following:

    a. "Have you recently gained weight?"

    b. "Have you recently lost weight?"

    c. "Over what period of time was the weight change?"

5. Assess medication usage (prescribed and over-the-counter [OTC]) and herbal supplement use as these may influence ability to eat or absorb nutrients, causing clients to be **underweight**; people may not purchase food because of a need to use money to purchase medication; ask client the following:

    a. "Do you take over-the-counter medications? If so, what?"

    b. "Do you use illegal drugs? If so, what do you use and how often?"

    c. "Do you use herbal supplements? If so, which ones and how often?"

6. Assess past medical history; this may give clues to prior eating habits or willingness to change diet; medical conditions may affect ability to eat; ask client the following:

    a. "Do you have cancer?" (may cause decreased ability to eat; steroid intake may cause weight gain)

    b. "Do you have cardiovascular disease?" (may need diet low in fat; heart failure may cause water weight gain or inability to eat from lack of energy)

    c. "Are you experiencing any metabolic problems?" (hypothyroidism may cause weight gain, whereas hyperthyroidism may cause weight loss; type 2 diabetes has been linked to obesity)

7. Evaluate client for recent foreign travel, which may expose client to food and water pathogens

8. Assess client for food intolerances or allergies:

    a. "Do you have any food intolerances or allergies? If so, what?"

    b. "What type of reaction do you experience when you consume the food to which you are allergic?"

9. Evaluate if client has psychosocial issues that may interfere with eating; food can become a substitute for relationships or depression may affect desire to eat; stress may cause loss of appetite; ask client the following:

    a. "Are relationships stressful or satisfying?"

Practice to Pass

After teaching the client about overnutrition, the nurse asks the client to describe the most common causes of overnutrition, which include what factors?

Practice to Pass

What problems will food intolerances or allergies cause in a client?

        b. "Describe the stressors in your life."

        c. "What are your normal coping mechanisms?"

   10. Assess self-care ability; people unable to care for themselves may not eat well to prevent causing additional work for caregiver; ask client the following:

        a. "Who does the shopping and cooking?"

        b. "Do you eat out frequently?"

   11. Assess activity level; inability to carry out activities of daily living (ADLs) may indicate nutritional deficiencies; ask client the following:

        a. "What activities do you do every day?"

        b. "What is your activity and exercise level?"

D. Family history related to nutrition

   1. Ask if client has a family history of genetic factors that influence nutritional intake; for example, "Are there any conditions in your family that affect your digestion, absorption, or metabolism?"

   2. Assess if client has family history of inflammatory bowel disease, which causes abdominal discomfort, weight loss, diarrhea, and affects nutritional intake

   3. Assess if there is a family history of cardiovascular disease, gout, obesity, or diabetes mellitus; all of these disease processes have familial tendencies and directly influence nutritional health

   4. Assess if client has a history of cancer, which interferes with adequate nutrition because of pathophysiology and gastrointestinal side effects of chemotherapy

III. PRESENT HEALTH HISTORY RELATED TO NUTRITION

A. Ask how client's health status has changed; health changes may influence nutrition

B. Evaluate if client is experiencing any illness; consider influence on client's ability to consume, digest, and metabolize nutrients

C. Assess if client has had any trauma, surgery, or new medications; these may stimulate stress response or otherwise influence nutritional intake

D. Vomiting or diarrhea affects health by decreasing nutrient intake and absorption

E. Infection accelerates metabolic needs, creating a need for additional nutrients

F. Ask client about changes in weight

   1. Changes in weight may be due to financial constraints or physical or social factors; also, weight loss may have been planned (anorexia, bulimia, dieting)

   2. Endocrine, cardiovascular, and respiratory problems or cancer may influence weight

G. Assess if client is experiencing any changes in taste, smell, chewing, or swallowing, which may affect ability to consume food; if so, ask the following:

   1. "When did this occur?"

   2. "What type of change have you experienced?"

H. Assess if client is able to prepare his or her own meals; ask client the following:

   1. "Are you able to prepare your meals? If not, who prepares them?"

   2. "Do you have a pleasant environment in which to dine?"

I. Assess what client eats each day; ask client the following:

   1. "What meals do you eat each day?"

   2. "How many and what snacks do you eat per day?"

IV. EQUIPMENT, PREPARATION, AND POSITIONING

A. Equipment

   1. Skin calipers: an instrument utilized to determine subQ fat measurements

   2. Tape measure: used to measure waist and hip circumferences

   3. Scale with **height** stick: used to obtain weight and height

   4. Height and weight tables: standardized table used to assess adequacy of weight by comparing it to height

B. **Preparation and positioning**
   1. Gather all equipment
   2. Ensure there is also adequate space to document data gathered; provide an area for writing and possibly one for client to complete a food questionnaire
   3. Since client will be answering many questions, provide a comfortable chair for use during first part of assessment
   4. An examination table is needed to obtain skin fold measurements
   5. Both client and nurse will stand when obtaining waist and hip measurements

V. NUTRITIONAL ASSESSMENT

A. **Purpose: to identify individuals who are at risk for developing nutritional deficiencies and to develop a nutritional plan of care**
B. **Components include weight, height, health history, *anthropometric measurements*, laboratory tests, nutritional screening tool(s), and physical assessment**
   1. Weigh client; obtain actual weight, as client may underreport; review weight history
      a. Appropriate questions include "How much did you weigh?" "How much did you gain or lose?" "Is there documentation of previous weight?"
      b. Calculate weight loss percentage by using this formula:
         [(Prior weight – current weight) / prior weight] $\times$ 100 = percentage of weight change
   2. Measure height (necessary to evaluate weight); if unable to measure height, note client's report of height; most clients perceive themselves as taller than they are
   3. Use **body mass index (BMI)** to evaluate appropriate weight for height through use of formula: body mass index = weight (kg) / height^2(meters^2) (See Table 4-1 for classification of nutritional status according to BMI value)
      a. BMI does not take into account individual body composition; individuals have different amounts of muscle mass, body fat, and bone density
         1) If body composition is not taken into account, then people may be viewed as **overweight**; an athlete may be classified as overweight because of mass muscle if the nurse uses only the BMI chart
         2) BMI charts do not take into account racial or ethnic differences
         3) Minimum body fat reference for men is 3%, for women is 12%
      b. Standard range of body fat for health is 12–20% in men and 20–30% in women
   4. Height-weight tables are no longer used unless they have a BMI indicator; these tables share the same limitations as BMI tables
   5. Waist circumference is a known risk factor for cardiovascular disease
      a. Measured at landmark of the ilium; to locate ilium stand behind client, palpate lateral ilium, and then mark it at midaxillary line; use a measuring tape parallel to floor and directly on skin (take care not to compress skin)
      b. Waist circumference greater than 102 cm in a male or 88 cm in a female is a risk factor for cardiovascular disease

Practice to Pass

The client weighed 165 pounds and lost 22 pounds in three months. The client's weight loss percentage is calculated to be ___%. (Show calculation.)

Table 4-1	BMI	Classification
Classification of Body Mass Index (BMI) in Adults	<16	Severe malnutrition
	16–16.99	Moderate malnutrition
	17–18.49	Mild malnutrition
	18.5–24.9	Normal
	25–29.9	Overweight
	30–34.9	Obese class 1
	35–39.9	Obese class 2
	>40	Obese class 3

Source: Department of Health and Human Services. National Heart, Lung, and Blood Institute. From http://www.nhlbisupport.com/bmi/bmicalc.htm; retrieved 02/07/2010

Practice to Pass

The nurse is assessing a client and calculates the BMI to be 16. How would the nurse classify this client's nutritional status based on this value?

Practice to Pass

A female client has a waist circumference of 96 cm. How should the nurse interpret this assessment data?

Practice to Pass

The client asks the nurse, "What is the purpose of taking these skinfold measurements?" How should the nurse respond?

6. **Skinfold measurements** are an estimate of amount of subQ body fat; obtain eight measurements from different body areas to obtain a full assessment
   a. Using skin calipers, pinch skin and subQ fat and hold gently between thumb and forefinger; be careful not to grasp muscle
   b. Hold calipers perpendicular to skinfold and leave in place for several seconds to permit for even compression after caliper tension released
   c. Take three measurements and then average the results
      1) Tricep skinfold measurement is taken at midpoint of arm equidistant from posterior aspect of acromium process to olecranon of elbow; use a measuring tape to determine midpoint of arm
      2) Measure client's arm when flexing elbow at a 90-degree angle; after midpoint is located, arm should hang at side so measurement can be taken
   d. Other sites to be used for skinfold measurements include chest, subscapular, midaxillary, suprailiac, abdomen, and upper thigh
   e. Take measurements and compare numbers to reference chart for gender, race, age, and fitness level
      1) Reference charts are for desired fitness levels for people over 20 years of age
      2) Skin elasticity is lost with aging and connective tissue changes affect skinfold measurements
7. **Mid-arm circumference** is also an estimate of body composition
   a. Mid-arm circumference is taken at same point as tricep skinfold
   b. Place measuring tape at mid-arm site without compressing skin and measure circumference in centimeters
8. **Calf circumference** is an estimate of body composition; measure all the way around calf in centimeters at widest part
9. **Bioelectrical impedance analysis** is a tool for assessing body composition using electroconduction through water, muscle, and fat
   a. Position client supine on a nonconductive surface and place electrodes on dorsal surfaces of right hand and foot
   b. Muscle and water have a higher concentration of electrolytes than fat and conduct electrical current differently
   c. Client must be adequately hydrated in order for measurements to be accurate
10. Near-Infrared Interactance (NIR) is a tool to measure body fat by passing infrared light through tissue and measuring reflected light at bicep; provides an estimate of body fat compared to gender, weight, height, frame size, and fitness level
11. Tools used for body composition analysis in laboratory research settings
    a. Dual x-ray absorptiometry (DEXA SCAN): measures a multi-component model of body composition by taking into account bone density through x-rays
    b. Underwater weighing: determines body composition by measuring the amount of water displaced when a client is fully submerged in water
    c. Plethysmography: measures air displaced by body when client is placed in a body pod; uses similar methodology as underwater weighing
12. Serum laboratory tests may aid assessment and ongoing monitoring of nutritional status; commonly used tests include serum albumin, prealbumin, and transferrin; these and other laboratory tests related to nutritional status are summarized in Table 4-2
13. Dietary intake data is obtained by performing a 24-hour dietary recall or using a food frequency questionnaire, interview, food diaries, or by direct observation
    a. **Diet recall** is a nutritional assessment in which client verbally recalls all food, beverages, and nutritional supplements or products ingested over a 24-hour period; also called a 24-hour diet recall
       1) Client can offer data if able or the clinician may ask open-ended questions in a non-judgmental way; appropriate questions include "What time did you first eat?" "What did you eat or drink?"

Table 4-2	Biochemical Assessment Laboratory Parameters	
Laboratory Measurement	**Significance**	**Values and Findings**
Albumin	Low albumin levels can be indicative of depleted visceral protein status and malnutrition. Dehydration or overhydration will lead to false levels due to hemoconcentration or hemodilution.	Expected 3.5 to 5 grams/L Half-life in days 14 to 20 Mild malnutrition 2.8 to 3.4 grams/L Moderate malnutrition 2.1 to 3.4 grams/L Severe malnutrition < 2.1 grams/L
Prealbumin	Also called thyroxine-binding prealbumin, has a long half-life and is therefore felt to provide a more current picture of protein status than albumin. Prealbumin is an acute-phase reactant protein and is affected by inflammation and infection. Hemoconcentration or hemodilution will cause false values.	Expected 150 to 350 mg/L Half-life in days 2 to 3 Mild malnutrition 110 to 150 mg/L Moderate malnutrition 50 to 109 mg/L Severe malnutrition < 50 mg/L
Transferrin	Responsible for iron binding and transport.	Expected > 200 mg/dL Half-life in days 8 to 10 Mild malnutrition 180 to 200 mg/L Moderate malnutrition 160 to 180 mg/L Severe malnutrition < 160 mg/L
Total Lymphocyte Count	Evaluates nutrition when confounding medical conditions such as cancer or immunosuppressive drugs interfere with nutritional assessment.	Expected TLC is 2,000 to 3,500 cells/mm³. Plasma level below 1,500 cells/mm³ may indicate malnutrition and poor immunocompetence.
Delayed Skin Hypersensitivity Testing	A delayed response to intradermal injection of foreign substances such as *Streptococcus* or *Candida*.	Delayed or no response may indicate malnutrition, poor immune system, or no previous exposure.
Cholesterol	High cholesterol may indicate overnutrition or undernutrition.	≥ 200 mg/dL is associated with cardiovascular disease. ≤160 mg/dL may indicate malnutrition.
Nutritional Anemia Assessment	Poor nutrition may be evidenced by low stores of iron, folic acid, vitamin B_{12}.	*Macrocytic anemia* is evidenced by deficient folic acid or vitamin B_{12} level. *Microcytic anemia* is evidenced by decreased red blood cell volume. *Iron deficiency anemia* is evidenced by low plasma hemoglobin and hematocrit.
Nitrogen Balance	Measured to estimate adequacy of dietary intake.	*Nitrogen balance* is evidenced by nitrogen intake equals nitrogen loss. *Catabolism* occurs when there is a negative nitrogen balance. *Anabolism* occurs when the intake of protein and calories exceeds the nitrogen loss.
Plasma Proteins Immunocompetence	Albumin, prealbumin, and transferrin are each used to assess visceral protein status. A depressed immune status can result from malnutrition, disease, medication, or other disease treatments.	

Source: D'Amico, D. & Barbarito, C. (2007). *Health & physical assessment in nursing.* Upper Saddle River, NJ: Pearson Education, Inc., p. 150, Table 9.6.

    2) Clinician must gather other data such as portion size and what is consumed on weekends versus weekdays (see Figure 4-1)

    3) Limitations include obtaining data from one day only, nurse's skills, inaccurate information because of poor recall ability, under-reporting of poor dietary habits, and over-reporting of good habits

  b. Food frequency questionnaire evaluates consumption of food type and amount per day and week

    1) May be a tool or informal discussion of dietary consumption; nurses often obtain additional information or insight into diet of individual

Figure 4-1

Using analogies to estimate portion size

Small potato or piece of fruit: computer mouse

2 tbsp: golf ball

3 oz. animal protein: deck of cards

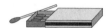

4 tbsp: four thumbs

1 oz. cheese: small box of wooden matches

1 cup dry measure: tightly clenched small woman's fist

      2) Use in addition to diet recall so further assessment can be made of dietary preferences, intolerances, and allergies

    c. Food diaries are useful when client is able to document all food consumed during a specific period of time (often 3 days); however, clients may often underreport dietary consumption and may include information they believe healthcare provider may want to hear

    d. Direct observation of client's eating habits is useful for the nurse to gather data as to what client is actually consuming

  14. Perform physical assessment to evaluate general health of individual; used in addition to nutritional assessment to indicate health

    a. Findings that may be pertinent to nutritional health include problems with dentition or swallowing, physical decline, change in mental status, fatigue, difficulty breathing, psychosocial issues, or problems with gastrointestinal system

    b. Nutritional deficiencies develop as a result of nutrients lacking in the diet; body utilizes tissue reserves to maintain metabolic processes; if body is depleted of nutrient reserves, blood levels drop and body begins to develop clinical manifestations

VI. EXPECTED FINDINGS

  A. Clients with normal nutritional status (i.e., absence of nutritional deficiencies) will exhibit a specific set of physical assessment and examination findings

  B. Clinical findings expected with normal nutritional status include the following:

    1. In a general health survey, client should have stable vital signs and no weight changes

    2. Skin, hair, and nails

      a. Skin should be dry and intact with smooth texture and even color; skin should have elasticity

      b. Hair should be evenly distributed with no alopecia or coarseness

      c. Nails should be smooth and pink with no ridges

    3. Eyes, nose, and mouth

      a. Eyes should be clear, bright, and evenly set in socket; eyes should not appear sunken nor should edema be present

      b. Sense of smell should be intact; nasal membranes should be pink and moist

      c. Oral mucosa should be pink, moist, and intact and without lesions; gums should not bleed; taste should be intact; gag reflex should be present

4. Client should be awake, alert, and oriented, and able to move all extremities without difficulty; sensation should be intact
5. Client should be free of dyspnea; breath sounds should be present in all lung fields and lungs should be clear to auscultation
6. In the cardiovascular system there should be no extra heart sounds, and rhythm should be regular; expected finding is absence of cyanosis
7. Abdomen should be soft, non-tender, non-distended and without masses; bowel sounds should be present in all quadrants and client should be able to pass soft brown stool regularly and without difficulty
8. Client should be producing urine without odor and that is light and pale in color in sufficient quantity (greater than 30 mL/hr or 0.5 mL/kg body weight)
9. Musculoskeletal system should have no deformities or tenderness

VII. UNEXPECTED FINDINGS

A. **Unexpected findings during physical assessment may be associated with nutritional deficiencies or weight or psychosocial issues**

B. **Clinical manifestations that may be present when there are nutritional deficits**

1. Weight changes may reflect fluid retention or dehydration; blood pressure (BP) may indicate dehydration if low, and elevated BP may reflect fluid overload, excessive sodium intake or obesity; an increase in respiratory and heart rate and/or cardiac murmurs result from iron deficiency anemia
2. Skin that is flaky and scaling could indicate deficiency or excess in vitamin A, zinc, and fatty acids
3. Protein deficits cause skin to be transparent and cracked; skin lesions may be due to a lack of protein and vitamin C; children who are not growing may be experiencing protein deficit
4. Lack of vitamin C may weaken immune system and may lead to petechiae and swollen bleeding gums; severe vitamin C deficits have also been linked to sudden cardiac death
5. Purpura may be caused by vitamin C and K deficiencies
6. Client experiencing dehydration will exhibit decreased skin turgor (tenting will be present)
7. Concave shape of nails may be due to iron deficiencies; nails with transverse ridges usually result from protein deficits
8. Papilledema may result from excessive vitamin A (although more common causes are hypertension and increased intracranial pressure); vitamin A excess may also cause headache, dizziness, and lethargy in clients
9. Deficiency in vitamin A may decrease night vision; pale conjunctiva may reflect iron deficiency
10. Dehydration will lead to sunken eyes, dark circles, and decreased or absent tears; client may also exhibit disorientation and confusion
11. Excessive cholesterol may cause yellow fat deposits around eyelids
12. Riboflavin deficiency may cause cracks in corners of mouth (cheilosis); if corners of mouth and ulcerated lips are inflamed, this is known as cheilitis
13. Lack of riboflavin, niacin, folic acid, vitamin B_{12}, protein, and iron may cause *atrophic lingual papillae* (of tongue); glossitis may be present if client has all of the above deficits and, in addition, a pyridoxine deficit
14. A client deficient in zinc may report lack of ability to taste
15. Vitamin D deficits may cause musculoskeletal deformities; if teeth do not erupt in infants, then suspect deficiency of vitamin D
16. Evaluate client's calcium and magnesium levels for low values if experiencing *tetany* (muscle twitches, cramps, and carpopedal spasm) and increased deep tendon reflexes (DTRs)

17. Vitamin B_{12} and niacin deficits may contribute to dementia
18. Ophthalmoplegia (a paralysis or weakness of one or more muscles that control eye movement) may develop as result of phosphorus and thiamine deficits
19. When evaluating a client in heart failure or with an S3 heart sound consider thiamine, phosphorus, or iron deficit
20. Potassium deficits may cause cardiac dysrhythmias
21. *Ascites* (accumulation of serous fluid in abdominal cavity) may indicate deficit of either protein or vitamin A

C. **Intact gag reflex is required for client to eat; it is essential to assess gag reflex prior to feeding client who may have impaired swallowing ability**

VIII. LIFESPAN CONSIDERATIONS

A. **Infants (birth to 12 months) have high metabolic needs; due to rapid growth, an infant needs high protein levels and fat intake essential to neurological development**
1. Caloric requirements begin at 100–200 kcal/day at birth and decrease at one year to 80–100 kcal; protein requirement is 2.5–3.5 grams at birth and decrease to 2 grams at 12 months
2. Infants require 30–55% of fat from caloric intake; solids are introduced between four and six months; iron reserves are depleted between four and six months when iron-rich cereal is introduced

B. **Toddlers' (1–3 years) growth rate decreases; they often develop food fads; fat remains essential to neurological development and iron deficiency remains potential problem**
1. Require whole milk and intake of all essential elements; should adhere to MyPyramid guidelines; require five grams of fiber per day; serving size is approximately one tablespoon per year of age
2. Protein deficiency malnutrition may occasionally occur in families because of insufficient income to buy adequate nutritious foods; families who eat a vegan diet and have not yet learned how to combine foods to get all necessary amino acids may also experience protein deficiency

C. **Preschool children (3–6 years) grow at a rate of 2 inches and 5 pounds per year**
1. Are learning lifelong eating habits
2. Need approximately 1800 calories per day; serving size remains at one tablespoon per year

D. **School-age children (6–12 years)**
1. Should be making healthy food choices
2. Caloric requirements are 2000 calories; require 800 mg of calcium

E. **Adolescents (12–20 years) have increased skeletal growth and need increased calcium for strong bones and teeth**
1. Males have increased need for calories, calcium, iron, water soluble vitamins and zinc to mature
2. Females need increased iron
3. All adolescents require four servings of dairy foods per day

F. **Adults need to continue healthy food choices and to consume foods from MyPyramid in serving size as recommended**

G. **Older adults**
1. May need to decrease caloric intake as a result of decreased activity and basal metabolic rate
2. May experience malnutrition due to lack of income or living on fixed income

IX. DOCUMENTATION

A. **Items to be documented should include past medical history that can affect nutrition**
B. **It is especially important to note weight changes**

C. Allergy and food intolerance provides essential information to develop a plan of care to eliminate nutritional deficiencies

D. Recording dietary intake, height, weight, and laboratory diagnostic tests assists in providing information on nutritional status

E. Subjective data includes food intake, ability to eat, ability to make meals, and dietary preference

F. Objective data includes vital signs (temperature, pulse, respirations, BP), height, weight, skin condition (integrity, lesions, turgor, dryness or moisture)

Case Study

A 70-year-old male client is seen at the health center for weight loss and poor dietary intake. He has been under a physician's care for heart failure and is taking 25 mg per day of hydrochlorothiazide and following a low sodium diet. The nurse notes the client is 5 feet, 11 inches tall, weighed 200 pounds during his annual checkup four months ago, and currently weighs 172 pounds. The client has skin tenting and examination of his mouth reveals oversized dentures. While obtaining the nutritional assessment the nurse ascertains that the client does not like to eat "since his wife died." The client also says "food does not taste good anymore." The client says it is easier to eat "frozen meals." The diet recall conducted by the nurse includes the following:

Breakfast:	*Coffee, cereal with milk*
Lunch:	*Egg salad on white toast*
	Soda
Midday Snack:	*Chips and soda*
Dinner:	*Frozen dinner*
	Soda
	Canned soup
Evening snack:	*Tea*
	Irish soda bread or scones

1. What problems is the client experiencing?

2. What is the client's weight loss percentage?

3. What is the client's current BMI? What was the previous BMI? What are the implications of the change for this client?

4. What dietary and other instruction should the nurse provide for this client?

5. How should the nurse document this assessment?

For suggested responses, see pages 308–309

POSTTEST

1 During a nutrition education class, the nurse discusses that which of the following objectives is a nutritional objective of Healthy People 2010?

1. Increase the number of people who are at a healthy weight.
2. Place all overweight adults on a calorie restricted diet.
3. Encourage low-carbohydrate diets.
4. Encourage all adults to eat two servings of fruit, vegetables, and grains.

2 The nurse is writing a grant to fund a nutrition education program. The nurse would plan the program for which group of people who are at risk for undernutrition?

1. Older adults
2. College students
3. School-age children
4. Working adults with busy schedules

3 The nurse is performing a nutritional assessment on an adult client. The nurse would obtain information on which parameters? Select all that apply.

1. Medical history
2. Medication and herbal use history
3. Water quality
4. Alcohol intake
5. Number of hours of sleep each night

4 The nurse is performing a nutritional assessment on a 75-year-old healthy woman who has lost 10 pounds in the last five months with no significant past medical history. The nurse should next investigate whether this weight loss is related to which of the following?

1. A change of respiratory status
2. Alternating bowel patterns due to changes associated with aging
3. Increased caloric needs
4. Possible financial difficulty due to existing on a fixed income

5 The nurse who is assessing both the adipose and muscle tissue of a client would perform which anthropometric measurement?

1. Height and weight
2. Body mass index
3. Tricep skinfold measurement
4. Mid-arm circumference

6 The nurse is evaluating clients for cardiovascular disease using waist circumference. The nurse would conclude that which client is at increased risk?

1. Male, waist circumference of 110 centimeters (cm)
2. Male, waist circumference of 64 cm
3. Female, waist circumference of 54 cm
4. Female, waist circumference of 75 cm

7 When assessing a young male who has been taking liquid protein supplements to increase his muscle mass when weight lifting, the nurse notes that the client has normal weight status. With further assessment, what would the nurse expect to find?

1. Waist circumference greater than 130 cm
2. Low iron levels
3. Increased serum albumin levels
4. Decreased mid-arm circumference measurements

8 A young male is being evaluated for weight loss and indigestion. When interviewing the client the nurse concludes that the client has not been eating well and is consuming foods from fast-food eateries and is drinking beverages containing sugar. What should the nurse do next to obtain more thorough nutritional assessment data on this client?

1. Have client see healthcare provider for possible lower gastrointestinal assessment.
2. Have client complete a 24-hour diet recall.
3. Ask client to complete a food diary.
4. Take anthropometric measurements on client.

9 The nurse is performing a nutritional assessment on a client who has newly immigrated to the United States. It is essential that the nurse question the client about which of the following?

1. Information about whether the client is happy here because, if not, the client may not eat well
2. Religious factors that may influence food intake
3. Information about whether new-culture foods are being introduced into the diet
4. Information about the client's knowledge of herbal supplementation

10 The client does not consume calcium products and is concerned with not having enough bone density. The nurse should plan to prepare the client for which prescribed diagnostic study?

1. Waist circumference measurements
2. Dual x-ray absorptiometry (Dexa Scan)
3. Venipuncture for albumin and iron levels
4. 24-hour diet recall

➤ *See pages 71–72 for Answers and Rationales.*

ANSWERS & RATIONALES

Pretest

1 **Answer: 1, 3, 4, 5** **Rationale:** The questions in options 1, 3, 4, and 5 are designed to gather data in a nonjudgmental manner about nutritional intake and dietary patterns. Options 1, 4, and 5 address food intake directly. Recall that nutritional supplements (option 3) could include protein-based and/or caloric products as well as vitamin, mineral, or herbal supplements, and thus option 3 is a useful question. The question "how much water did you drink yesterday?" (option 2) provides information about hydration status but not about caloric nutrient intake. **Cognitive Level:** Application **Client Need:** Health Promotion and Maintenance **Integrated Process:** Nursing Process: Assessment **Content Area:** Foundational Sciences: Nutrition **Strategy:** Consider that interviewing techniques need to obtain information about the full range of options for dietary intake. This would include all food items as well as when the client ate. Next eliminate option 3, recalling that water aids in hydration but provides no calories or nutrients to the body. **Reference:** D'Amico, D. & Barbarito, C. (2007). *Health & physical assessment in nursing.* Upper Saddle River, NJ: Pearson Education, Inc., p. 138.

2 **Answer: 20** **Rationale:** The weight loss percentage is calculated by using the formula
[(Prior weight – current weight) / prior weight] × 100
The weight loss percentage for this client is then calculated as

$$150 - 120 = 30$$
$$30 \div 150 = 0.20$$
$$0.20 \times 100 = 20\%$$

Cognitive Level: Application **Client Need:** Health Promotion and Maintenance **Integrated Process:** Nursing Process: Assessment **Content Area:** Foundational Sciences: Nutrition **Strategy:** Specific knowledge of the formula used to determine weight loss percentage is needed to answer the question. Double check your answer by calculating that the weight change needs to be divided by the original weight and then converted from a decimal to a percentage by multiplying by 100. **Reference:** D'Amico, D. & Barbarito, C. (2007). *Health & physical assessment in nursing.* Upper Saddle River, NJ: Pearson Education, Inc., p. 140.

3 **Answer: 3** **Rationale:** Waist circumference should be obtained when the client has risk factors for cardiovascular disease (option 3). A large, centrally located abdominal fat deposit is considered to be an independent risk factor for cardiovascular disease by the National Heart, Lung, and Blood Institute (NHLBI). Specifically, a waist circumference greater than 102 cm

for men or 88 cm for women is considered to place the client at risk. Weight (option 1) is assessed for evidence of gain or loss. Body mass index (option 2) is used to assess the extent to which weight is appropriate for height. Skinfold measurements (option 4) are used to obtain data related to body fat stores. **Cognitive Level:** Application **Client Need:** Health Promotion and Maintenance **Integrated Process:** Nursing Process: Assessment **Content Area:** Foundational Sciences: Nutrition **Strategy:** Consider the measurements listed in each option and recall the benefit of each. Recall that centrally located abdominal fat is an independent risk factor for heart disease and then focus on the critical word *waist* in the correct option to choose correctly. If this question is difficult for you to answer, review techniques to calculate anthropometric measurements. **Reference:** D'Amico, D. & Barbarito, C. (2007). *Health & physical assessment in nursing.* Upper Saddle River, NJ: Pearson Education, Inc., p. 142.

4 **Answer: 4** **Rationale:** To obtain skinfold measurements grasp the subcutaneous fat and skin layers and measure at the midpoint between the posterior edge of the acromium process of the scapula and the olecranon process of the elbow using skinfold calipers. The calipers do not measure muscle tissue (options 2 and 3), and the nurse should measure in the area of the triceps muscle at the back of the arm, not the biceps muscle anteriorly (option 1). **Cognitive Level:** Application **Client Need:** Health Promotion and Maintenance **Integrated Process:** Nursing Process: Implementation **Content Area:** Foundational Sciences: Nutrition **Strategy:** The critical word in the question is *tricep*. Visualize the location of the tricep muscle to eliminate option 1. Then recall that this technique measures only skin and fat layers to eliminate options 2 and 3. **Reference:** D'Amico, D. & Barbarito, C. (2007). *Health & physical assessment in nursing.* Upper Saddle River, NJ: Pearson Education, Inc., p. 142.

5 **Answer: 2** **Rationale:** Common causes of weight loss include poor dentition, swallowing and chewing difficulties, as well as physical and functional difficulties. Issues in the mouth, physical limitations, and functional difficulties could cause or contribute to weight loss. The incorrect options (1, 3, and 4) provide partial assessments but are not as comprehensive to evaluate this client thoroughly. **Cognitive Level:** Application **Client Need:** Physiological Integrity: Reduction of Risk Potential **Integrated Process:** Nursing Process: Assessment **Content Area:** Foundational Sciences: Nutrition **Strategy:** The critical word in the question is *essential*. This indicates that the correct option is one that contains the key information needed to further evaluate the client's concern. Next recall the various causes of weight loss, and eliminate each of the incorrect options because they are partial answers only. Option 2 is the most comprehensive or global option. Recall that poor dentition, swallowing and chewing difficulties, and physical and functional decline are all causes of weight loss. **Reference:** D'Amico, D. & Barbarito, C. (2007). *Health & physical assessment in nursing.* Upper Saddle River, NJ: Pearson Education, Inc., p. 96.

6 **Answer: 4** **Rationale:** The school-age child is most at risk for overnutrition due to an increasing societal trend toward frequent use of take-out meals because of many extracurricular activities (option 4). These foods tend to be higher in calories and fat overall. School-age children are not usually at risk for undernutrition unless they are experiencing a chronic illness (options 1 and 3) and fortified foods are readily available in supermarkets and other food stores. Adolescents are most likely to engage in fad dieting (option 2).

Cognitive Level: Application **Client Need:** Health Promotion and Maintenance **Integrated Process:** Nursing Process: Assessment **Content Area:** Foundational Sciences: Nutrition **Strategy:** Focus on the age of the clients in the question (school-age children) since age is added to the question for a specific reason. Eliminate option 2 because this age group does not engage in fad dieting. Next eliminate option 3 because lack of access to fortified food would not be age-specific. Next choose option 4 over option 1 since hunger in children would trigger food intake to prevent option 1. **Reference:** D'Amico, D. & Barbarito, C. (2007). *Health & physical assessment in nursing.* Upper Saddle River, NJ: Pearson Education, Inc., p. 136.

7 **Answer: 4** **Rationale:** A high cholesterol level may cause subcutaneous fat deposits around the eyes (option 4). Albumin levels are used as one measure of circulating protein levels (option 1). Iron levels are used to indicate the total iron binding capacity of hemoglobin (option 2). The complete blood count is used to evaluate the red and white blood cell counts (option 3).

Cognitive Level: Application **Client Need:** Physiological Integrity: Reduction of Risk Potential **Integrated Process:** Nursing Process: Analysis **Content Area:** Foundational Sciences: Nutrition **Strategy:** Review the indications for various laboratory tests listed in the question. Recall that cholesterol is a sticky yellow substance and associate this with the word *yellow* in the stem of the question. **Reference:** D'Amico, D. & Barbarito, C. (2007). *Health & physical assessment in nursing.* Upper Saddle River, NJ: Pearson Education, Inc., p. 146.

8 **Answer: 3** **Rationale:** Spongy, bleeding gums are consistent with a vitamin C deficiency. Vitamin C is necessary for healing (option 3). Stomatitis is usually due to a deficiency of riboflavin (option 2). Biting the inside of

the mouth (option 1) would not cause the gums to be spongy. A protein deficiency (option 4) would be evidenced by muscle wasting.

Cognitive Level: Application **Client Need:** Health Promotion and Maintenance **Integrated Process:** Nursing Process: Analysis **Content Area:** Foundational Sciences: Nutrition **Strategy:** Specific knowledge of the manifestations of vitamin C deficiency is needed to answer this question. If this question is difficult, review various nutritional deficiencies and their causes to assist in this area. **Reference:** D'Amico, D. & Barbarito, C. (2007). *Health & physical assessment in nursing.* Upper Saddle River, NJ: Pearson Education, Inc., p. 146.

9 **Answer: 2** **Rationale:** Macrocytic anemia is caused by a deficiency in folic acid or vitamin B_{12} and usually indicates poor nutrition (option 2). Iron deficiency anemia is often associated with a low hemoglobin level (option 1). Macrocytic anemia can result from malnutrition (option 3), but this answer is less specific than the correct option. Poor nutrition due to cancer may result in a decreased lymphocytic count, a specific subgroup of white blood cells (WBCs), but not an overall decreased WBC count (option 4).

Cognitive Level: Application **Client Need:** Physiological Integrity: Physiological Adaptation **Integrated Process:** Communication and Documentation **Content Area:** Foundational Sciences: Nutrition **Strategy:** The critical words in the question are *best response.* This tells you that more than one option may be technically correct but that one answer is better than the others. Consider the etiologies of macrocytic anemia to help you choose correctly. **Reference:** D'Amico, D. & Barbarito, C. (2007). *Health & physical assessment in nursing.* Upper Saddle River, NJ: Pearson Education, Inc., p. 150.

10 **Answer: 2** **Rationale:** MyPyramid is an individualized approach to nutrition (option 2). The client can enter personal data into an interactive website and receive dietary recommendations that, when followed, lead to proper nutrition. The pyramid is designed for individuals, not group education (option 1), as it requires the client to enter personalized data into the website. The pyramid recommends proportionality and variety so it would not suggest low carbohydrates (option 3). It would recommend six servings of grain (not two) for an active adult (option 4).

Cognitive Level: Application **Client Need:** Health Promotion and Maintenance **Integrated Process:** Nursing Process: Evaluation **Content Area:** Foundational Sciences: Nutrition **Strategy:** Note that options 3 and 4 both involve low carbohydrate intake so those cannot be correct and must be eliminated first. Next recall the features of the MyPyramid website and focus on the critical words *group* in option 1 and *individualized* in option 2 to choose option 2 over option 1. **Reference:** D'Amico, D. & Barbarito, C. (2007). *Health & physical assessment in nursing.* Upper Saddle River, NJ: Pearson Education, Inc., p. 152.

ANSWERS & RATIONALES

Posttest

1 **Answer: 1** **Rationale:** The main subject of concern in nutrition is overweight status and obesity, so one of the Healthy People 2010 goals is to increase the number of people who are at a healthy weight (option 1). Healthy People 2010 indicators suggest eating two servings of fruit, three servings of vegetables, and six servings of grain (options 2, 3, and 4).
Cognitive Level: Comprehension **Client Need:** Health Promotion and Maintenance **Integrated Process:** Nursing Process: Implementation **Content Area:** Foundational Sciences: Nutrition **Strategy:** The wording of the question indicates that the correct answer is also a true statement. Eliminate options 2 and 4 first because of the word *all* in those options. This word makes it unlikely for these options to be correct because it is so encompassing. Choose option 1 over option 4 because overweight status and obesity are rampant nationally, while two servings each in three main food groups are insufficient for most adults. **Reference:** D'Amico, D. & Barbarito, C. (2007). *Health & physical assessment in nursing.* Upper Saddle River, NJ: Pearson Education, Inc., p. 152.

2 **Answer: 1** **Rationale:** The populations most at risk for undernutrition include infants, young children, immigrants, pregnant females, the economically disadvantaged, and older adults (option 1). College students and school-age children have access to food through school programs and meal plans (options 2 and 3). Working adults who have busy schedules are not necessarily too busy to eat (option 4).
Cognitive Level: Application **Client Need:** Health Promotion and Maintenance **Integrated Process:** Nursing Process: Planning **Content Area:** Foundational Sciences: Nutrition **Strategy:** First eliminate option 4, since this population is not likely to be economically deprived and a busy schedule does not preclude eating. Next recall that school-age children have access to school food programs and college students generally have access to meal programs to eliminate options 2 and 3. Alternatively, recall that older adults are often economically disadvantaged to choose option 1. **Reference:** D'Amico, D. & Barbarito, C. (2007). *Health & physical assessment in nursing.* Upper Saddle River, NJ: Pearson Education, Inc., pp. 136–137.

3 **Answer: 1, 2, 4** **Rationale:** The nutritional history should include information about the client's medical history (option 1) because illness can adversely affect nutritional intake. The medication history is essential as medications can interact with nutrient absorption or utilization; additionally, many herbal medication preparations interfere with nutritional health (option 2). Alcohol intake may interfere with nutrition intake as well as provide empty calories (option 4). Water quality (option 3) and hours of sleep (option 5) are not part of a nutritional assessment.
Cognitive Level: Application **Client Need:** Health Promotion and Maintenance **Integrated Process:** Nursing

Process: Assessment **Content Area:** Foundational Sciences: Nutrition **Strategy:** The words *select all that apply* indicate that the correct answer will include more than one option but not all of them. To answer the question correctly it is necessary to recall that the components of the nutrition assessment include diet recall, physical assessment, and laboratory diagnostics. **Reference:** D'Amico, D. & Barbarito, C. (2007). *Health & physical assessment in nursing.* Upper Saddle River, NJ: Pearson Education, Inc., pp. 136–138.

4 **Answer: 4** **Rationale:** Living on a fixed income may decrease the older adult's ability to procure food (option 4). As a healthy person ages there should be no change in respiratory status that affects nutritional intake (option 1). An older adult should not have a change in bowel patterns unless there is underlying pathophysiology (option 2). As people age there is a decrease in caloric needs (option 3).
Cognitive Level: Application **Client Need:** Health Promotion and Maintenance **Integrated Process:** Nursing Process: Assessment **Content Area:** Foundational Sciences: Nutrition **Strategy:** First eliminate options 2 and 3 since they would not be responsible for weight loss over the five-month period in the question. Since the question provides no clues that there are physiological reasons for the weight loss, select a social or environmental option that negatively impacts nutrition such as poverty or the inability to procure or prepare food. In this question, this line of thinking would lead you to select option 4. **Reference:** D'Amico, D. & Barbarito, C. (2007). *Health & physical assessment in nursing.* Upper Saddle River, NJ: Pearson Education, Inc., pp. 137, 151.

5 **Answer: 4** **Rationale:** The mid-arm circumference is used to determine adipose and muscle mass (option 4). Height and weight measurements do not directly determine adipose and muscle mass (option 1). Body mass index is used to evaluate whether a client is considered to be overweight or underweight (option 2). The skinfold tricep measurement calculates skin layers and subcutaneous fat (option 3).
Cognitive Level: Application **Client Need:** Health Promotion and Maintenance **Integrated Process:** Nursing Process: Assessment **Content Area:** Foundational Sciences: Nutrition **Strategy:** Recall that anthropometric measurements that accurately provide standard information include arm circumference, bioelectrical impedance, near infrared interactance, and Dexa Scan. With this in mind, eliminate options 1, 2, and 3 since only option 4 is included in the list of anthropometric measurements. **Reference:** D'Amico, D. & Barbarito, C. (2007). *Health & physical assessment in nursing.* Upper Saddle River, NJ: Pearson Education, Inc., pp. 136–145.

6 **Answer: 1** **Rationale:** Males with a waist circumference of greater than 102 cm are at risk for cardiovascular disease (options 1), while a measurement of 64 cm is acceptable (option 2). A female with a waist circumference of greater than 88 cm is at risk for cardiovascular disease, which does not place the females in options 3 and 4 at increased risk for cardiovascular disease. **Cognitive Level:** Application **Client Need:** Nursing Process: Assessment **Integrated Process:** Nursing Process: Evaluation **Content Area:** Foundational Sciences: Nutrition **Strategy:** Specific information is needed to answer this question. Specifically it is necessary to know that a waist circumference greater than 102 cm for men and 88 cm for women indicates increased risk. Alternatively, since the question associates waist circumference with increased risk, choose the option that indicates the largest overall weight circumference as the answer to the question. **Reference:** D'Amico, D. & Barbarito, C. (2007). *Health & physical assessment in nursing*. Upper Saddle River, NJ: Pearson Education, Inc., p. 142.

7 Answer: 3 Rationale: The client who is taking protein supplements may experience elevated serum albumin levels (option 3). A weight lifter would most likely have a small waist circumference (option 1). Protein supplements would have no effect on the iron levels (option 2). A weight lifter should have an increased mid-arm circumference due to increased muscle mass (option 4). **Cognitive Level:** Application **Client Need:** Physiological Integrity: Reduction of Risk Potential **Integrated Process:** Nursing Process: Assessment **Content Area:** Foundational Sciences: Nutrition **Strategy:** The critical words in the question are *protein supplements* and *normal weight status*. Because of normal weight status, eliminate options 1 and 4, which are the opposites of what would be expected in this client. Correlate the word *protein* in the question with the word *albumin* in the correct option to help you choose correctly. **Reference:** D'Amico, D. & Barbarito, C. (2007). *Health & physical assessment in nursing*. Upper Saddle River, NJ: Pearson Education, Inc., p. 136.

8 Answer: 3 Rationale: A food diary is kept for three days to provide nutritional history data (option 3). Lower gastrointestinal assessment does not provide the information necessary to evaluate this client (option 1). Additionally, the question asks what the nurse would do next, and this option defers the assessment to another healthcare provider. A 24-hour diet recall will not provide enough data to evaluate this client's eating habits due to the erratic patterns (option 2). Anthropometric measurements will not provide data as to the etiology of this client's problem (option 4). **Cognitive Level:** Application **Client Need:** Physiological Integrity: Physiological Adaptation **Integrated Process:** Nursing Process: Implementation **Content Area:** Foundational Sciences: Nutrition **Strategy:** The critical words in the question are *foods from fast-food eateries* and *beverages containing sugar*. This

indicates that the client has suboptimal nutrient intake and that the next best action of the nurse is to focus further immediate assessment on the client's diet. Eliminate option 1 first because it defers assessment to another healthcare provider and because it focuses on the lower GI system, while indigestion is an upper GI symptom. Eliminate option 4 because it does not address the dietary intake issue. Choose option 3 over option 2 because it provides more thorough and complete data because it is done over three days instead of 24 hours. **Reference:** D'Amico, D. & Barbarito, C. (2007). *Health & physical assessment in nursing*. Upper Saddle River, NJ: Pearson Education, Inc., p. 139.

9 Answer: 3 Rationale: It is essential that the nurse gather data about whether or not the client is introducing the new culture's food, as it may or may not be as healthy as the original culture (option 3). It is not essential that the nurse ask the client if the client is happy (option 1). A client's religion would not change so no additional information is needed (option 2). A new immigrant is not at any greater nutritional risk for religious factors or herbal supplementation that influences diet (option 4). **Cognitive Level:** Application **Client Need:** Health Promotion and Maintenance **Integrated Process:** Nursing Process: Assessment **Content Area:** Foundational Sciences: Nutrition **Strategy:** The critical words in the question are *nutritional assessment* and *newly immigrated*. From there, select the option that addresses food intake in the new cultural setting. **Reference:** D'Amico, D. & Barbarito, C. (2007). *Health & physical assessment in nursing*. Upper Saddle River, NJ: Pearson Education, Inc., p. 151.

10 Answer: 2 Rationale: Dual x-ray absorptiometry is used to evaluate bone density as well as lean body mass (option 2). Waist circumference is used to assess for the risk of cardiovascular disease (option 1). Albumin measures protein stores and iron levels evaluate binding capacity of hemoglobin (option 3). A 24-hour recall will provide information on the dietary intake for a day (option 4). **Cognitive Level:** Application **Client Need:** Physiological Integrity: Reduction of Risk Potential **Integrated Process:** Nursing Process: Planning **Content Area:** Foundational Sciences: Nutrition **Strategy:** Recall that bone density is used to provide information about body composition. Waist circumference is considered an accurate measure of cardiovascular risk. Diet recall provides a quick view of dietary intake. **Reference:** D'Amico, D. & Barbarito, C. (2007). *Health & physical assessment in nursing*. Upper Saddle River, NJ: Pearson Education, Inc., pp. 138, 142, 145.

References

Bickley, L. (2010). *Bates guide to physical examination and history taking* (10th ed.). Philadelphia: Lippincott Williams & Wilkins.

Capra, S. (2007). Nutrition assessment – How much information is enough to make a diagnosis of malnutrition in acute care. *Nutrition, 23*(4), 356–357.

D'Amico, D. & Barbarito, C. (2007). *Health & physical assessment in nursing.* Upper Saddle River, NJ: Pearson Education, Inc.

Jarvis, C. (2008). *Physical examination and health assessment* (5th ed.). St. Louis, MO: Elsevier Saunders.

Kubrack, C. (2007). Malnutrition in acute care patients: A narrative review. *International Journal of Nursing Studies. Aug: 44*(6), 1036–1054.

Mini Nutrition Assessment Tool and information on usage. Retrieved June 20, 2007, from www.mna-elderly.com

National Heart, Lung, and Blood Institute. *Trans Fat Promotes Risky Weight Gain.* Retrieved October 20, 2009, from http://www.nhlbi.nih.gov/public/sept06/newsitms.htm

United States Department of Health and Human Services. (2000). *Healthy People 2010.* Retrieved June 20, 2007, from www.healthypeople.gov/document/tableofcontents.html#vol1

U.S. Department of Agriculture and Department of Health and Human Services. *Dietary Guidelines for Americans, 2005.* Retrieved June 20, 2007, from www.HealthierUS.gov/dietaryguidelines. Washington, D.C.

Zator Estes, M. (2009). *Health assessment and physical examination* (4th ed.). Clifton Park, NY: Delmar Cengage Learning.

5 Cardiovascular Assessment

Chapter Outline

NCLEX-RN® Test Prep

Visit the Companion Website for this book
at www.pearsonhighered.com/hogan to
access additional practice opportunities
and more.

Objectives

➤ Review the anatomy and physiology of the cardiovascular system.
➤ Conduct a cardiovascular health history.
➤ Prepare the client for a cardiovascular assessment.
➤ Utilize the techniques of cardiovascular assessment.
➤ Describe expected and unexpected findings associated with the
cardiovascular system.

Review at a Glance

aortic aneurysm a ballooning of
aortic wall due to weakness in wall
of artery

apical pulse a rhythmic pulsation felt
or heard over apex of heart

bruit a loud blowing sound, most often
associated with atherosclerotic plaque
that obstructs blood flow

cardiac catheterization
percutaneous intravascular insertion of a
catheter in any chamber of heart or great
vessels for diagnosis, assessment of
abnormalities or treatment

dyspnea air hunger resulting in
labored breathing

**electrocardiogram (ECG or
EKG)** a record of electrical activity of
heart, measured by waves providing

important information about spread of
electricity to different parts of heart

echocardiography a noninvasive
diagnostic study that uses ultrasound to
visualize cardiac structures

infective endocarditis a condition caused by bacterial infiltration of lining of heart's chambers

lift (or heave) a forceful rising or
thrusting of ventricle during systole

Marfan's syndrome a degenerative
disease of connective tissue that can be
accompanied by cardiovascular defects
such as aortic aneurysm and mitral valve
prolapse

myocardial infarction (MI)
death of cardiac muscle cells as a result
of coronary artery occlusion

periorbital edema excessive
accumulation of serous fluid in tissue
surrounding eyes

stenosis narrowing of a passage or
orifice; can refer to cardiac valves or
blood vessels in cardiovascular system

stress test an exercise tolerance test
that uses exercise and/or pharmacologic
agents as metabolic stressors to evaluate
cardiovascular dynamics and how well
body adapts to metabolic demands that
exceed resting energy requirements

thrill a palpable vibration signifying
turbulent blood flow; accompanies loud
cardiac murmurs

xanthelasma yellow cholesterol
deposits seen on the eyelids; indicative of
premature atherosclerosis

PRETEST

1 The nurse is assessing a client who has a low-pitched murmur. What is the most appropriate way for the nurse to position the client to auscultate this murmur?

1. Supine using the bell of the stethoscope
2. Supine using the diaphragm of the stethoscope
3. On the left lateral side using the bell of the stethoscope
4. On the left lateral side using the diaphragm of the stethoscope

2 During a cardiovascular assessment the nurse finds a bluish tinge on the client's lips, fingers, and toes. What is the appropriate documentation for this finding?

1. Central cyanosis
2. Peripheral cyanosis
3. Central and peripheral cyanosis
4. Cyanosis

3 When evaluating a client's circulation the nurse should include which assessments? Select all that apply.

1. Palpation of pulses
2. Skin temperature of bilateral extremities
3. Skin color
4. Skin dryness
5. Hair on the legs and feet

4 During a cardiovascular assessment the nurse notes that the client has a heart rhythm with a pause after each beat and a skip every third beat. What is the appropriate interpretation of this finding?

1. Asystole
2. Normal
3. Regular
4. Regularly irregular

5 When obtaining a cardiovascular health history the nurse should ask the client which questions? Select all that apply.

1. "Are you able to perform your activities of daily living?"
2. "Do you have musculoskeletal aches?"
3. "Have you had any weight changes?"
4. "Have you been treated for cardiovascular disease?"
5. "Do you know your cholesterol and triglyceride levels?"

6 When performing a dietary history on a client with a cardiovascular history, the nurse should obtain information related to which items?

1. Dairy consumption
2. Sodium intake
3. Whole grain intake
4. Vitamin supplements

7 In preparing to perform a cardiovascular assessment, the nurse should initially place the client in which position?

1. Supine
2. Lithotomy
3. Sitting upright
4. Prone

8 The nurse performing a cardiovascular assessment observes splinter hemorrhages. The nurse should evaluate this client for which of the following?

1. Endocarditis
2. An aneurysm
3. Bruits
4. Poor circulation

9 When palpating the carotid arteries it is essential that the nurse do which of the following?

1. Palpate the carotids while the client is supine
2. Avoid palpating the carotids simultaneously
3. Determine if there is a heave
4. Palpate for an enlarged heart

10 Before assessing the client's carotid arteries for pulsations, the nurse would raise the client's head of bed to how many degrees elevation for proper positioning? Provide a numerical response.

➤ *See pages 94–95 for Answers and Rationales.*

I. HEALTH HISTORY

A. Anatomy and physiology review

1. Structures of the heart (see Figure 5-1a and 5-1b)
   a. Hollow muscular organ enclosed in a protective sac, divided into four chambers—two atria and two ventricles—divided by septum into right and left sides
   b. Heart wall has three layers: the *epicardium*, fibrous outside protective layer; the *myocardium*, middle layer of specialized cardiac muscle; and the *endocardium*, endothelial lining of chambers
   c. *Pericardium:* protective sac encasing the heart
   d. Valves of the heart
      1) Atrioventricular (AV) valves (tricuspid on right and mitral on left) separate atria from ventricles and control blood flow between atria and ventricles
      2) Semilunar valves (pulmonic on right and aortic on left) separate ventricles from great vessels and control blood flow from heart
      3) S1, first heart sound ("lub"), is heard when AV valves close during systole
      4) S2, second heart sound ("dub"), is heard when semilunar valves close during diastole
   e. Coronary circulation (see Figure 5-2)
      1) Left anterior descending (LAD) artery supplies anterior left ventricle, anterior ventricular septum, and left ventricle apex; circumflex artery supplies left atrium and lateral and posterior left ventricle

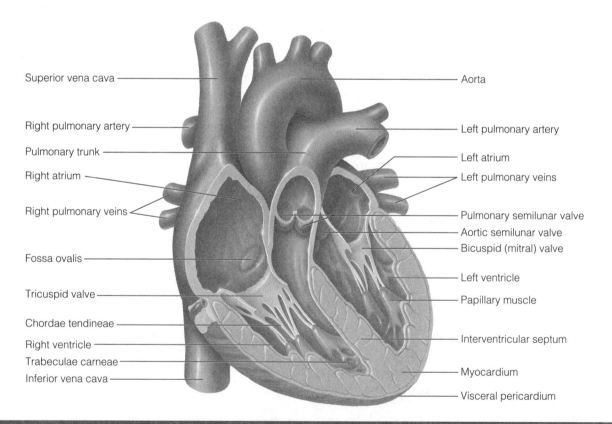

Figure 5-1a

Structural anatomy of the heart

Figure 5-1b

Cardiac valves

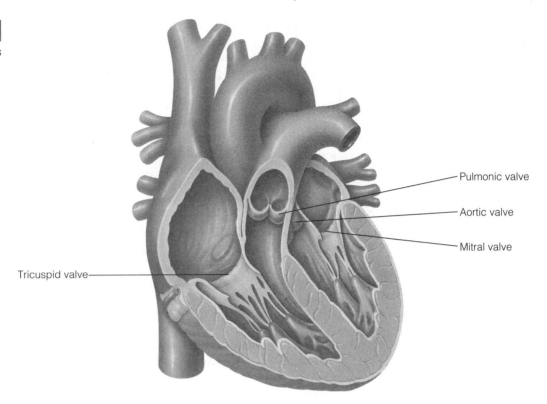

Pulmonic valve

Aortic valve

Mitral valve

Tricuspid valve

    2) Right coronary artery (RCA) supplies right atrium and ventricle, inferior left ventricle, posterior septal wall, and sinoatrial (SA) and atrioventricular (AV) nodes

  2. Functions of heart

    a. Circulation: right side circulates deoxygenated blood to lungs; left side pumps oxygenated blood throughout body to perfuse tissues

    b. Coronary arteries branch off aorta to supply oxygenated blood to heart

Figure 5-2

Coronary circulation

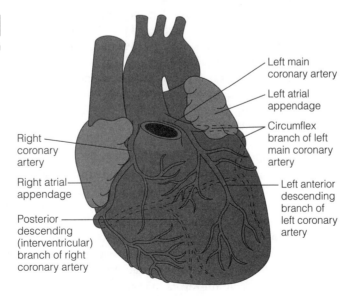

Left main coronary artery

Left atrial appendage

Circumflex branch of left main coronary artery

Right coronary artery

Right atrial appendage

Left anterior descending branch of left coronary artery

Posterior descending (interventricular) branch of right coronary artery

    c. Cardiac conduction system transmits electrical impulses and stimulates depolarization and cardiac muscle contraction; cells have electrophysiologic properties: *automaticity* (ability to initiate an electrical impulse), *excitability* (ability of a cell to respond to a stimulus), and *conductivity* (ability to transmit impulses from one cell to another)

        1) Sinoatrial (SA) node: natural pacemaker; generates heart rate normally at 60 to 100 beats per minute (bpm)

        2) Internodal pathways: carry impulse from SA node to AV node; depolarization results in myocardial contraction of both atria

        3) AV node: slows electrical impulse; allows atria to fully empty before initiating depolarization of ventricles; when SA node is not functioning, AV node can initiate an impulse at rate of 40 to 60 bpm

        4) Bundle of His: short branch of conductive cells connecting AV node to bundle branches at intraventricular septum

        5) Bundle branches: right (RBB) and left (LBB) split off on either side of intraventricular septum; carry impulses to Purkinje fibers

        6) Purkinje fibers: terminal branches of conduction system that initiate rapid depolarization wave throughout myocardium causing ventricular contraction; when SA and AV nodes fail, they can initiate impulses at rate of 20 to 40 bpm

    d. Cardiac cycle: one complete heartbeat; includes two parts—systole (ventricular contraction) and diastole (relaxation and ventricular refilling)

    e. Cardiac output (CO): volume of blood in liters ejected by heart each minute; indicator of pumping function of heart; normal adult CO is 4 to 8 L/min

$$CO = HR \times SV$$

        1) Heart rate (HR): number of complete cardiac cycles per minute

        2) Stroke volume (SV): volume of blood ejected from left ventricle with each cardiac cycle; SV and ultimately CO are influenced by preload, afterload, and contractility

        3) Preload: degree of myocardial fiber stretch at end of ventricular diastole; influenced by ventricular filling volume and myocardial compliance

        4) Afterload: resistance that ventricles must overcome to eject blood into systemic circulation; directly related to arterial blood pressure (BP)

        5) Contractility: strength of contraction regardless of preload; decreased by hypoxia and some drugs (e.g., beta-blockers and calcium channel blockers); increased by other drugs (e.g., digoxin [Lanoxin] and dopamine [Intropin])

    f. Autonomic nervous system responds to chemoreceptors, baroreceptors, and stretch receptors in the body

        1) Sympathetic: produces epinephrine and norepinephrine; results in increased heart rate (HR), myocardial contractility, peripheral vasoconstriction, and arterial BP

        2) Parasympathetic: produces acetylcholine; results in decreased HR and contractility

3. Structure and function of blood vessels

    a. Distribute blood to body tissues

    b. Walls of an artery or vein consist of three layers: tunica intima, tunica media, and tunica adventitia; the amount of pressure in a vessel determines thickness of the walls and amount of connective tissue and smooth muscle

    c. Arterial system consists of high-pressure vessels, beginning with aorta, then arteries, arterioles, and ending with capillaries; delivers blood to various tissues for nourishment and contributes to tissue temperature regulation

    d. Venous system begins after capillaries and consists of venules and veins (large diameter, thin-walled vessels) under much less pressure; some veins, most commonly in legs, contain valves to regulate one-way flow; returns blood from capillaries to right atrium and acts as a reservoir for blood volume

4. Regulation of BP
    a. Autonomic nervous system
    b. Baroreceptors in aortic arch and carotid sinus; chemoreceptors in large arteries of thorax and neck
    c. Antidiuretic hormone (ADH)
    d. Renin-angiotensin-aldosterone system; angiotensin I is converted to angiotensin II, a powerful vasoconstrictor
    e. Others: temperature (cold results in vasoconstriction, heat results in vasodilation); substances such as nicotine (vasoconstrict) and alcohol (vasodilate); diet (sodium and fat intake); and factors such as age, gender, ethnicity, weight, physical health, and emotional state

B. **Gather data related to cardiovascular illness, including questions such as the following; ask further follow-up questions (such as those labeled a., b., etc.) if client responds affirmatively to the initial question (labeled 1., 2., etc.)**
    1. "Have you ever been diagnosed with a heart problem?"
        a. "When were you diagnosed with the problem?"
        b. "What treatment was prescribed?"
        c. "Did the treatment alleviate the problem?"
        d. "Have you found any alternative/nonprescribed treatment that has been beneficial?"
        e. "What are your current health practices?"
    2. "Did you ever have an infection or viral illness that affected your heart?"
        a. "When was the infection diagnosed?"
        b. "What treatment was prescribed?"
        c. "Was the treatment beneficial?"
        d. "Have you had any recurrent infections?"
        e. "Do you do anything to prevent infections?"
    3. "Have you ever had any diagnostic studies (**electrocardiogram [ECG or EKG]**, a record of the electrical activity of the heart, **echocardiography** [a noninvasive diagnostic study that uses ultrasound to visualize cardiac structures], **stress test** [an exercise tolerance test that uses exercise and/or pharmacologic agents as metabolic stressors to evaluate cardiovascular dynamics], **cardiac catheterization** [percutaneous intravascular insertion of a catheter in any chamber of the heart or great vessels for diagnosis, assessment of abnormalities or treatment]) or surgical procedures related to the heart?"
    4. "Do you have a history of hypertension, diabetes, thyroid disorders, high cholesterol or triglyceride levels, a heart murmur, congenital heart disease, **periorbital edema** (excessive accumulation of serous fluid in the tissue surrounding the eyes), rheumatic fever, unexplained joint pains as a child, recurrent sore throats or tonsillitis, **stenosis** (constriction or narrowing of a passage or orifice) of the cardiac valves, or anemia?"
    5. "Have you had any surgical procedures on the heart or any blood vessels?"
        a. "When did you have this surgery?"
        b. "What type of surgery was done?"
        c. "Have your lifestyle and daily living activities changed since the surgery? If so, in what way?"
        d. "Did you ever receive one or more blood transfusions? If so, did you ever have a blood transfusion reaction? What did you experience?"
    6. "Have you ever had childhood illnesses such as German measles, streptococcal throat infections, or rheumatic fever?" (all can affect cardiovascular health in adulthood)
        a. "When did this illness/infection occur? How old were you?"
        b. "Have you been diagnosed with any subsequent health problems that occurred as a result of this illness/infection?"
    7. "Are your immunizations up to date, as far as you know?" (verify with an actual review of immunization history)

> **Practice to Pass**
>
> The nurse is obtaining the health history of a client. What health problems should the nurse inquire about to assess for childhood illnesses or infections that could cause cardiac problems during adulthood?

8. Allergies
  a. "Do you have any allergies? If so, what are you allergic to?"
  b. "What triggers the allergy and how often does it occur?"
  c. "What treatment(s) or medication(s), if any, are you using for this allergy? Does it work sufficiently?"

II. PRESENT HEALTH HISTORY

A. Focus initial questions on data related to chest pain or tightness
  1. Onset
    a. "When did the symptoms begin?"
    b. "Have you had these symptoms before?"
  2. Location
    a. "Where is the pain?"
    b. "Is the pain localized or does it radiate to other areas?"
  3. Character and intensity
    a. "How would you describe the pain?"
    b. "Does it feel like a crushing, stabbing, or burning sensation, or some other sensation?"
    c. "On a scale of 1 to 10 ranging from minimal to maximal discomfort, how would you rate the pain?"
  4. Precipitating factors
    a. "Did the pain occur suddenly or in relation to any activity, or emotional stress?"
    b. "What happened when you stopped the activity?"
  5. Associated symptoms
    a. "Did you experience any dizziness, shortness of breath, nausea, or vomiting?"
    b. "Have you experienced any changes in your energy level?"
    c. "Describe any other symptoms."
  6. Alleviating factors
    a. "Was there anything that helped relieve the pain?"
    b. "Did you take nitroglycerin? If so, how many tablets and how often?"

B. Data related to *dyspnea* (air hunger resulting in labored breathing)
  1. "Were you aware of any difficulty with your breathing?"
  2. "Does it occur unexpectedly or is it constant?"
  3. "Have you noticed any change in your facial color such as blue or ashen gray?"
  4. "Is your breathing pattern affected by activity? If so, what type?"
  5. "Do you find it more difficult to breathe lying down?"
  6. "Do you awaken from sleep at night?"
  7. "How many pillows do you use when sleeping or lying down?"

C. Data related to cough
  1. "Do you have a cough?"
  2. "When did you first notice the cough?"
  3. "How would you describe your cough (dry, hacking, hoarse, moist, barking)?"
  4. "Does the cough change at different times of the day?"
  5. "Do you have any pain when you cough? If so, describe the type and severity of the pain."
  6. "Do you produce any sputum when you cough? If so, what color is the sputum? Have you noticed any change in color throughout the day? Any odor?"

D. Data related to edema
  1. "Have you noticed any swelling in your feet, ankles, and legs? If so, are both legs equally swollen? Are you able to wear shoes? How long has this been present?"
  2. "Does the swelling decrease with rest, elevation, or after sleep?"

3. "Do you awaken during the night with urgency to urinate? If so, how long has this been occurring?"
4. "Are there other associated symptoms such as shortness of breath?"
5. "Have you noticed whether you have had any weight gain or loss that seems to coincide with increase or decrease in the amount of edema?"

E. **Data related to lifestyle**
1. "Describe your diet. Do you use table salt? If so, how much, and how frequent?"
2. "Have you had a problem with your weight? Do you diet? If so, what type of diet have you tried? Do you take supplemental vitamins, protein supplements, or antioxidants?"
3. "Do you exercise regularly? What type of exercise do you perform? How often, and for what length of time?"
4. "Do you smoke? Type of product? For how long? How many packs per day? Are you exposed to second-hand smoke? How frequently?"
5. "Do you take street drugs or drink alcohol? If so, describe the type, amount, frequency, and duration of use."

F. **Age-related questions**
1. Infants
   a. "Were there any health occurrences during pregnancy such as unexplained fever, infections, hypertension, swelling of the face and hands, protein in the urine, and any use of substances?"
   b. "Is the infant able to finish nursing or feeding without becoming fatigued? Is there any cyanosis while the infant is nursing or feeding, or when the infant cries?"
   c. "Has the infant progressed as expected according to growth and development charts?"
   d. "How long does the infant nap each day?"
2. Children
   a. "Has the child developed as expected according to growth charts?"
   b. "Does the child have any difficulty during activities such as walking, or climbing stairs? What position does the child assume during activities, or have there been any changes in skin color?" (a child with a congenital heart problem can be cyanotic, mottled, ashen, or pale)
   c. "Has the child ever experienced unexplained fever or joint pain?"
   d. "Does the child complain of frequent headaches or experience nosebleeds?"
   e. "Has the child had frequent respiratory infections? What treatment did he or she receive? Have any of the infections been streptococcal?"
   f. "Does the child have a sibling with any heart problems or defects?"
3. Pregnancy
   a. "What was your blood pressure before pregnancy?"
   b. "Have you ever had high blood pressure during previous pregnancies?"
   c. "What treatment did you receive for high blood pressure?"
   d. "Did you experience other symptoms such as weight gain, swelling in your feet, legs, or face, or any reports of protein in your urine?"
   e. "Have you experienced any faintness or dizziness during this pregnancy?"
4. Older adults
   a. "Do you have a history of heart or lung disease such as high blood pressure, coronary artery disease (CAD), chronic bronchitis, or emphysema?"
   b. "What treatment do you receive? What medications do you take?"
   c. "What symptoms have you had? Have they worsened?"
   d. "Have you noticed any changes in your activity level?"

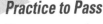

Practice to Pass

The nurse assessing an adult client notes the presence of bilateral edema in the lower legs. What information should the nurse gather regarding this sign as part of the cardiovascular assessment?

III. FAMILY HISTORY

A. Provides information about client's risk factors for diseases

1. "Do you have a family history of disorders affecting the heart such as coronary artery disease, angina, **myocardial infarction** (death of cardiac muscle cells as a result of coronary artery occlusion) or heart attack, heart murmurs, or congestive heart failure?"

2. "Do you have a family history of disorders affecting blood vessels such as diabetes, arteriosclerotic disease, or peripheral vascular disease?"

B. Have client review as many family generations as possible

1. This will provide maximal data; many individuals can provide information about parents, grandparents, and possibly great-grandparents

2. Information about adopted family members does not provide genetic information for client; however, it does provide information about environmental factors, since all individuals residing in the home will share exposure to the same toxins

IV. EQUIPMENT, PREPARATION, AND POSITIONING

A. To perform cardiovascular assessment, gather the following equipment:

1. Examination gown
2. Drape
3. Stethoscope: diaphragm for high-pitched sounds, and the bell for low-pitched sounds
4. Good lighting (natural light is best) and a strong flashlight

B. Positioning and preparation

1. Conduct assessment in a warm, quiet, private environment with good lighting
2. Use proper hand hygiene and warm the hands and stethoscope prior to examination
3. Provide adequate coverage to prevent unnecessary exposure of breasts in female clients
4. Introduce self and explain purpose of examination
5. Explain that you will be touching the neck, tapping the chest, and listening to heart sounds with a stethoscope
6. Inform client that he or she can breathe regularly throughout examination
7. Tell client to inform you of any discomfort during examination
8. Explain to a female client that left breast will need to be displaced upward and that she may be asked to hold breast during that part of the examination
9. Explain various position changes (sitting and lying down)
10. Stand on client's right side to facilitate hand placement and auscultation
11. Begin examination with client in an upright position, then proceed to place client in a supine position with head elevated 45 degrees

Practice to Pass

The nurse is preparing to conduct a cardiovascular assessment. What items should the nurse gather before beginning the assessment?

V. PHYSICAL EXAMINATION

A. Inspection and palpation

1. Face, lips, ears, and scalp
   a. Observe facial skin color
   b. Examine eyes and tissue surrounding eyes (periorbital area) and eyelids
   c. Inspect lips, buccal mucosa, gums, and tongue for color changes
   d. Assess structure of skull in proportion to face
2. Carotid arteries
   a. Place client supine with head of exam table raised about 45 degrees
   b. Inspect carotid arteries (located lateral to trachea in a groove medial to sternocleidomastoid muscle) for pulsations; use good lighting and a flashlight to identify visible pulsations

      c. Palpate each carotid artery medial to sternocleidomastoid muscle in neck one at a time; avoid excessive pressure on carotid sinus area higher in neck, as excessive vagal stimulation could slow heart rate, especially in older adults

      d. Auscultate using diaphragm and bell of stethoscope; ask client to hold breath briefly

3. Jugular veins

      a. Maintain same position as for examining carotid arteries

      b. Turn client's head slightly away from examined side, and direct strong light onto neck to highlight pulsations and shadows; note that jugular veins are not normally visible when client sits upright

4. Anterior chest (see Figures 5-3a and 5-3b for anterior thoracic landmarks useful in cardiac assessment)

      a. Observe respiratory pattern and inspect for veins on chest

      b. Inspect chest for bulges and masses

Figure 5-3

A. Cardiac assessment landmarks

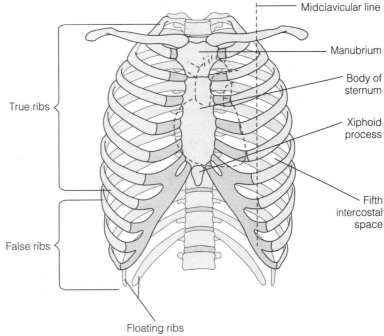

- Midclavicular line
- Manubrium
- Body of sternum
- Xiphoid process
- Fifth intercostal space
- True ribs
- False ribs
- Floating ribs

B. Precordial assessment landmarks

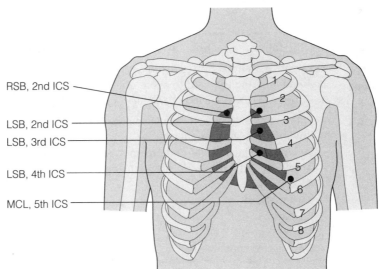

- RSB, 2nd ICS
- LSB, 2nd ICS
- LSB, 3rd ICS
- LSB, 4th ICS
- MCL, 5th ICS

!

    c. Inspect each cardiac landmark systematically; begin with client in upright position, then proceed to a low- to mid-Fowler's position (30- to 45-degree angle)
       1) Aortic area: at 2nd intercostal space (ICS), right sternal border (RSB)
       2) Pulmonic area: at 2nd ICS, left sternal border (LSB)
       3) Precordial area or Erb's Point: at 3rd ICS, LSB
       4) Tricuspid area: at 4th ICS, LSB
       5) Mitral area: over apex, at 5th ICS, left mid-clavicular line (LMCL)

!

    d. Specifically palpate apical area located at left 5th intercostal space, mid-clavicular line for point of maximal impulse (PMI)

5. Abdomen
    a. Observe for pulsations and fat distribution in abdominal area
    b. Location of major arteries:
       1) Aorta: located superior to umbilicus to left of midline
       2) Left renal artery: located to left of umbilicus in left upper quadrant
       3) Right renal artery: located to right of umbilicus in right upper quadrant
       4) Right iliac artery: located to right of umbilicus in right lower quadrant
       5) Left iliac artery: located to left of umbilicus in left lower quadrant

6. Hands, fingers, and legs
    a. Inspect nail beds of hands and feet for color, shape, splinter hemorrhages
    b. Assess for **Marfan's syndrome** (a degenerative disease of connective tissue that can be accompanied by cardiovascular defects) by asking client to make a fist and wrap fingers over thumb; an alternative method is to ask client to wrap thumb and little finger around opposite wrist
    c. Inspect skin color and hair distribution on legs

!

    d. Palpate peripheral pulses bilaterally, first on one side and then the other; note the rate, rhythm, symmetry, and amplitude of each set of pulses (see Box 5-1)
       1) Radial pulses: ask client to extend each hand with palm up and palpate with two fingers over radial bone
       2) Brachial pulses: ask client to extend arm and palpate just superior to antecubital region
       3) Allen's test: may be done if obstruction or insufficiency is suspected in arm; ask client to place hands on knees with palms up; compress radial arteries of both hands with examiner's thumbs; ask client to open and close fist several times; next ask client to open hands while still compressing radial arteries and look for color to become pink immediately (this indicates patent ulnar arteries); may repeat process compressing ulnar arteries to assess patency of radial arteries

---

Box 5-1	Use the following techniques to accurately assess peripheral pulses:

Peripheral Pulse Assessment	**1.** Palpate peripheral pulses using gentle pressure over each artery
	2. Avoid pressing too hard to avoid obliterating the pulse
	3. Determine the following characteristics for each pulse:
	
	• Rate: number of pulsations per minute (should coincide with cardiac rate)
	• Rhythm: regularity of pulsations
	• Symmetry: similarity of findings for a specific pulse on each side of body
	• Amplitude: strength of pulsation, using a range of 0 to 4
	    4 = Bounding
	    3 = Increased
	    2 = Normal
	    1 = Weak
	    0 = Absent, nonpalpable

4) Femoral pulses: ask client to flex knee, externally rotate hip, and palpate inferior and medial to the inguinal ligament; if femoral artery is deep, the examiner may need to place one hand on top of the other to locate pulse

5) Popliteal pulses: ask client to flex knee and relax leg and palpate deep in popliteal fossa lateral to midline

6) Dorsalis pedis pulses: expose foot and palpate on medial side of dorsum of foot, placing fingers lateral to extensor tendon of great toe

7) Posterior tibial pulses: expose foot and palpate behind and slightly below medial malleolus of ankle (in groove between malleolus and Achilles' tendon)

e. Inspect for edema in upper and lower extremities; to palpate edema in legs, press for at least 5 seconds over tibia, behind medial malleolus, and on dorsum of each foot; look for depression (called pitting) and grade edema if found (see Figure 5-4)

7. Skeletal structure

a. With client standing, observe skeletal structure for any deformities

b. Observe neck and extremities, which should be in proportion to chest

B. Percussion: percuss heart using thoracic and cardiac landmarks to determine cardiac border

1. Place client in a reclining position at lowest angle that can be tolerated

2. Percuss at 5th intercostal space (ICS), left anterior axillary line

3. Continue to percuss at 5th ICS toward left mid-clavicular line (MCL) and left sternal border (LSB)

4. Repeat process at 3rd and 2nd ICS on left side of thorax

C. Auscultation

1. Use diaphragm of stethoscope with client in an upright position

a. Right sternal border (RSB), 2nd ICS (aortic areas)

b. Left sternal border (LSB), 2nd ICS (pulmonic area)

c. LSB, 3rd ICS (Erb's Point)

d. LSB, 4th ICS (tricuspid area)

e. Apex at 5th ICS, left MCL (mitral area)

2. Use bell of stethoscope lightly over five key landmark positions

3. Use diaphragm and bell of stethoscope to auscultate carotid arteries; instruct client to hold his or her breath briefly

4. Compare **apical pulse** (a rhythmic pulsation felt or heard over apex of heart) to carotid pulse; auscultate apical pulse while simultaneously palpating carotid pulse

Practice to Pass

The nurse conducting a cardiovascular examination would use the skill of palpation during which components of the exam?

Figure 5-4

Grading system for peripheral edema

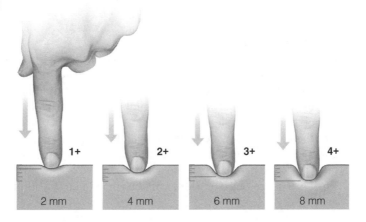

VI. EXPECTED FINDINGS

A. Face, lips, ears, and scalp

1. Facial color should be uniform
2. Eyes should be uniform, periorbital areas should be flat, and eyelids smooth
3. Lips, buccal mucosa, gums, and tongue should be uniform in color without any underlying tinge of blueness
4. Earlobes should be smooth and without creases
5. Structure of skull should be in proportion with face

B. Carotid arteries

1. Carotid pulsations should be visible bilaterally
2. Apical and carotid pulses should be synchronous

C. Jugular veins: normal jugular venous pulsation is 2 cm or less above sternal angle

D. Anterior chest

1. Respiratory pattern should be regular, even, and unlabored with no retractions
2. Veins on chest should be evenly distributed and flat
3. Intercostal spaces on chest area should be even and free of bulges or masses
4. Pulsation may be visible at mitral or apical areas; is more noticeable in children or in thinner individuals
5. Percussion tone in anterior thorax area should range from resonance (area over lungs) to dull
6. Heart sounds
   a. S2 is louder than S1 at aortic and pulmonic areas
   b. S1 and S2 are equal in intensity at Erb's point
   c. S1 is louder than S2 at tricuspid and mitral (apex) areas

E. Abdomen

1. Epigastric area is a common area where pulsations may be visible in thin individuals
2. Peristaltic waves may also be seen in thin individuals and should not be confused with pulsations

F. Hands, fingers, and legs

1. Shape of nail beds should be rounded and even
2. Color should be pink with white crescents at base of each nail
3. Skin color of legs should be even and uniform
4. Hair distribution on legs should be even and without bare patches
5. Pulses should be regular and even, symmetrical side to side, with an amplitude of 2 (normal)

G. Skeletal structure

1. Skeletal structure should be free of deformities
2. Neck and extremities should be in proportion to chest

VII. UNEXPECTED FINDINGS

A. Face, lips, ears, and scalp

1. Flushed skin may indicate rheumatic heart disease or presence of a fever
2. Protruding eyes are associated with hyperthyroidism; excessive hormone secretion in hyperthyroidism results in increased CO and rapid HR
3. Puffiness or edema around periorbital area may be caused by fluid retention or valvular heart disease
4. **Xanthelasma** (yellow deposits on eyelids) indicate premature atherosclerosis
5. Changes in color, especially blue-tinged lips, may indicate cyanosis, which often is a late sign of inadequate tissue perfusion
6. Presence of creases in earlobes bilaterally in a young adult client may indicate coronary artery disease

7. A protruding skull is associated with Paget's disease resulting in thickened distorted contours of skull; also characterized by increased CO, which can lead to cardiac muscle fatigue and heart failure

B. Carotid arteries

1. Carotid pulsations that are bounding may indicate fever; an absence of pulsation may indicate an obstruction

2. Bruit is a loud, blowing sound that could be caused by narrowing or stricture of carotid artery

3. An apical pulse rate that is greater than carotid rate indicates a pulse deficit, and may indicate a cardiac dysrhythmia

4. A **thrill** (a palpable vibration signifying turbulent blood flow) accompanies loud cardiac murmurs

C. Jugular veins

1. Distention of neck veins indicates elevation of central venous pressure and is commonly seen with heart failure, fluid overload, or increased pressure in superior vena cava

2. Unilateral distention may be associated with an aneurysm

D. Anterior chest

1. Pulmonary edema is a severe complication of cardiovascular disease and would cause respiratory distress

2. Veins on chest that are dilated or distended may indicate an obstructive process, such as obstructed superior vena cava

3. A bulge noted on chest may indicate obstruction or aneurysm; a mass may indicate obstruction or presence of tumor

4. Pulsations visible with every heartbeat over entire precordial area may indicate valvular regurgitation or shunting; pulsations present at pulmonic area may indicate pulmonary artery dilation or excessive blood flow; pulsations present at LSB from 3rd to 5th ICS may indicate right ventricular overload; a **lift (or heave)** (a forceful rising or thrusting of ventricle during systole) visible at LSB, 3rd to 5th intercostal spaces, may indicate right ventricular hypertrophy or respiratory disease, such as pulmonary hypertension

5. A dull sound percussed over a larger area than a heart of normal size would indicate cardiomegaly, which could ultimately lead to heart failure

6. Low-pitched extra sounds such as S3 (heard immediately after S2 and called a ventricular gallop), S4 (heard immediately before S1 and called an atrial gallop), and murmurs are best auscultated with bell of stethoscope (see Table 5-1 for information on distinguishing heart murmurs and Table 5-2 for classification of heart murmurs)

7. A pericardial friction rub is due to irritation of pericardium; it is heard with either bell or diaphragm of stethoscope and sounds like fingers rubbing hair at the ear

E. Abdomen

1. Visible, prominent pulsations located in areas outside of gastric area may be potentially life-threatening

2. Abnormal pulsations may indicate presence of **aortic aneurysm** (a ballooning of aortic arterial wall due to weakness in wall of artery)

F. Hands, fingers, and legs

1. Clubbed fingertips and nails are consistent with congenital heart disease because of chronic reduced oxygenation

2. Thin red lines or splinter hemorrhages in nail beds are associated with **infective endocarditis** (a condition caused by bacterial infiltration of lining of heart's chambers)

3. Fingernails and tips that are stained yellow can be related to smoking, one of main contributors to development of atherosclerosis

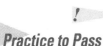

Practice to Pass

The nurse is assessing a client's heart sounds to detect a murmur. What should the nurse be alert for as an indicator that a murmur is present?

Table 5-1 Distinguishing Heart Murmurs	
Ask Yourself	**Information**
1. How loud is the murmur?	Murmurs are graded on a rather subjective scale of 1–6: • Grade 1: Barely audible with stethoscope, often considered physiologic not pathologic. Requires concentration and a quiet environment. • Grade 2: Very soft but distinctly audible. • Grade 3: Moderately loud; there is no thrill or thrusting motion associated with the murmur. • Grade 4: Distinctly loud, in addition to a palpable thrill. • Grade 5: Very loud, can actually hear with part of the diaphragm of the stethoscope off the chest; palpable thrust and thrill present. • Grade 6: Loudest, can hear with the diaphragm off the chest; visible thrill and thrust.
2. Where does it occur in the cardiac cycle: systole, diastole, or both?	Location in cardiac cycle: • Systole: early systole, midsystole, late systole • Diastole: early diastole, mid-diastole, late diastole • Both
3a. Is the sound continuous throughout systole, diastole, or only heard for part of the cycle?	Duration of murmur: • Continuous through systole only • Continuous through diastole only • Continuous through systole and diastole *Systolic murmurs* may be of two types: • Midsystolic: Murmur is heard after S_1 and stops before S_2. • Pansystolic/holosystolic: Murmur begins with S_1 and stops at S_2. *Diastolic murmurs* may be one of three types: • Early diastolic: Murmur auscultated immediately after S_2 and then stops. There is a gap where this murmur stops and S_1 is heard. • Mid-diastolic: Murmur begins a short time after S_2 and stops well before S_1 is auscultated. • Late diastolic: This murmur starts well after S_2 and stops immediately before S_1 is heard.
3b. What does the configuration of the sound look like? *Potential configurations:* S_1 S_2 **Pansystolic/holosystolic** S_1 S_2 S_1 **Continuous** S_1 S_2 **Crescendo (Systolic represented)**	S_2 S_1 **Decrescendo (Diastolic represented)** S_1 S_2 **Crescendo Decrescendo (Systole represented)** S_2 S_1 **Rumble**
4. What is the quality of the sound of the murmur?	• Blowing • Harsh • Musical • Raspy • Rumbling

Table 5-1 **Distinguishing Heart Murmurs (Continued)**

Ask Yourself	Information
5. What is the pitch or frequency of the sound?	• Low • Medium • High
6. In which landmark(s) do you best hear the murmur?	Use the five landmarks for auscultation: • Pulmonic areas 1 and 2 • Aortic area • Tricuspid area • Mitral area • Apex
7. Does it radiate?	• To the throat? • To the axilla?
8. Is there any change in pattern with respirations?	• Increases/decreases with inspiration • Increases/decreases with expiration
9. Is it associated with variations in heart sounds?	• Associated with split S_1? • Associated with split S_2? • Associated with S_3? • Associated with S_4? • Associated with a click or ejection sound?
10. Does intensity of murmur change with position?	• Increases/decreases with squatting? • Increases/decreases with client in the left lateral position? (Do not have the client perform the Valsalva maneuver or any abrupt positional changes, because some clients do not tolerate position changes well.)

Source: D'Amico, D. & Barbarito, C. (2007). *Health & physical assessment in nursing.* Upper Saddle River, NJ: Pearson Education, Inc., pp. 432–433, Table 17.3.

Table 5-2 **Classifications of Heart Murmurs**

Murmur	Cardiac Cycle Timing	Auscultation Site	Configuration of Sound	Continuity
Aortic stenosis	Midsystolic	RSB, 2nd ICS	S_1 ——— S_2	Crescendo-decrescendo, continuous
Pulmonary stenosis	Midsystolic	LSB, 2nd to 3rd ICS	S_1 ——— S_2	Crescendo-decrescendo, continuous
Mitral regurgitation	Systole	Apex	S_1 ——— S_2	Holosystolic, continuous
Tricuspid regurgitation	Systole	4th ICS, LSB	S_1 ——— S_2	Holosystolic, continuous

(continued)

Table 5-2 **Classifications of Heart Murmurs (Continued)**

Murmur	Cardiac Cycle Timing	Auscultation Site	Configuration of Sound	Continuity
Mitral stenosis	Diastole	Apical	S_2 ———— S_1	Rumble that increases in sound toward the end, continuous
Tricuspid stenosis	Diastole	Lower LSB	S_2 ———— S_1	Rumble that increases in sound toward the end, continuous
Ventricular septal defect (left-to-right shunt)	Systole	3rd, 4th, 5th ICS, LSB	S_1 ———— S_2	Holosystolic, continuous
Aortic regurgitation	Diastole (early)	3rd ICS, LSB	S_2 ———— S_1	Decrescendo, continuous
Pulmonic regurgitation	Diastole (early)	3rd ICS, LSB	S_2 ———— S_1	Decrescendo, continuous
Aortic stenosis	Usually harsh, coarse	Medium	Most commonly into neck into carotid area and down left sternal border, possibly apex	Expiration may intensify the murmur
Pulmonary stenosis	Usually harsh	Medium	Toward the left upper neck and shoulder areas	Inspiration may intensify the murmur
Mitral regurgitation	Blowing and can be harsh in sound quality	High	Usually to left axilla, LSB, and base	Expiration may intensify the murmur
Tricuspid regurgitation	Blowing	High	May radiate to LSB and MCL but not to axilla	Inspiration may intensify the murmur
Mitral stenosis	Rumbling	Low and best heard with bell	Rare	Expiration may intensify the murmur
Tricuspid stenosis	Rumbling	Low	Rare	Inspiration may intensify the murmur
Ventricular septal defect (left-to-right shunt)	Harsh	High	May radiate across precordium but not to axilla	Expiration may intensify the murmur
Aortic regurgitation	Blowing	High, best auscultated with diaphragm unless client is sitting up and leaning forward	May radiate to 2nd ICS, RSB and may proceed to apex	Expiration may intensify the murmur if the client leans forward and sits up
Pulmonic regurgitation	Blowing	High, best auscultated with diaphragm	May radiate to 2nd ICS, RSB and may proceed to apex	Inspiration may intensify the murmur

Source: D'Amico, D. & Barbarito, C. (2007). *Health & physical assessment in nursing.* Upper Saddle River, NJ: Pearson Education, Inc., pp. 433–434, Table 17.4.

4. Marfan's syndrome should be suspected when thumb is readily visible outside of clenched fist or if little finger extends at least 1 cm beyond thumb

5. Reduced or absent pulses in legs accompanied by pale, cool skin, and possibly ulcers, are characteristic of arterial insufficiency, also commonly called peripheral vascular disease

6. Patches of lighter skin color on legs and cooler skin may indicate compromised circulation such as arterial insufficiency; mottling indicates severe hemodynamic compromise

! ➤ 7. Thickened nails, hair loss on extremities, and thin, shiny skin on legs are called trophic changes, and these are also consistent with arterial insufficiency

! ➤ 8. Leg edema accompanied by brown skin discoloration is consistent with venous insufficiency; edema is aggravated by prolonged standing

! ➤ 9. Pain in iliac vessels, popliteal space, or calf muscle in leg may indicate deep vein thrombosis; pain is worsened or triggered by sharp dorsiflexion of foot (Homan's sign)

10. Dilated, twisting veins that are visible under skin in legs is characteristic of varicose veins

! ➤ 11. Blood vessel spasms in fingers leading to pallor or cyanosis, followed by rubor, is characteristic of Raynaud's disease; circulatory changes may be accompanied by numbness and/or burning or throbbing pain during episode

12. Gross unilateral swelling of one limb is consistent with lymphedema, an obstruction in lymph nodes

G. Skeletal structure

1. Scoliosis is associated with prolapsed mitral valve
2. Tall height in combination with elongated neck and extremities suggests Marfan's syndrome (a connective tissue disorder that could lead to aortic enlargement or dissection over time) and requires correlation with other supporting data such as bluish color to sclera of eyes and elongated thumb that is partially visible when fingers curled over thumb into a fist

VIII. LIFESPAN CONSIDERATIONS

A. Infants and children

1. Listen carefully to data that parents present about child and observe child; if an infant is crying during examination, a pacifier may quiet him or her

! ➤ 2. Expected heart rate findings:
   a. Newborn: 115–180 beats per minute (highest if crying, coughing)
   b. 1 year old: 80–160 beats per minute
   c. 5 years old: 80–130 beats per minute
   d. 10 years old: 70–110 beats per minute
   e. 14 years old: 60–105 beats per minute

! ➤ 3. Unexpected findings: cyanotic skin color, shortness of breath during play, assuming a squatting position during play, and distress during a crying episode

B. Pregnant women

1. Due to uterine enlargement related to fetal growth, client should be placed in a comfortable position throughout exam

2. Findings may include the following:
! ➤ a. Increased heart rate of 10 to 15 beats per minute
   b. Slight decrease in blood pressure from pre-pregnancy unless there are complications due to pregnancy
   c. S1 heart sound may be louder with exaggerated splitting
   d. Systolic murmur related to pregnancy may be heard, which will resolve following delivery

C. Older adults

1. Assessment should include a thorough medical examination and medication review, as older adults are at greater risk for developing toxicities because of an overall decline in kidney and liver function

2. Findings may include the following:
    a. Increase in systolic blood pressure
    b. Increase in anterior–posterior (AP) chest wall diameter, which makes it more difficult to palpate PMI and general precordium
    c. Heart sounds may be more distant when auscultating, and splitting of S2 heart sound may be more difficult to hear
    d. When assessing cardiac system it's important to include peripheral vascular and respiratory systems, as a problem usually affects all three systems
    e. Obtain baseline electrocardiogram

IX. DOCUMENTATION

A. Neck
1. Note if carotid pulsation is observed
2. Note rate, rhythm, symmetry, and amplitude of carotid pulse
3. Estimate jugular venous pressure

B. Anterior chest/precordium
1. Inspection and palpation
    a. Describe location of apical impulse
    b. Note any visible pulsations or thrills and their location
    c. Note that S1 and S2 are audible
    d. Identify rate and rhythm of heart
    e. Note any extra heart sounds or murmurs

C. Abdomen: note any visible pulsations or abdominal bruits

D. Hands, fingers, and legs
1. Note skin color and temperature, and specify areas where skin has pallor, rubor, or cyanosis
2. Note presence and degree of edema and whether associated with brownish skin discoloration of venous disease and whether unilateral or bilateral
3. Note and describe any leg ulcers
4. Note rate, rhythm, symmetry, and amplitude of peripheral pulses
5. Note trophic changes, pain, or any other unexpected findings

Case Study

A male client, age 48, is a traveling salesman with a strong family history of heart disease. As he was getting ready for work one day, he suddenly became weak, short of breath, and complained of pressure in the midsternal area of his chest. After resting for 10 minutes, he described the pain as an "elephant sitting on my chest." His wife calls for an ambulance and he is brought to a local emergency department, where is he admitted by a registered nurse.

1. Why was it important to call emergency medical services for this client?

2. What are the components of a thorough pain assessment?

3. What health history questions should the nurse ask during and after treatment of the chest pain?

4. What would the nurse include in an examination of the heart?

5. What would the nurse include in an examination of the vascular system?

For suggested responses, see page 309

POSTTEST

1. What approach would the nurse use to elicit the cooperation of a school-age child during a cardiovascular assessment?

1. Explain procedure to the child
2. Explain procedure to the parents
3. Permit the child to listen to his or her parent's chest with stethoscope
4. Sedate the child

2. The client has a history of aortic stenosis and an S3 murmur. What action would the nurse take to auscultate this murmur?

1. Listen at the pulmonic area
2. Use the diaphragm of stethoscope
3. Listen at the 2nd intercostal space
4. Use the bell of the stethoscope

3. In the client with mitral regurgitation the nurse would confirm the presence of a murmur at which location on the anterior chest?

1. Apex
2. Aortic area
3. Pulmonic area
4. Second intercostal space

4. To detect the presence of an ascending aortic aneurysm, the nurse would palpate which area on the client's chest? Select the correct area in the figure shown.

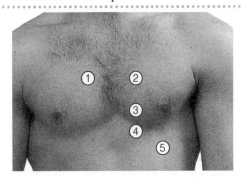

5. When auscultating the apical pulse the nurse should assess for which characteristics? Select all that apply.

1. Rate
2. Intensity
3. Temperature
4. Regularity
5. Rhythm

6. The nurse caring for a client experiencing chest discomfort should obtain which assessment data from the client?

1. Presence of a fever
2. Description of the pain and location
3. Recent weight gain
4. Whether the client smokes

7. The nurse is performing a cardiovascular assessment and notes creases in the client's earlobes. Based on this finding the nurse would conclude that the client may be experiencing which condition?

1. Endocarditis
2. Pericarditis
3. Coronary artery disease
4. Fluid overload

8. During inspection of the carotid arteries the nurse assesses a bounding pulse. The nurse should evaluate the client for which additional finding?

1. Fever
2. Bruits
3. Chest pain
4. Cyanosis

9. The nurse is performing a cardiovascular assessment. To evaluate the client for pulmonary edema the nurse would assess the client for which manifestation?

1. Edema in the lower extremities
2. Shortness of breath
3. A thrill
4. Splinter hemorrhages

10 The nurse assessing a client who has a history of hypertension would assess the client for pulsations by palpating which cardiac landmark?

1. Fifth intercostal space, midclavicular line
2. Second intercostal space, right sternal border
3. Pulmonic area
4. Tricuspid area

➤ *See pages 95–97 for Answers and Rationales.*

ANSWERS & RATIONALES

Pretest

1 **Answer: 3** **Rationale:** The nurse should use the bell of the stethoscope with the client on the left lateral side to hear low-pitched sounds (option 3). Placing the client supine while using the bell does not enhance the ability to hear the murmur as much as placing the client on the lateral side (option 1). Placing the client supine while using the diaphragm does not enhance the ability to hear a low-pitched murmur (option 2). Even if the client is placed on the left lateral side the diaphragm of the stethoscope is used to hear high-pitched sounds (option 4). **Cognitive Level:** Application **Client Need:** Health Promotion and Maintenance **Integrated Process:** Nursing Process: Assessment **Content Area:** Adult Health: Cardiovascular **Strategy:** Recall that lateral positioning brings the heart closer to the chest wall. Then use the process of elimination, remembering the bell of the stethoscope is for low-pitched sounds, while the diaphragm is for high-pitched sounds. **Reference:** D'Amico, D. and Barbarito, C. (2007). *Health & physical assessment in nursing.* Upper Saddle River, NJ: Pearson Education, Inc., p. 461.

2 **Answer: 3** **Rationale:** The most appropriate method of documentation is to fully describe the findings. Central and peripheral cyanosis describes cyanosis of the lips, hands, and feet (option 3). Central cyanosis is cyanosis of the lips (option 1). Peripheral cyanosis is a bluish tinge to the hands and/or feet (option 2). Documenting cyanosis alone does not describe the location of the cyanosis (option 4). **Cognitive Level:** Application **Client Need:** Health Promotion and Maintenance **Integrated Process:** Communication and Documentation **Content Area:** Adult Health: Cardiovascular **Strategy:** Recall basic definitions to aid in answering this question. Cyanosis is a bluish tinge to the mucous membranes. Central cyanosis is a blue tinge to the lips. Peripheral cyanosis is a bluish tinge to the extremities. **Reference:** D'Amico, D. and Barbarito, C. (2007). *Health & physical assessment in nursing.* Upper Saddle River, NJ: Pearson Education, Inc., p. 190.

3 **Answer: 1, 2, 3, 5** **Rationale:** To evaluate the circulation of the lower extremities the nurse should palpate the pulses of the lower extremities (option 1). Warm skin is consistent with adequate circulation (option 2). The color of the skin should be pink and not dusky; duskiness may indicate poor circulation (option 3). Circulation is needed for hair growth (option 5). Skin dryness is an indicator of general skin condition (option 4). **Cognitive Level:** Application **Client Need:** Health Promotion and Maintenance **Integrated Process:** Nursing Process: Assessment **Content Area:** Adult Health: Cardiovascular **Strategy:** The critical word in the question is *circulation.* Evaluate each of the options to determine whether they are consistent with assessments that reflect circulatory status. Eliminate option 4 since it reflects skin condition primarily, rather than functioning of the circulatory system. **Reference:** D'Amico, D. and Barbarito, C. (2007). *Health & physical assessment in nursing.* Upper Saddle River, NJ: Pearson Education, Inc., p 190.

4 **Answer: 4** **Rationale:** The heart rhythm that skips every third beat is regularly irregular (option 4). Asystole is no rate or rhythm (option 1). Normal rhythm is when every beat occurs as expected (option 2). Regular rhythm is when every beat comes as expected (option 3). **Cognitive Level:** Application **Client Need:** Health Promotion and Maintenance **Integrated Process:** Nursing Process: Analysis **Content Area:** Adult Health: Cardiovascular **Strategy:** Recall that the rhythm is regular when each beat occurs when expected. Regularly irregular is a rhythm that occurs in a patterned irregularity but abnormal heart rhythm. Asystole has the prefix *a-,* which means without. **Reference:** D'Amico, D. and Barbarito, C. (2007). *Health & physical assessment in nursing.* Upper Saddle River, NJ: Pearson Education, Inc., p. 459.

5 **Answer: 1, 3, 4, 5** **Rationale:** When obtaining a health history the nurse should ask the client if he or she is able to perform activities of daily living because inability to do so may indicate a cardiovascular problem (option 1). Weight gain is a risk factor for cardiovascular disease (option 3), while weight loss may be associated with other disease processes. When obtaining information for a cardiovascular history the nurse needs to know if the client has been diagnosed with a cardiovascular disease and what treatment was selected (option 4). Elevated triglyceride and cholesterol levels are associated with cardiovascular disease (option 5). Musculoskeletal aches (option 2) may indicate a health problem, but it would not be associated with the cardiovascular system. **Cognitive Level:** Application **Client Need:** Health Promotion and Maintenance **Integrated Process:** Nursing Process:

Assessment **Content Area:** Adult Health: Cardiovascular **Strategy:** Recall indicators of cardiovascular function to answer the question. Choose ability to carry out activities of daily living, history of cardiovascular disease, cholesterol and triglyceride levels and weight changes, because all are indicators of cardiovascular disease. Do not include option 2 because of the word *musculoskeletal*, which indicates another body system. **Reference:** D'Amico, D. and Barbarito, C. (2007). *Health & physical assessment in nursing.* Upper Saddle River, NJ: Pearson Education, Inc., pp. 444–445.

6 **Answer: 2** **Rationale:** The nurse should obtain a dietary history to aid the client with dietary changes to slow the progression of cardiovascular (CV) disease. Sodium intake is directly related to hypertension and other CV diseases (option 2). Vitamin supplements, fiber, and diary consumption are essential components of the diet, but they support general health, not just CV health (options 1, 3, and 4). **Cognitive Level:** Application **Client Need:** Health Promotion and Maintenance **Integrated Process:** Nursing Process: Assessment **Content Area:** Adult Health: Cardiovascular **Strategy:** Review each of the options. Note that the only negative cardiovascular health risk used as a distracter is sodium intake, so eliminate the essential nutritional elements. **Reference:** D'Amico, D. and Barbarito, C. (2007). *Health & physical assessment in nursing.* Upper Saddle River, NJ: Pearson Education, Inc., pp. 446–447.

7 **Answer: 3** **Rationale:** The nurse should position the client upright to perform inspection of the chest and skin (option 3). Positioning the client supine will not permit inspection of the posterior chest (option 1). Lithotomy is the position used for examination of the female genitalia (option 2). Positioning the client prone will not permit the examination of the anterior chest (option 4). **Cognitive Level:** Application **Client Need:** Health Promotion and Maintenance **Integrated Process:** Nursing Process: Implementation **Content Area:** Adult Health: Cardiovascular **Strategy:** Eliminate options that will not permit access to the chest wall. **Reference:** D'Amico, D. and Barbarito, C. (2007). *Health & physical assessment in nursing.* Upper Saddle River, NJ: Pearson Education, Inc., p. 452.

8 **Answer: 1** **Rationale:** The client experiencing endocarditis may have splinter hemorrhages of the fingernails (option 1). Aneurysms would be assessed by inspecting for pulsations or auscultating for bruits (option 2). A bruit is assessed by listening over an artery with a stethoscope for turbulent blood flow (option 3). Poor circulation would be evaluated by inspecting for hair distribution changes on the lower extremities as well as skin color changes or palpating for pulses (option 4). **Cognitive Level:** Application **Client Need:** Health Promotion and Maintenance **Integrated Process:** Nursing Process: Assessment **Content Area:** Adult Health: Cardiovascular **Strategy:** Eliminate the options with bruit and aneurysm as they are similarly assessed. For an aneurysm the nurse would inspect for heaves, palpate for pulsations, or

auscultate for bruits. Poor circulation manifests through lack of hair distribution and color changes on the lower extremities. **Reference:** D'Amico, D. and Barbarito, C. (2007). *Health & physical assessment in nursing.* Upper Saddle River, NJ: Pearson Education, Inc., p. 455.

9 **Answer: 2** **Rationale:** The nurse should never palpate the carotid arteries simultaneously because applying pressure to both sets of baroreceptors will decrease cerebral blood flow and, therefore, cerebral blood pressure (option 2). The nurse can palpate the carotid arteries one at a time while the client is in the supine position (option 1). Heaves are assessed by inspecting over major arteries (option 3). An enlarged heart is evaluated through the use of an echocardiogram (option 4). **Cognitive Level:** Application **Client Need:** Health Promotion and Maintenance **Integrated Process:** Nursing Process: Assessment **Content Area:** Adult Health: Cardiovascular **Strategy:** The critical word in the question is *essential.* With this in mind, look for an option that is highly important and/or relates to safety. Recall that palpation causes partial occlusion to a blood vessel and select option 2 because of the words *avoid* and *simultaneously.* **Reference:** D'Amico, D. and Barbarito, C. (2007). *Health & physical assessment in nursing.* Upper Saddle River, NJ: Pearson Education, Inc., pp. 458, 459.

10 **Answer: 45** **Rationale:** The client should be lying at a 45-degree angle for accurate assessment of pulsation of the carotid artery on each side of the neck. The pulsation should be noted lateral to the trachea in a groove that is medial to the sternocleidomastoid muscle. This position is also used to measure in centimeters the amount of jugular vein distention. **Cognitive Level:** Application **Client Need:** Health Promotion and Maintenance **Integrated Process:** Nursing Process: Assessment **Content Area:** Adult Health: Cardiovascular **Strategy:** Specific knowledge of proper positioning is needed to answer this question. As a memory aid, recall that the 45-degree head of bed elevation is the same degree of elevation used to measure the amount of jugular vein distention in a client. **Reference:** D'Amico, D. and Barbarito, C. (2007). *Health & physical assessment in nursing.* Upper Saddle River, NJ: Pearson Education, Inc., p. 454.

Posttest

1 **Answer: 3** **Rationale:** To elicit cooperation of a school-age child the nurse should allow the child to listen to the parent's heart sounds with the stethoscope (option 3). Permitting the child to listen to his or her parent's chest will help reduce the child's fear. Explaining the procedure to the child (option 1) or the child's parents (option 2) will not eliminate the child's fear nor will it make the child familiar with the procedure. Sedation is not necessary (option 4). **Cognitive Level:** Application **Client Need:** Health Promotion and Maintenance **Integrated Process:** Nursing Process: Implementation **Content Area:** Child Health **Strategy:** Note that questions that refer to the developmental age of a client include the age for a specific reason. To choose correctly, recall that children are usually more cooperative when they are familiar with the procedure and equipment. **Reference:** D'Amico, D. and Barbarito, C. (2007). *Health & physical assessment in nursing.* Upper Saddle River, NJ: Pearson Education, Inc., p. 460.

2 Answer: 4 Rationale: The nurse should use the bell of the stethoscope to auscultate the low pitched sounds of the heart (option 4). The pulmonic area provides information about pulmonic stenosis murmurs (option 1). The diaphragm of the stethoscope is used to hear high-pitched sounds (option 2). At the 2nd intercostal space the S2 sound is heard more prominently then S1 (option 3). **Cognitive Level:** Application **Client Need:** Health Promotion and Maintenance **Integrated Process:** Nursing Process: Assessment **Content Area:** Adult Health: Cardiovascular **Strategy:** Select from the options that are opposites. There are only two aspects of the stethoscope that can be used for the purpose of hearing sounds: the bell and the diaphragm. Recall that low-pitched sounds are heard best with the bell. **Reference:** D'Amico, D. and Barbarito, C. (2007). *Health & physical assessment in nursing.* Upper Saddle River, NJ: Pearson Education, Inc., pp. 460, 461.

3 Answer: 1 Rationale: In the client with mitral regurgitation the nurse would expect to hear the murmur at the apex of the heart (option 1). Aortic stenosis murmurs are heard at the aortic area at the 2nd intercostal space at the right sternal border (option 2). Pulmonic murmurs are heard at the pulmonic area (option 3). The second intercostal is where an aortic murmur will be heard (option 4). **Cognitive Level:** Application **Client Need:** Health Promotion and Maintenance **Integrated Process:** Nursing Process: Implementation **Content Area:** Adult Health: Cardiovascular **Strategy:** To answer this type of question think about the various cardiac valvular disorders and visualize on the chest where the murmurs would be heard using knowledge of landmarks. Recall that sounds of a valve are heard best in the area toward which the blood the flowing after passing through the valve. **Reference:** D'Amico, D. and Barbarito, C. (2007). *Health & physical assessment in nursing.* Upper Saddle River, NJ: Pearson Education, Inc., p. 465.

4 Answer: The correct area is indicated as 1 in the diagram. Rationale: The nurse should inspect and palpate the 2nd intercostal space at the right sternal border. The presence of pulsations or heaves in this area may indicate an ascending aortic enlargement or aneurysm, aortic stenosis, or systemic hypertension. **Cognitive Level:** Application **Client Need:** Health Promotion and Maintenance **Integrated Process:** Nursing Process: Analysis **Content Area:** Adult Health: Cardiovascular **Strategy:** Specific information is needed to answer this question. Recall that the landmark for detecting ascending aortic problems is the same area as for detecting aortic valvular problems. **Reference:** D'Amico, D. and Barbarito, C. (2007).

Health & physical assessment in nursing. Upper Saddle River, NJ: Pearson Education, Inc., p. 456.

5 Answer: 1, 4, 5 Rationale: The nurse should assess the rate, regularity, and rhythm of the apical pulse. Rate is the number of beats per minute (option 1). Regularity and rhythm are the terms used to describe that the beat is occurring when expected (options 4 and 5). Intensity is a term to describe the strength of a murmur (option 2). If there is a pulse the extremity should be warm to touch (option 3). **Cognitive Level:** Application **Client Need:** Health Promotion and Maintenance **Integrated Process:** Nursing Process: Assessment **Content Area:** Adult Health: Cardiovascular **Strategy:** Recall that pulses are always evaluated for rate, rhythm, and regularity. **Reference:** D'Amico, D. and Barbarito, C. (2007). *Health & physical assessment in nursing.* Upper Saddle River, NJ: Pearson Education, Inc., p. 461.

6 Answer: 2 Rationale: It is essential that the nurse obtain data related to the type, quality, and location of pain (option 2). While a fever may indicate endocarditis the nurse would take the temperature rather than asking about one, and would not focus on temperature when a description of an acute problem such as pain is needed (option 1). While weight gain may provide data for a cardiac disorder such as congestive heart failure, it does not provide information about an acute problem such as myocardial infarction (option 3). Asking the client if he or she smokes is not useful when the client is experiencing chest pain. Smoking data can be obtained after the acute pain is resolved (option 4). **Cognitive Level:** Analysis **Client Need:** Health Promotion and Maintenance **Integrated Process:** Nursing Process: Assessment **Content Area:** Adult Health: Cardiovascular **Strategy:** When a client is experiencing chest discomfort it is essential that the nurse obtain information about the characteristics, quality, location, and radiation of the pain. The nurse should also obtain information about the precipitating factors if any, as well as any factor that relieves the pain. **Reference:** D'Amico, D. and Barbarito, C. (2007). *Health & physical assessment in nursing.* Upper Saddle River, NJ: Pearson Education, Inc., p. 446.

7 Answer: 3 Rationale: Earlobe creases in an adult may indicate coronary artery disease (option 3). Endocarditis manifests with fever, fatigue, and murmur (option 1). Pericarditis manifests with fatigue, shortness of breath, and pericardial friction rub (option 2). Fluid overload manifests as shortness of breath, edema, and increased jugular vein distention (option 4). **Cognitive Level:** Analysis **Client Need:** Health Promotion and Maintenance **Integrated Process:** Nursing Process: Analysis **Content Area:** Adult Health: Cardiovascular **Strategy:** Eliminate options ending in -*itis* as these conditions imply inflammation or infection. Eliminate option 4 as fluid overload is manifested as edema in the periphery or in the lungs. **Reference:** D'Amico, D. and Barbarito, C. (2007). *Health & physical assessment in* *nursing.* Upper Saddle River, NJ: Pearson Education, Inc., p. 453.

8 **Answer: 1** **Rationale:** The client who is experiencing bounding pulses may be experiencing fever, which increases the body's need for oxygen and blood flow (option 1). Bruits are turbulent blood flow and usually indicate blockage (option 2). Chest pain is not associated with bounding pulse (option 3). Cyanosis is a blue tinged color to the mucous membranes or skin and is associated with decreased oxygenation (option 4). **Cognitive Level:** Application **Client Need:** Health Promotion and Maintenance **Integrated Process:** Nursing Process: Assessment **Content Area:** Adult Health: Cardiovascular **Strategy:** Eliminate chest pain and bruits as these symptoms are not observed through inspection. Cyanosis implies color, therefore, it is not related to a bounding pulse. **Reference:** D'Amico, D. and Barbarito, C. (2007). *Health & physical assessment in nursing.* Upper Saddle River, NJ: Pearson Education, Inc., p. 454.

9 **Answer: 2** **Rationale:** The client with pulmonary edema will experience respiratory symptoms such as shortness of breath and dyspnea (option 2). Edema in the lower extremities may indicate lymphedema or heart failure (option 1). A thrill is palpated and indicates turbulent blood flow (option 3). Splinter hemorrhages are red lines in the nails due to endocarditis (option 4). **Cognitive Level:** Application **Client Need:** Health Promotion and Maintenance **Integrated Process:** Nursing Process:

Assessment **Content Area:** Adult Health: Cardiovascular **Strategy:** Recall that pulmonary edema occurs when the left ventricle fails and that the vascular system "behind" the failing ventricle consists of the pulmonary vessels in the lungs. To choose correctly, next consider that congestion in these blood vessels produces shortness of breath, dyspnea, tachypnea, and possibly cyanosis. **Reference:** D'Amico, D. and Barbarito, C. (2007). *Health & physical assessment in nursing.* Upper Saddle River, NJ: Pearson Education, Inc., pp. 454–455.

10 **Answer: 2** **Rationale:** The client with hypertension may exhibit pulsations at the right sternal border at the 2nd intercostal space (option 2). A murmur at the 5th intercostal space, midclavicular line (apical area) may be the result of mitral regurgitation (option 1). A murmur of the pulmonic area may be the result of pulmonary stenosis (option 3). A murmur of the tricuspid area may be the result of tricuspid stenosis (option 4). **Cognitive Level:** Application **Client Need:** Health Promotion and Maintenance **Integrated Process:** Nursing Process: Assessment **Content Area:** Adult Health: Cardiovascular **Strategy:** Recall that pulsations or heaves at the 2nd intercostal space at the right sternal border are the result of hypertension, aortic aneurysm, or aortic stenosis. **Reference:** D'Amico, D. and Barbarito, C. (2007). *Health & physical assessment in nursing.* Upper Saddle River, NJ: Pearson Education, Inc., p. 458.

References

Bickley, L. (2010). *Bates guide to physical examination and history taking* (10th ed.). Philadelphia: Lippincott Williams & Wilkins.

D'Amico, D. and Barbarito, C. (2007). *Health and physical assessment in nursing.*

Upper Saddle River, NJ: Pearson Education, Inc., pp. 426–509.

Jarvis, C. (2008). *Physical examination and health assessment* (5th ed.). St. Louis, MO: Elsevier Saunders.

Zator Estes, M. (2009). *Health assessment and physical examination* (4th ed.). Clifton Park, NY: Delmar Cengage Learning.

6 Respiratory Assessment

Chapter Outline

Health History
Past Medical History
Present Health History
Family History

Equipment, Preparation, and
Positioning
Physical Examination
Expected Findings

Unexpected Findings
Lifespan Considerations
Documentation

 NCLEX-RN® Test Prep

Visit the Companion Website for this book
at www.pearsonhighered.com/hogan to
access additional practice opportunities
and more.

Objectives

➤ Identify the anatomy and physiology of the respiratory system.
➤ Conduct a respiratory health history.
➤ Prepare the client for a respiratory assessment.
➤ Utilize the techniques of respiratory assessment.
➤ Describe expected and unexpected findings associated with the
respiratory system.

Review at a Glance

adventitious breath sounds
abnormal sounds heard in the lungs that
include crackles, rhonchi, and wheezes
bradypnea slow rate of breathing,
usually less than 10 to 12 breaths per
minute in an adult (normal 12–20)
bronchial breath sounds loud
high-pitched breath sounds normally
heard over the trachea; signifies consolidation of lung tissue if heard elsewhere
in the lungs
bronchophony abnormal sounds
produced when client is asked to say
"99"; in areas of consolidation, sounds
produced are more distinct when listening with stethoscope
**bronchovesicular breath
sounds** medium-pitched and loud
breath sounds normally heard around the
areas of tracheal bifurcation; signifies consolidation if heard elsewhere in the lungs
crackles abnormal breath sounds
indicating fluid in air passages that are
classified as fine crackles when soft, high-
pitched, and brief; classified as coarse
when sound is louder and low-pitched

dullness flat sound produced during
percussion by fluid or solid organs
dyspnea difficulty during respiratory
effort that is observable
egophony abnormal sound produced
when client is asked to say "E"; normally
when listening with stethoscope, nurse
should hear "E" and not "aaay," which is
found over areas of consolidation
eupnea normal breathing without
difficulty at a respiratory rate of 12 to
20 breaths per minute in an adult
fremitus palpable vibration when
client speaks; decreased fremitus occurs
when the client is experiencing chronic
obstructive pulmonary disease, pneumothorax, pleural effusion, tumors, and
fibrosis of the lung; increased fremitus
occurs with consolidation of lung tissue
such as in lobar pneumonia
orthopnea dyspnea while lying
flat that is resolved or reduced by
sitting upright
**paroxysmal nocturnal dyspnea
(PND)** a sudden awakening during
the night with the feeling of an inability
to breathe

resonance sound heard over an air-
filled space during percussion
rhonchi sonorous low-pitched sound
occurring over major airways because
of mucus
stridor loud high-pitched crowing
sound produced by obstructed airway
tachypnea rapid breathing at rate
greater than 20 breaths per minute in
an adult
vesicular breath sounds soft
low-pitched sounds audible over peripheral lung fields
wheezes high-pitched sounds produced by blocked air flow because of
narrowing of airways; may be described
as inspiratory, expiratory, or both
whispered pectoriloquy sound
produced by asking the client to whisper
"one, two, three"; sound is indistinguishable when listening with a stethoscope in
a client without disease process; sound
is clear and audible in the client experiencing consolidation (such as lobar
pneumonia)

PRETEST

1 When performing respiratory assessment of an adult client the nurse notes hyperresonance on percussion. The nurse would conclude that this is due to which client condition?

1. Pulmonary disease
2. Scoliosis
3. A mass
4. Pain

2 A client who has been diagnosed with a myocardial infarction presents with a complaint of "awakening in the middle of the night with a feeling of not being able to breathe." What is the appropriate action for the nurse to take?

1. Have the client keep a log of number and length of awakenings with a heart and respiratory rate to provide data for evaluation
2. Instruct the client to sleep in semi-Fowler's position because of paroxysmal nocturnal dyspnea
3. Instruct the client to cough and deep breathe as client is experiencing chronic obstructive pulmonary disease (COPD)
4. Encourage the client to use a CPAP machine for sleep apnea

3 During a respiratory assessment, the nurse would elicit fremitus by doing which of the following during the examination?

1. Placing the hands over anterior and posterior lung fields, asking the client to say "ninety-nine"
2. Asking the client to say "ninety-nine" while listening to the lungs with a stethoscope
3. Palpating the anterior and posterior chest and costal margins
4. Percussing over the anterior and posterior chest

4 The nurse is performing a respiratory assessment on a client who is presenting with an underlying obstructive respiratory disease. What is the most important question for the nurse to ask the client during the interview to provide information about contributing risk factors?

1. "Have you ever smoked tobacco products?"
2. "Have you had your immunizations?"
3. "Do you experience dyspnea?"
4. "Are you currently using over-the-counter medications for your cough?"

5 The nurse has auscultated the client's lungs and hears bubbling sounds bilaterally in the lower lung fields. The nurse would document which finding in the client's medical record?

1. Bilateral rhonchi at the bases
2. Expiratory wheezing at the bases
3. Inspiratory wheezing at the bases
4. Bilateral crackles at the bases

6 The client is admitted to the hospital unit reporting inability to sleep because of shortness of breath. The nurse should take which preferred action?

1. Reassure the client that this will resolve shortly
2. Evaluate the client for history of asthma
3. Position the client in right lateral Sim's position
4. Have the client sleep on two pillows

7 The nurse is performing a respiratory assessment on a client and finds unequal chest excursion. The nurse would conclude that this may be caused by which of the following factors?

1. Client's physical stature
2. Chronic obstructive pulmonary disease
3. Collapse or obstruction of part of the lung
4. Diaphragmatic breathing

8 The client has a history of chronic obstructive pulmonary disease (COPD). The nurse should expect to document which clinical manifestations following physical examination? Select all that apply.

1. Increased tactile fremitus
2. Asymmetrical excursion
3. Decreased bilateral excursion
4. Fine crackles
5. A transverse to anteroposterior diameter of 1:1

9 A client who has been in a motor vehicle accident (MVA) has decreased lung sounds on the right side of the chest, decreased fremitus, tracheal deviation to the left, and pain and hyperresonance on the left. The nurse should prepare to implement which nursing intervention?

1. Prepare chest tube drainage setup
2. Administer a pulmonary bronchodilator
3. Prepare client for emergency tracheostomy
4. Administer low flow oxygen via nasal cannula

10 In what order would the nurse complete the following components of a respiratory assessment on an assigned client? Place numbers that correspond to the options in correct sequence.

1. Percuss the anterior thorax
2. Palpate the anterior thorax
3. Position the client
4. Explain the procedure to client
5. Auscultate the anterior thorax

➤ *See pages 115–117 for Answers and Rationales.*

I. HEALTH HISTORY

A. Respiratory assessment is an integral aspect of physical assessment to prevent or control disease

1. Use assessment to identify pulmonary disorders, detect unhealthy behavior, and recognize when a client's respiratory status is changing

2. An ideal time to teach health promotion and disease prevention related to the respiratory system is during a respiratory assessment; clients with chronic respiratory disease benefit from information about basic anatomy and physiology of the respiratory system prior to learning disease management

   a. Explain that the respiratory system consists of the nose (nasal cavity and nares), nasopharynx, pharynx, oropharynx, larynx, laryngopharynx, trachea, bronchi, bronchioles, and alveoli (see Table 6-1)

   b. Explain in simple terms the physiological concepts of oxygen and carbon dioxide exchange and the effects of bronchoconstriction and bronchodilation on ease of breathing

   c. In all clients, identify risks to respiratory system (such as smoking cigarettes/tobacco or inhalation of other irritants, and how to avoid them)

B. Consider client's physical ability to participate in interview and assessment

1. Client may be experiencing **dyspnea** (difficulty in breathing) and have difficulty speaking

2. Improve oxygenation ability of the client prior to conducting the interview

C. A focused interview encompasses questions to obtain information about respiratory system symptoms and risk factors

Table 6-1	Structure	Function
Respiratory Structures and their Functions	Nasal cavity	Warms, filters, and moistens air from the environment
	Nasopharynx	Passage posterior to the nasal cavity; houses adenoids and tonsils
	Pharynx	Passage for air to move between nose and larynx
	Oropharynx	Passage for food and air behind the mouth
	Larynx	Passage between pharynx and trachea that houses vocal cords
	Laryngopharynx	Distal portion of pharynx that anteriorly conducts air into trachea and posteriorly conducts food into the esophagus
	Trachea	Conducts air from larynx to bronchi
	Bronchi	Conducts air to lung
	Bronchioles	Conducts air into alveoli
	Alveoli	Area of lung in which gas exchange takes place
	Lung	Right and left; each houses bronchioles and alveoli

D. Health history includes information that can be used to direct physical assessment

1. Biographical data will assist with obtaining information related to respiratory dysfunction
   a. How old is the client?
   b. Is the respiratory symptom or problem an expected change with aging?
   c. Is the respiratory change associated with environmental factors?
   d. Is the respiratory change associated with occupational factors?
2. Current health status begins with the client's current complaint (may be termed *chief complaint*)
   a. Is the client experiencing dyspnea?
   b. Is the client experiencing **paroxysmal nocturnal dyspnea (PND)** (a sudden awakening during the night with the feeling of the inability to breathe)?
   c. Is the client experiencing **orthopnea** (dyspnea while lying flat that is resolved or reduced by sitting upright)?
   d. Is the client experiencing a cough?
   e. Is the client experiencing pain?

Practice to Pass

What information will the health history provide?

II. PAST MEDICAL HISTORY

Practice to Pass

What is the purpose of obtaining the client's past medical history?

A. Purpose

1. Provides a review of the respiratory system and previous respiratory problems
2. Compares current health status and habits to factors that may be predisposing the client to respiratory disorders

B. Questions to obtain past medical history of the respiratory system

1. "As a child did you have frequent respiratory infections, a history of tuberculosis, or asthma?" (may indicate underlying disease)
2. "Have you ever been hospitalized for respiratory problems?" (obtains baseline data and may provide access to medical records)
3. "Can you describe any respiratory trauma or surgeries you have had?"
4. "Do you have heart or renal disease?" (may produce respiratory symptoms)
5. "Have you had immunizations for pneumonia, influenza, or Bacille Calmette-Guerin (BCG) for tuberculosis?" (positive purified protein derivative [PPD] test result may be due to previous BCG inoculation to prevent tuberculosis)
6. "Do you have a history of allergies to food, pollen, drugs, or environmental factors? If so what type of reaction do you experience?"
7. "Have you traveled recently?" (traveling by plane exposes the individual to recirculated air and staying in a hotel may expose the individual to inadequate or unclean filtration systems)
8. "Have you been in the military? If so, where were you located?" (may provide information related to exposure to disease, infections, or environmental toxins)
9. Review of systems evaluation enables the nurse to determine whether there is anything in the client's previous medical history that has influenced the current health of the individual
   a. "Have you experienced any changes in mental capability?" (changes in mental status may indicate hypoxia or hypercarbia)
   b. "Have you experienced any confusion?" (confusion or restlessness may indicate hypoxia)
   c. "Have your eyes been tearing?" (tearing of eyes may be clinical manifestation of allergies)
   d. "Have you had postnasal drip, pain in the facial area, or a sore throat?" (these symptoms may indicate sinus infection, allergies, or other infection)
   e. "Have you had swelling of the throat or difficulty swallowing?" (dysphagia places client at risk for aspiration)

    f. "Have you experienced chest pain?" (chest pain may be a clinical manifestation of cardiac dysfunction or dysrhythmia)

    g. "Have you experienced nausea, gastrointestinal upset, or gastric reflux?" (these manifestations may be related to congestive heart failure)

    h. "Have you lost weight?" (weight loss may be sign of chronic obstructive pulmonary disease [COPD])

    i. "Have you had frequent urination at night?" (nocturia may indicate congestive heart failure)

    j. "Have you experienced any changes in skin color?"

    k. "Does your skin feel tight and swollen?"

    l. "Have you experienced any medical issues that you can remember that may be influencing your health?"

III. PRESENT HEALTH HISTORY

    A. Focus questions on current respiratory system problems; it is important to identify risk factors as well as any health promotion activities in which the client engages

    B. Questions to obtain current health history information include the following:

      1. "Do you take any medications for your respiratory problem?"

      2. "What are the medications you are taking?"

      3. "Do you have any cardiac problems?"

      4. "Do you have chest pain?"

      5. "Do you have shortness of breath? If so, does anything precipitate it?"

      6. "Do you have a cough? Is it precipitated by anything? Please tell me about it."

      7. "Do you use tobacco? If so, what type and for how long?"

      8. "Do you use street drugs?"

      9. "Do you seek healthcare for any respiratory problems?"

     10. "Have you lost or gained weight?"

     11. "Do you exercise? If so, what type and how long are the sessions?"

     12. "Do you sleep through the night? If not, what wakes you up?"

     13. "Do you take naps throughout the day?"

     14. "Do you feel rested when you wake in the morning or after a nap?"

     15. "Do you clean or have hobbies that require use of chemicals or materials with noxious fumes?"

     16. "Do you breathe through your nose or mouth? If you breathe through the mouth, what caused you to breathe through your mouth?" (mouth breathing associated with disorders of the nose or hypoxia)

     17. "Do you have any problems with your nose or mouth? If so, how long have you had this problem?"

     18. "Have you received any treatments for breathing problems? If so, what?"

     19. "Tell me about the breathing difficulties you experience when engaged in activity. How long have you had difficulty?" (respiratory rate and depth should increase with activity)

     20. "What do you do to stop the difficulty breathing when exercising?" (stopping activity should stop difficulty)

     21. "When you lie down flat do you have difficulty breathing?"

     22. "How many pillows do you need for sleep? How long have you slept on this many pillows?"

     23. "Do you use pillows for comfort or to ease your breathing?"

     24. "Does the position or number of pillows effectively help with breathing?"

     25. "Do you need to sit upright at night?"

     26. "What is your occupation?"

     27. "Are you exposed to chemicals at work?"

     28. "Where do you live? Are you exposed to environmental hazards? If so, what type?"

IV. FAMILY HISTORY

    A. Provides data about genetic predisposition, and can aid in identifying risk factors; data will assist in differentiating disease processes; questions include the following:

        1. "Has anyone in your family been diagnosed with cystic fibrosis?" (cystic fibrosis is caused by an autosomal recessive gene)

        2. "Does anyone in your family have allergies?" (will provide information about potential exposure)

        3. "Does anyone in your family have asthma or obstructive respiratory disease?" (has tendency to run in families and has been linked to stress, allergies, and environmental conditions)

        4. "Has anyone in your family been tested for an alpha antitrypsin deficiency?" (has been linked to chronic obstructive pulmonary disease)

        5. "Does anyone living in your home smoke?" (second-hand smoke is linked to many respiratory diseases such as chronic obstructive pulmonary disease and asthma, and is a causative factor in cancer)

        6. "How long have you been exposed to second-hand smoke?"

        7. "Has anyone living in your home been diagnosed with tuberculosis? If so what type?"

    B. Have the client review as many family generations as possible to provide maximal data; most individuals can provide information about parents, grandparents, and possibly great-grandparents

    C. Information about adopted family members does not provide genetic information for client; however, it does provide information about environmental factors, since all individuals residing in the home will share exposure to the same toxins

V. EQUIPMENT, PREPARATION, AND POSITIONING

    A. To perform respiratory assessment gather the following equipment:

        1. Examination gloves

        2. Drape or blanket to cover client

        3. Gown as client will need to undress

        4. Stethoscope

        5. Skin marker

        6. Ruler

        7. Alcohol wipe for cleaning the stethoscope to decrease the risk of transmitting organisms to others

        8. Tissues for the client when he or she is coughing

    B. Preparation and positioning

        1. Provide an environment that is private and comfortable

        2. Provide adequate lighting to be able to discern color changes

        3. Explain each step of the procedure to the client to decrease anxiety

        4. Explain to the client that additional instructions will be provided throughout the examination

        5. When explaining procedure, inform the client of any discomfort associated with that aspect of the assessment

        6. Observe the client continually for signs of discomfort

        7. Instruct the client to inform you if experiencing discomfort

        8. Be aware that the ideal position for performing a respiratory examination is sitting; if the client is unable to sit, have him or her lie down but provide for maintenance of airway

        9. Complete the respiratory assessment just after examination of the neck and thyroid; position yourself behind the client to examine his or her posterior thorax (see Figure 6-1) and lateral aspects of chest wall, and then examine anterior thorax

        10. Minimize position changes for the client

Figure 6-1

Pattern for palpating the
posterior thorax

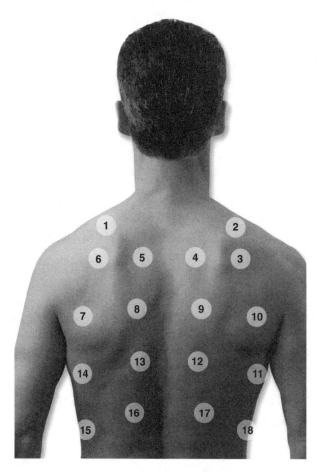

VI. PHYSICAL EXAMINATION

A. Inform the client that that you will be looking at chest structures of the posterior thorax

B. Observe skin color; color varies with individual pigmentation; look for pink mucous membranes and nail beds as these are consistent with adequate oxygenation

C. Observe the client's thoracic structures; all structures should be compared bilaterally and should be consistent in size, shape, and anatomical level

1. Compare the body for symmetry, such as scapulae and clavicles
2. Compare transverse anteroposterior diameter; transverse aspect of chest should be two times anteroposterior aspect
3. Observe respiratory pattern

D. Inspect the posterior chest wall

1. Explain to the client that you will be "looking at chest wall"; provide instructions; tell the client to breathe normally throughout the assessment
2. Count respiratory rate over one minute
   a. Do not tell the client you are counting his or her respiratory rate as this often makes it difficult for the client to breathe using his or her normal patterns
   b. Look for use of intercostal muscles (often called accessory muscle use)
3. Observe skin color
4. Inspect structure of thorax; look for symmetry and respiratory excursion

E. Palpate posterior thorax

1. Inform the client that you will be touching his or her thorax
2. Ask the client to indicate any areas of discomfort or tenderness

Practice to Pass

The nurse is inspecting the thorax. It is essential that the nurse document what assessments?

3. Ask the client to breathe normally throughout the assessment
4. Palpate posterior thorax by using finger pads to lightly touch thorax; compare side to side
   a. Assess muscle structure
   b. Palpate for lesions or masses
   c. Palpate for tenderness
   d. Palpate ribs and intercostal muscles
   e. Palpate for respiratory excursion (see Figure 6-2a)
      1) Tell the client you will be placing your hands on his or her lower chest and asking the client to breathe deeply
      2) Place palmar surface of hands on back with thumbs close to vertebrae at the 10th rib
      3) Ask the client to breathe; movement should be symmetrical and thumbs should move evenly as he or she inhales
5. Palpate for tactile **fremitus**; fremitus is vibration of the thorax when the client speaks
   a. Instruct the client that you will be feeling his or her thorax while asking that he or she repeat "ninety-nine" or "one, two, three" (see Figure 6-2b)
   b. Using palmar surface of hand, place on posterior thorax and move hand side to side comparing for symmetry
   c. May use both hands by placing one hand on each side of thorax and comparing one side of thorax to next; this method facilitates speed and may be easier to identify areas of asymmetry

F. Percuss posterior thorax
   1. Explain to the client that you will be tapping on the posterior thorax
   2. Instruct the client to breathe normally and to lean forward while you percuss thorax

Practice to Pass

When assessing for fremitus the nurse should also palpate for what characteristic?

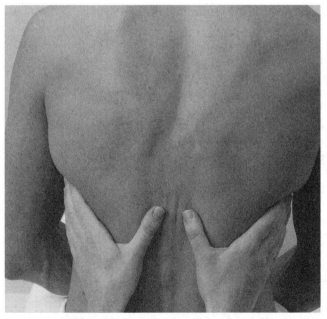

A. Palpation for respiratory expansion

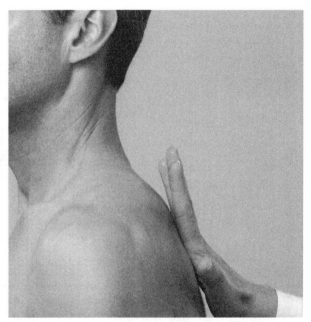

B. Palpation for tactile fremitus using metacarpophalangeal joint area

Figure 6-2

Palpation of the posterior thorax

3. Percuss lungs by placing the second finger of your non-dominant hand firmly on posterior thorax and tapping that finger with the second finger of your dominant hand
4. Percuss from apex of lung to distal aspect of lung; proceed from side to side comparing sounds bilaterally
5. Percuss for diaphragmatic excursion
    a. Explain to the client that you will continue to tap on posterior aspect of thorax and you will ask him or her to exhale while you place a mark on the back with skin marker; inform the client that marker will not leave permanent marks
    b. Find the diaphragm around the T10 or T12 level of the thorax by percussing for **dullness** (flat sound produced by fluid or solid organs) at midscapular line during normal respirations; begin to percuss downward until you hear dullness, instead of **resonance** (sound heard over an air-filled space); repeat bilaterally; mark those areas; marks should be parallel and approximately at the level of the 10th intercostal space
    c. Measure diaphragmatic movement by instructing the client to exhale, begin percussing at skin marking, and assess from areas of resonance to dullness; mark that area
    d. Ask the client to fully inhale and hold his or her breath as you percuss from the level of diaphragm distally going from resonance to dullness; measure distance in centimeters; repeat bilaterally

G. Auscultate posterior thorax

1. Auscultation involves listening to sounds produced by air being inhaled and exhaled by placing diaphragm of stethoscope firmly on the thorax; if sounds are distorted from normal, the degree of change will be based on the amount of fluid or secretions in airways and lungs
2. Become an expert in listening for breath sounds in order to detect changes in client's condition; it is important to listen to inspiration and expiration for loudness, pattern, location, pitch, and duration (see Table 6-2)
3. Normal breath sounds are categorized into bronchial, bronchovesicular, and vesicular sounds
    a. **Bronchial breath sounds** are those from the level of the trachea downward and are usually high-pitched and loud; usually longer on exhalation
    b. **Bronchovesicular breath sounds** are those over bronchi posteriorly between scapulae and anteriorly near the sternum and 2nd intercostal space; sounds are medium in terms of loudness and pitch
    c. **Vesicular breath sounds** are those heard over peripheral lung fields and are soft, low-pitched sounds that are longer on inspiration then exhalation
    d. A global term for abnormal breath sounds is **adventitious sounds**; these abnormal breath sounds include **crackles** (classified as fine crackles when soft, high-pitched, and brief; classified as coarse when sound is louder and low-pitched), **rhonchi** (sonorous low-pitched sound occurring over major airways because of mucus), and **wheezes** (high-pitched sounds produced by blocked air flow because of narrowing of airways; may be described as inspiratory, expiratory,

Table 6-2	Characteristic	Description
Characteristics of Breath Sounds	Loudness	Describes intensity of sound; usually described as soft (audible but faint), medium (easy to hear), and loud (easy for novice to differentiate)
	Location	Describes area where sound is best heard
	Pitch	Described as loud, medium, or soft
	Pattern	Describes whether sound occurs during inspiration or expiration; does sound occur throughout the respiratory phase?

or both); in certain disease processes you may also hear **stridor** (loud, high-pitched crowing sound produced by obstructed airway) and friction rubs

4. Instruct the client that you will be listening with a stethoscope to posterior thorax
5. Instruct the client to take a breath, when asked, through his or her mouth
6. Inform the client to report if he or she becomes tired or short of breath and you will stop the assessment for a pause
7. Use the same space landmarks for auscultation as were used for percussion; proceed from apex distally to bases of lungs (see Figure 6-3)
8. Move bilaterally from side to side comparing sounds
9. Assess voice sounds, also called vocal resonance; vocal resonance includes assessing for abnormal sounds such as the following:
   a. **Bronchophony** is assessed by having the client say "ninety-nine" while listening to a stethoscope over all landmarks; in areas of consolidation, sound produced is more distinct when listening with a stethoscope
   b. **Egophony** is assessed by having the client say "E" while listening with a stethoscope over all landmarks; normally when listening with a stethoscope, the nurse should hear "E" and not "aaay," which is found over areas of consolidation
   c. **Whispered pectoriloquy** is assessed by having the client whisper "one, two, three"; sound is indistinguishable when listening with a stethoscope in a client with no disease process; sound is clear and audible in a client experiencing consolidation
   d. The presence of bronchophony, egophony, or whispered pectoriloquy is abnormal and indicates consolidation of lung tissue in that area

Figure 6-3

Pattern for auscultation of the posterior thorax

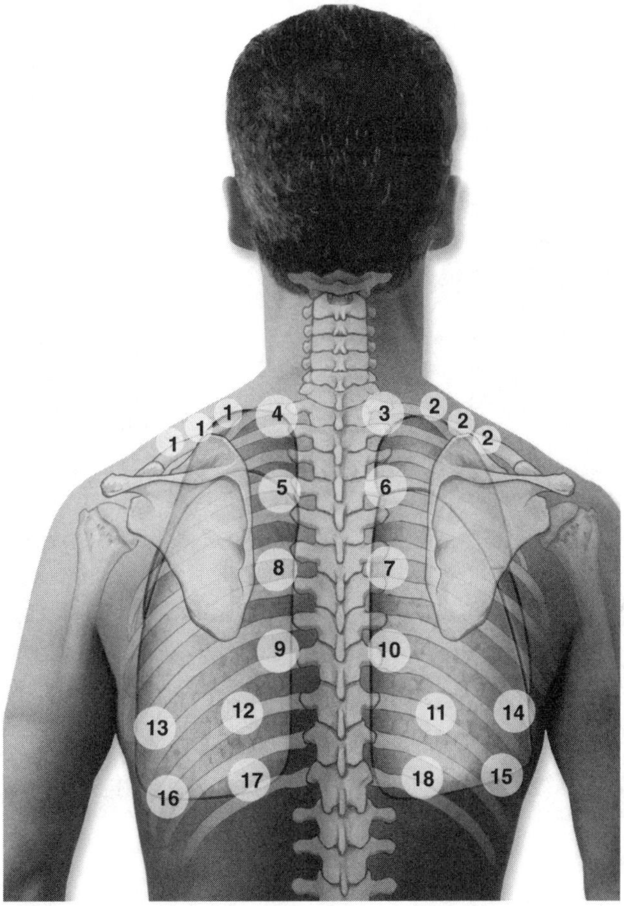

H. Inspect and then palpate anterior thorax

1. Position the client sitting upright
2. Inspect for symmetry and accessory muscle use and palpate for respiratory excursion as was done for the posterior thorax (see Figure 6-4a)
3. Instruct the client to breathe normally as you move through thorax landmarks during the assessment comparing one side to another
4. Have the client inform you of any pain or discomfort during the assessment
5. Palpate anterior chest by palpating chest wall beginning at anterolateral wall at suprasternal notch and proceeding downward to xiphoid process for symmetry, tactile fremitus, tenderness, lesions, and/or masses (see Figure 6-4b)

I. Percuss anterior thorax

1. Instruct the client that you will be tapping his or her anterior chest and to try to breathe normally
2. Begin percussion at apex of lung and proceed distally to bases, moving from one side to another; do not percuss clavicle; begin at midclavicular line and proceed to midaxillary line
3. Do not percuss over breast tissue; for large breast you may ask the client if he or she wishes to hold his or her breast out of area to be percussed or if you may move breast tissue; often in females with a large amount of breast tissue little data will be obtained

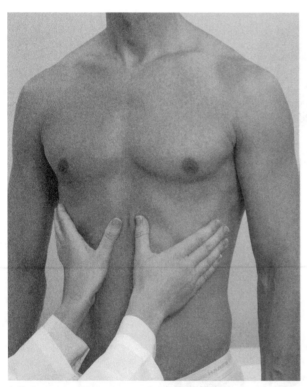

A. Palpation for respiratory expansion, anterior view

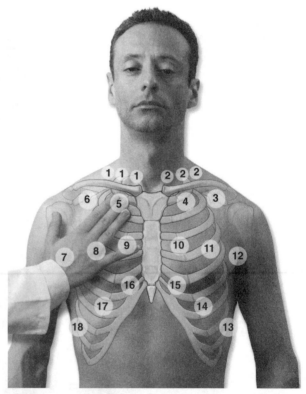

B. Pattern for palpation of anterior thorax

Figure 6-4

Palpation of anterior thorax

J. Auscultate anterior lungs

1. Instruct the client that you will be listening to the thorax with the diaphragm of stethoscope
   a. Lung sounds can be confused with environmental noises; the client's clothing or gown can create sounds; it is important to place the stethoscope directly on the skin and avoid listening through the gown
   b. Client noises make it difficult for the nurse to identify lung sounds
      1) The client may have a hairy chest, which can create extraneous sounds; shivering may cause extraneous noises
      2) The nurse may create extra sounds by banging stethoscope or excessive movement of tubing
2. Instruct client to breathe through his or her mouth each time stethoscope is placed on his or her chest when asked and to inform you if he or she becomes fatigued or short of breath
3. Auscultate in the following sequence (see Figure 6-5):
   a. Place stethoscope over trachea above the suprasternal notch to listen for tracheal (T) breath sounds
   b. Move stethoscope to the left and right side of trachea above each sternoclavicular joint to hear bronchial (B) breath sounds
   c. Place stethoscope in triangular area above each clavicle to auscultate the apices for vesicular (V) breath sounds
   d. Auscultate at the 2nd and 3rd intercostal spaces at the left and right sternal borders for bronchovesicular (BV) breath sounds
   e. Continue auscultating over lung fields left to right (side to side) in a descending pattern
4. Auscultate for normal and adventitious breath sounds (abnormal breath sounds such as crackles, rhonchi, and wheezing; further described in section VIII)

Figure 6-5

Auscultation of anterior thorax with accompanying expected sounds

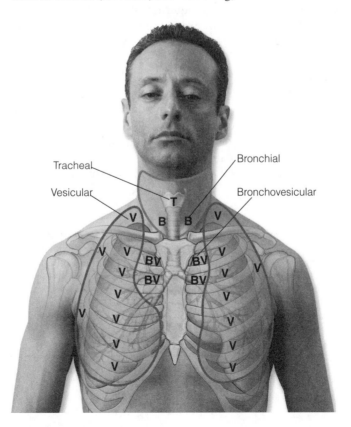

VII. EXPECTED FINDINGS

A. Inspection

1. During inspection of the thorax expect the client to have pink mucous membranes to reflect adequate oxygenation
2. Clavicles and scapulae should be of same height and sternum and vertebrae midline
3. Chest movement should be smooth with no use of intercostal muscles
4. Transverse diameter of the chest is twice the anteroposterior diameter in an adult; chest should be elliptical in shape
5. Respiratory rate should be 12 to 20 breaths per minute; respirations should be smooth and even
6. In males, breaths should originate in abdomen, whereas in females breaths tend to be more costal

B. Palpation

1. During palpation of thorax no masses, nodules, or lesions should be felt
2. Thorax should feel smooth without tenderness or pain
3. Crepitus should not be felt under the skin
4. All ribs and vertebrae should be in alignment and no deviations felt
5. Respiratory excursion should feel smooth and even
6. When assessing for tactile fremitus, strongest palpable vibration should be over the mainstem bronchus bifurcation (2nd intercostal space anteriorly or the level of T4 posteriorly), and vibrations should decrease as you palpate distally to the base of the lungs

C. Percussion

1. When using percussion over the thorax, the usual finding is resonance (which is a low-pitched hollow sound) over air filled structures
2. Percussion over a solid or bony structure elicits flat sound
3. During assessment of diaphragmatic excursion, the diaphragm should be symmetrical; measurement of excursion should be three to five centimeters; due to anatomical location of liver, right excursion measurement may be one to two centimeters higher

D. Auscultation

1. Expected findings to anticipate when assessing the respiratory system with a stethoscope is to hear a variety of sounds, including tracheal, bronchial, bronchovesicular, and vesicular (see Table 6-3)
2. Breath sounds should be heard bilaterally; sounds should be equal and have the same pitch and quality
3. There should be no adventitious breath sounds

Practice to Pass

When assessing for bronchophony, what sounds should the nurse anticipate?

Table 6-3	Sound	Location	Ratio Inspiration to Expiration	Quality
Normal Breath Sounds	Tracheal	Over trachea	I < E	Harsh, high-pitched
	Bronchial	Next to trachea	E > I	Loud, high-pitched
	Bronchovesicular	Sternal border between scapula	I = E	Medium loudness, medium pitch
	Vesicular	Remainder of lungs	I > E	Soft, low-pitched

Source: D'Amico, D. & Barbarito, C. (2007). *Health & physical assessment in nursing.* Upper Saddle River, NJ: Pearson Education, Inc., Table 15.1, p. 377.

4. During assessment of voice sounds, the nurse should hear muffled sounds when testing for bronchophony

5. When testing for egophony, the nurse should clearly hear sound of EEE

6. In lungs without disease process, the nurse should hear a muffled sound when assessing for whispered pectoriloquy

7. Tracheal and bronchial sounds should be heard in the area of the trachea; bronchovesicular sounds should be heard along sternum and vertebrae; vesicular should be heard over lung fields

VIII. UNEXPECTED FINDINGS

A. Inspection

1. During inspection of thorax, unexpected or abnormal findings include cyanosis, pallor, rubor, erythema, duskiness, or gray coloring

2. Clavicles should be at an equal height and sternum and vertebrae should be midline; if structures are not at correct anatomical position (asymmetry) then evaluate for further abnormal findings; asymmetry may indicate musculoskeletal deformity or respiratory disease process

   a. Abnormal chest shapes may cause impaired respiratory processes

   1) Barrel chest usually results from chronic obstructive pulmonary disease (COPD); in this condition the anteroposterior diameter of the chest is equal to the transverse diameter

   2) Another congenital musculoskeletal deformity is *pectus excavatum*, known as funnel chest; with this deformity the sternum is depressed in the area of xiphoid process; the deformity may cause respiratory dysfunction and/or cardiac compression

   3) *Pectus carinatum* (pigeon chested) is a congenital deformity in which the lower aspect of the sternum is displaced anteriorly; it will not cause respiratory compromise

   4) Scoliosis is a lateral deviation of the spine; deviation may cause individual body image disturbances as shoulder and hip may elevate, and will cause respiratory compromise

   5) Kyphosis is a posterior curvature of the vertebrae at the thoracic level and is usually due to aging; long-term effects include respiratory and cardiac dysfunction

3. Anteroposterior: transverse diameter not consistent with a 1:2 ratio may be caused by aging or chronic obstructive disease process

4. When assessing respiratory rate expect a regular unlabored pattern with a rate of 12 to 20, which is termed **eupnea**; any finding greater or less than expected range is considered abnormal

5. **Bradypnea**: term used to describe regular unlabored pattern of respirations with a rate less than 10 breaths per minute; often precipitated by narcotics use and increased intracranial pressure

6. **Tachypnea**: term used to describe abnormally high regular unlabored respiratory rate of greater than 24 breaths per minute; often precipitated by fever, anxiety, respiratory insufficiency, pain, and respiratory diseases where there is inadequate oxygenation

7. Hypoventilation: term used to describe slow, shallow respirations with a rate of less than 10 breaths per minute; may be due to narcotic overdose and chest trauma

8. Hyperventilation: term used to describe rapid, deep respirations with a rate greater than 24 breaths per minute; may be precipitated by fear, hypoxia, hypoglycemia, acidosis, and infection

9. Biot's breathing is characterized by shallow breaths with periods of apnea

10. Cheyne-Stokes respirations are deep respirations accompanied by apnea

Practice to Pass

What intervention would the nurse anticipate in a client experiencing a dusky color?

Practice to Pass

What respiratory pattern would the nurse expect to observe in a client who is experiencing fever and anxiety?

Table 6-4	Adventitious Sound	Description	Quality
Adventitious Breath Sounds	Crackles (formerly rales)	Crackling noises	Loud, high-pitched crackling or bubbling
	Rhonchi	Sonorous	Low-pitched sounds
	Wheezes	Musical	High-pitched sounds
	Stridor	Crowing	Loud, high-pitched sound
	Friction rub	Rubbing or grating	Low-pitched sound

B. Palpation
  1. Palpation should not yield findings of pain or tenderness, which would indicate inflammation
  2. Crepitus should not be felt under fingertips during palpation as it is caused by air in subcutaneous tissue, called subcutaneous emphysema
  3. There should be no deviation in the spine
  4. Uneven respiratory excursion is an abnormal finding that indicates COPD or pneumothorax
  5. Tactile fremitus that is decreased may be the result of COPD, pleural effusion, pneumothorax, or a mass; increased tactile fremitus may indicate infection (pneumonia) or fluid in lungs

C. Percussion
  1. Do not expect the client to exhibit hyperresonance on percussion; this would be caused by pneumothorax (air) or emphysema (because of hyperinflation of the lungs)
  2. Dullness is elicited when the nurse percusses over the area of fluid or the mass
  3. Uneven diaphragmatic excursion is significant as it may indicate pleural effusion on the side of diaphragm that is elevated
  4. Diaphragmatic excursion distance that is shortened would indicate pain, increased abdominal pressure, respiratory depression, COPD, or atelectasis

D. Auscultation
  1. Adventitious breath sounds that may be auscultated include crackles, rhonchi, and wheezes
    a. Crackles may be classified as fine or coarse
      1) Fine crackles are soft and high-pitched, whereas coarse crackles are louder, longer, and lower in pitch
      2) Crackles are due to fluid in air passage and will not disappear if client coughs; if the client is sitting upright then crackles must be at bases and are usually heard near end of inspiration
    b. Rhonchi may be described as sonorous low-pitched sounds
      1) Sounds may disappear with coughing and may be the result of fluid or exudates in larger airways
      2) May be heard on inspiration or expiration
    c. Wheeze is a term used to describe a high-pitched sound; it is produced due to an obstructed airway; it is found on inspiration or expiration
    d. Stridor is a sound described as a low-pitched crowing sound; it can be heard without a stethoscope as result of obstructed airway on inspiration
    e. Friction rub is a low-pitched sound; it may be heard on inspiration or expiration (see Table 6-4)

Practice to Pass

A client is reported to have crackles in the right base. When conducting an initial shift assessment, during what phase of the respiratory cycle should the oncoming nurse expect to hear these adventitious lung sounds?

IX. LIFESPAN CONSIDERATIONS

A. Infants

Practice to Pass

How should the nurse position an infant for a respiratory assessment?

1. During the first few hours after birth, fetal circulation closes and the respiratory rate may be 40 to 80 breaths per minute and irregular
2. When assessing infants, parents may the hold the infant in their arms; the order of assessment may be reordered to auscultate the lungs of a quiet infant; breath sounds would be difficult to hear clearly in an infant who is crying
3. With a crying infant it is beneficial to palpate fremitus
4. The shape of the chest in an infant is circular
5. Because of a thin chest wall, lung sounds are louder and hyperresonance is noted upon percussion
6. When assessing for excursion, suspect hernia or pneumothorax if movement is asymmetrical
7. Stridor upon auscultation is a sign of upper airway obstruction, croup, or epiglottitis; wheezing is sign of asthma

B. Children

1. May be held in parent's arms if that provides consolation; child should be positioned upright
2. Child should be permitted to handle equipment to reduce anxiety
3. Children are abdominal breathers until approximately the age seven; it is easier to count respirations in abdomen
4. Children like games, so having them "blow out" a penlight will assist in auscultating breath sounds
5. Shape of chest in child will be elliptical around age six
6. By age six respiratory rate should be less than 35 breaths per minute

C. Older adults

1. If older adult is ill, he or she may need assistance in sitting upright; a second examiner may provide support; if a second person unavailable to support the client then the nurse would need to roll the client side to side
2. The older adult may need to have rest periods built into the assessment
3. Lungs should be clear without adventitious sounds
4. Excursion should be smooth and symmetrical
5. Kyphosis may develop, which can lead to hypoventilation
6. Hyperresonance becomes more predominant with age because of overinflation of the lungs

X. DOCUMENTATION

A. Inspection

1. Shape of thorax should be documented as well as skin color and contour
2. Respiratory rate and pattern is essential

B. Palpation

1. Document diaphragmatic expansion and fremitus
2. Document masses, nodules, pain, or tenderness

C. Percussion

1. Document percussion of lung fields
2. Include excursion documentation

D. Auscultation

1. Note breath sounds
2. If abnormal breath sounds are heard, document voice fremitus

Case Study

A male client who was in a motor vehicle accident is reporting shortness of breath. The client has no other apparent signs of distress. At the beginning of the assessment of the client the nurse finds decreased breath sounds on the right as well as an increased respiratory rate of 22 breaths/minute.

1. What subjective data should the nurse document?

2. How should the nurse position this client to perform the assessment?

3. Due to decreased breath sounds on the right, the nurse should perform what additional aspects of the respiratory assessment?

4. When percussing the client's chest, what sound should the nurse expect to document?

5. What is the most appropriate nursing diagnosis for this client?

For suggested responses, see page 309

POSTTEST

1 The nurse is caring for a client who has curvature of the thoracic and lumbar spine. The nurse should develop a plan of care based on which priority risk nursing diagnosis?

1. Impaired gas exchange
2. Impaired comfort
3. Disturbed body image
4. Ineffective social relationships

2 The client is admitted to the hospital. During the assessment the nurse notes dyspnea, decreased fremitus, dullness over the right lung, and decreased breath sounds on the right with a pleural friction rub. The nurse would prepare the client for diagnostic tests to evaluate the client for which health problem?

1. Pneumothorax
2. Pleural effusion
3. Congestive heart failure
4. Pneumonia

3 The nurse is assessing the client and notes shallow breathing with periods of apnea. When participating in interdisciplinary care rounds the nurse should report that the client is experiencing which of the following?

1. Bradypnea
2. Cheyne-Stokes respirations
3. Hyperventilation
4. Biot's breathing

4 The nurse is caring for a client who is coughing up greenish-yellow mucus. Based on this clinical manifestation the nurse would conclude that the client is experiencing which respiratory condition?

1. Tuberculosis
2. Hemoptysis
3. Lung infection
4. Pleural effusion

5 The nurse is caring for an older adult client who states, "It is more difficult for me to breathe when I clean the house." To what would the nurse relate this clinical manifestation?

1. Deconditioning of the cardiac system
2. A normal age-related change
3. A respiratory infection
4. Environmental exposure

6 The nurse is teaching a client with allergies about work related allergens. To prevent respiratory distress the nurse should instruct the client to avoid which of the following?

1. Eating lunch with co-workers who are eating foods to which the client is allergic
2. Having allergy testing to prevent anaphylaxis
3. Contact with people who are smoking
4. Exercise to decrease dyspnea

7 The nurse is a assessing a client whose respiratory rate is 20 breaths per minute with symmetrical chest movement. The nurse will interpret this to be a normal finding in which client?

1. Infant
2. Pregnant female in the third trimester
3. Middle-aged client
4. An older adult client with lung disease

8 When assessing a client who reports a cough, it is essential that the nurse evaluate the cough by asking which of the following questions? Select all that apply.

1. "How long do you think you will be able to tolerate this cough?"
2. "How long have you been coughing?"
3. "Can you describe your cough?"
4. "Are you coughing up mucus?"
5. "Do you have pain when you cough?"

9 The nurse is performing a respiratory assessment on an older adult client who has a history of dizziness and is at risk for falls. Which aspect of the respiratory assessment is *most important* for the nurse to complete in determining contributing factors that could enhance risk for falls?

1. Position of comfort to detect orthopnea
2. Respiratory rate to detect hyperventilation
3. Apical-radial pulse to determine pulse deficits
4. Lung sounds to assess for bibasilar crackles

10 After percussing the client's thorax and hearing dullness in the right middle lobe, the nurse would conclude that this assessment finding is consistent with which health problem?

1. Chronic obstructive pulmonary disease (COPD)
2. Pneumothorax
3. Tumor
4. Bronchitis

➤ *See pages 117–119 for Answers and Rationales.*

ANSWERS & RATIONALES

Pretest

1 Answer: 1 Rationale: Hyperresonance on percussion may be caused by chronic obstructive pulmonary disease (COPD) or emphysema (option 1). Scoliosis, a lateral curvature of the spine, may produce respiratory difficulty in individuals but not hyperresonance (option 2). A mass or a consolidation in the lungs of the client may produce adventitious sounds, dullness, and bronchial or bronchovesicular sounds but not hyperresonance (option 3). Pain does not produce hyperresonance (option 4).
Cognitive Level: Application Client Need: Physiological Integrity: Physiological Adaptation Integrated Process: Nursing Process: Analysis Content Area: Adult Health: Respiratory Strategy: Eliminate option 2 as scoliosis does not produce a sound on percussion. Eliminate option 4 as pain does not produce a respiratory sound on percussion. Recall that masses are solid and therefore produce dullness to eliminate option 3. An air fluid area will produce hyperresonance. COPD is a condition characterized by a hyperinflated lung (option 1). Reference: D'Amico, D. & Barbarito, C. (2007). *Health & physical assessment in nursing.* Upper Saddle River, NJ: Pearson Education, Inc., p. 374.

2 Answer: 2 Rationale: Paroxysmal nocturnal dyspnea (PND) is the experience of waking up at night with dyspnea. Placing the client in an upright position will facilitate air exchange. A log of the number and length of awakenings (option 1) will not provide data to improve the client's ability to sleep. Coughing and deep breathing (option 3) may increase the client's dyspnea. The client should slow his or her breathing. For the client experiencing COPD, the nurse should instruct the client to use diaphragmatic or purse lipped breathing. The purpose of the CPAP machine (option 4) is to keep the alveoli open by increasing positive pressure.
Cognitive Level: Application Client Need: Physiological Integrity: Reduction of Risk Potential Integrated Process: Nursing Process: Implementation Content Area: Adult Health: Respiratory Strategy: Recall that a client with respiratory disease should always be positioned upright to assist with breathing, while a client with normal respiratory status may remain supine. Associate the critical words *middle of the night* in the question and the word *nocturnal* in the correct option to help assure you of this selection. Reference: D'Amico, D. & Barbarito, C. (2007). *Health & physical assessment in nursing.* Upper Saddle River, NJ: Pearson Education, Inc., p. 362.

3 Answer: 1 **Rationale:** Fremitus, also called tactile fremitus, is elicited by feeling for vibration while the client is saying "99." Auscultating with a stethoscope while the client is saying "99" (option 2) elicits bronchophony. The anterior and posterior aspects of the chest are palpated for masses, chest expansion, and fremitus, but the costal margins are not palpated (option 3). The anterior and posterior aspects of the chest are percussed to determine resonance, not fremitus (option 4). **Cognitive Level:** Application **Client Need:** Health Promotion and Maintenance **Integrated Process:** Nursing Process: Implementation **Content Area:** Adult Health: Respiratory **Strategy:** Remember that fremitus (also called tactile fremitus) involves palpation, while auscultation involves the use of the stethoscope. This will help to eliminate option 2. Next recall that percussion is a procedure utilizing tapping to produce body sounds to eliminate option 4. Finally, note the words *costal margins* in option 3 as incorrect to eliminate this option. **Reference:** D'Amico, D. & Barbarito, C. (2007). *Health & physical assessment in nursing.* Upper Saddle River, NJ: Pearson Education, Inc., p. 381.

4 Answer: 1 **Rationale:** Tobacco use has been linked to obstructive airway disease (option 1). Information related to immunizations (option 2) will inform the nurse of risk reduction for flu or pneumonia. Asking questions about clinical manifestations (option 3) will provide information about symptoms but not risk. Asking about over-the-counter medications (option 4) will provide information about substances that relieve clinical manifestations. **Cognitive Level:** Analysis **Client Need:** Health Promotion and Maintenance **Integrated Process:** Nursing Process: Assessment **Content Area:** Adult Health: Respiratory **Strategy:** Read the question to determine critical words such as *most important question* and *risk*. This tells you that more than one option may be plausible but that one of them is better than the others. To choose correctly, recall that the most significant risk factor for chronic lung disease is smoking. **Reference:** D'Amico, D. & Barbarito, C. (2007). *Health & physical assessment in nursing.* Upper Saddle River, NJ: Pearson Education, Inc., pp. 364–366.

5 Answer: 4 **Rationale:** Fluid-filled space produces crackling, bubbling sounds, which are known as crackles (option 4). In the lung fields, fluid always pools to the center of gravity. Wheezing is produced by constriction in the airway. Rhonchi are sonorous sounds that may clear with coughing (option 1). Wheezes are high pitched adventitious musical sounds usually found in the upper airways (options 2 and 3). **Cognitive Level:** Application **Client Need:** Health Promotion and Maintenance **Integrated Process:** Communication and Documentation **Content Area:** Adult Health: Respiratory **Strategy:** Applying principles of gravity, fluid always pools toward the bases when the client is sitting upright. Recall that crackles are sounds produced when fluid has accumulated. **Reference:** D'Amico, D. & Barbarito, C. (2007). *Health & physical assessment in nursing.* Upper Saddle River, NJ: Pearson Education, Inc., p. 378.

6 Answer: 4 **Rationale:** The client is experiencing orthopnea. A more upright position using pillows should decrease the feeling of not being able to breathe (option 4). The nurse should never offer a client false reassurance (option 1). Asthma produces wheezing and a feeling of inability to get air into the lungs (option 2). The lateral Sim's position will increase the effort it takes to breathe (option 3). **Cognitive Level:** Application **Client Need:** Physiological Integrity: Basic Care and Comfort **Integrated Process:** Nursing Process: Implementation **Content Area:** Adult Health: Respiratory **Strategy:** Recall that an upright position eases the effort of breathing in a client experiencing respiratory difficulty. Another strategy to eliminate option 1 is to remember that false reassurance is a block to communication. **Reference:** D'Amico, D. & Barbarito, C. (2007). *Health & physical assessment in nursing.* Upper Saddle River, NJ: Pearson Education, Inc., p. 362.

7 Answer: 3 **Rationale:** When part of the lung is collapsed or obstructed the client experiences unequal chest excursion (option 3). Unequal chest excursion may also result from guarding to prevent pain. Physical stature (option 1) has no bearing on excursion. Chronic obstructive pulmonary disease would not cause unequal chest excursion, but it could lead to hyperinflation if the client has emphysema (option 2). Diaphragmatic breathing (option 4) is used in clients who have obstructed airway disease to increase air exchange. **Cognitive Level:** Application **Client Need:** Health Promotion and Maintenance **Integrated Process:** Nursing Process: Assessment **Content Area:** Adult Health: Respiratory **Strategy:** Recall that respiratory effort should be even and effortless. Then recall that, when assessing a client, there should always be symmetry. Associate the words *part of the lung* in option 3 with the words *unequal chest excursion* in the question because they both imply a localized or one-sided problem rather than a general one. **Reference:** D'Amico, D. & Barbarito, C. (2007). *Health and physical assessment in nursing.* Upper Saddle River, NJ: Pearson Education, Inc., p. 373.

8 Answer: 3, 5 **Rationale:** The client with a history of COPD will have a barrel chest appearance in which the anteroposterior diameter to transverse diameter is 1:1 instead of 1:2 (option 5). The nurse should expect decreased excursion (option 3) that is symmetrical (eliminating option 2). The client will not have crackles (option 4) but will demonstrate wheezing. Because of the increased diameter and decreased air velocity the client will have decreased fremitus (option 1). **Cognitive Level:** Application **Client Need:** Physiological Integrity: Physiological Adaptation **Integrated Process:** Communication and Documentation **Content Area:** Adult Health: Respiratory **Strategy:** Recall that gas exchange is impaired with COPD to help choose option 3. Next recall that COPD causes increased alveoli size, causing air accumulation in the alveoli and increased AP diameter of the chest. This will help you to select option 5. **Reference**: D'Amico, D. & Barbarito, C. (2007). *Health & physical assessment in nursing*. Upper Saddle River, NJ: Pearson Education, Inc., p. 373.

9 **Answer: 1** **Rationale**: The chest tube drainage system must be set up as the client is experiencing a medical emergency caused by pneumothorax (option 1). The pneumothorax is causing the decreased breath sounds on the affected side and the tracheal deviation to the opposite side. The client is having difficulty breathing but does not have a constricted airway so a bronchodilator (option 2) will not assist this client. A tracheostomy (option 3) will not remedy the airway problem this client is experiencing unless the client requires an airway and an endotracheal tube cannot be placed. The client will need high dose oxygen, not low flow (option 4) via a non-rebreather mask.
Cognitive Level: Analysis **Client Need**: Physiological Integrity: Physiological Adaptation **Integrated Process**: Nursing Process: Implementation **Content Area**: Adult Health: Respiratory **Strategy**: To answer this question correctly, you must first draw the correct conclusion about the significance of the client's symptoms. Recall that pneumothorax produces tracheal deviation to the opposite side of the damaged lung, absent or decreased breath sounds, decreased fremitus and asymmetrical chest movement. Then you can recall that this is a medical emergency requiring treatment by chest tube insertion. **Reference**: D'Amico, D. & Barbarito, C. (2007). *Health & physical assessment in nursing*. Upper Saddle River, NJ: Pearson Education, Inc., p. 378.

10 **Answer: 4, 3, 2, 1, 5** **Rationale**: The correct procedure for performing a respiratory assessment would be to explain the procedure to the client (option 4), provide for client privacy, interview the client, wash hands, position the client (option 3), inspect the client's anterior thorax, palpate the anterior thorax (option 2), percuss the anterior thorax (option 1), then auscultate the anterior thorax (option 5). The final step of the procedure is to discuss the findings with the client. Note that a posterior chest assessment is also done on the client but is not reflected in this question.
Cognitive Level: Analysis **Client Need**: Health Promotion and Maintenance **Integrated Process**: Nursing Process: Implementation **Content Area**: Adult Health: Respiratory **Strategy**: Begin by recalling that the first step of any procedure is to explain it to the client. Next determine that the client needs to be properly positioned to do the exam. Finally, recall that the correct sequence for respiratory assessment is inspection, percussion, palpation, and auscultation. **Reference**: D'Amico, D. & Barbarito, C. (2007). *Health & physical assessment in nursing*. Upper Saddle River, NJ: Pearson Education, Inc., pp. 361–384.

Posttest

1 **Answer: 1** **Rationale**: The client with a curvature of the spine may experience difficulty breathing and exchanging gases due to decreased lung volume (option 1). This would be the priority using airway, breathing, and circulation (ABCs) as a guide. The client may experience pain (option 2), difficulty with body image (option 3), or difficulty with social relationships (option 4), but these diagnoses are not the highest priority. Airway is always a priority.
Cognitive Level: Analysis **Client Need**: Physiological Integrity: Physiological Adaptation **Integrated Process**: Nursing Process: Analysis **Content Area**: Adult Health: Respiratory **Strategy**: Remember the ABCs (airway, breathing, circulation) to recall that airway is always the priority. **Reference**: D'Amico, D. & Barbarito, C. (2007). *Health & physical assessment in nursing*. Upper Saddle River, NJ: Pearson Education, Inc., pp. 386–387.

2 **Answer: 2** **Rationale**: Based on these clinical manifestations the nurse would prepare the client for testing to confirm a medical diagnosis of pleural effusion. The client with pleural effusion will have dyspnea, decreased fremitus, dullness over the fluid filled lung, decreased breath sounds on the affected sound, a pleural friction rub, and in severe cases a tracheal shift to the unaffected side (option 2). Pneumothorax results in tachypnea, tracheal shift to the unaffected side, decreased excursion on the affected side, decreased fremitus, hyperresonance, and decreased breath sounds (option 1). Congestive heart failure leads to tachypnea, dyspnea, shortness of breath, peripheral edema, cool clammy skin, wheezing, and crackles at the bases (option 3). Pneumonia produces tachypnea, productive cough, chills, dullness over the affected side, bronchophony, egophony, whispered pectoriloquy, and bronchial breath sounds (option 4).
Cognitive Level: Application **Client Need**: Physiological Integrity: Reduction of Risk Potential **Integrated Process**: Nursing Process: Planning **Content Area**: Adult Health: Respiratory **Strategy**: Understanding pathophysiology, clinical manifestations, and care priorities will guide the plan of care strategies. **Reference**: D'Amico, D. & Barbarito, C. (2007). *Health & physical assessment in nursing*. Upper Saddle River, NJ: Pearson Education, Inc., pp. 390–391.

3 **Answer: 4** **Rationale**: The client experiencing Biot's breathing will have shallow breathing with periods of apnea (option 4). Bradypnea is slow respirations of less than 10 breaths per minute (option 1). The client who is experiencing Cheyne-Stokes will have deep breathing with periods of apnea (option 2). Hyperventilation is rapid deep respirations of greater than 24 breaths per minute (option 3).
Cognitive Level: Application **Client Need**: Health Promotion and Maintenance **Integrated Process**: Nursing Process: Implementation **Content Area**: Adult Health: Respiratory

Strategy: Recall the characteristics of the respiratory patterns in the options and recall also that it is essential to accurately report and document the client's clinical manifestations, such as tachypnea, bradypnea, hyperventilation, hypoventilation, Cheyne-Stokes, and Biot's respirations. **Reference:** D'Amico, D. & Barbarito, C. (2007). *Health & physical assessment in nursing.* Upper Saddle River, NJ: Pearson Education, Inc., p. 385.

4 **Answer: 3** **Rationale:** The client with a lung infection will have a greenish yellow productive cough (option 3). Tuberculosis will produce a cough with rust colored sputum (option 1). Hemoptysis is the term given to blood tinged sputum (option 2). Pleural effusion does not cause a productive cough (option 4). **Cognitive Level:** Analysis **Client Need:** Physiological Integrity: Reduction of Risk Potential **Integrated Process:** Nursing Process: Evaluation **Content Area:** Adult Health: Respiratory **Strategy:** Eliminate option 4, pleural effusion, as it does not cause sputum production. To choose the correct answer, recall the following: tuberculosis causes rust-colored sputum, hemoptysis is bloody color to the sputum, and infection usually produces greenish-yellow drainage regardless of the location of the infection. **Reference:** D'Amico, D. & Barbarito, C. (2007). *Health & physical assessment in nursing.* Upper Saddle River, NJ: Pearson Education, Inc., p. 364.

5 **Answer: 2** **Rationale:** As a person ages there is a loss of elasticity in the lung that makes it more difficult to take deep breaths (option 1), as well as a loss of vital capacity. As long as the older adult client stays active there should be little deconditioning (option 2). A respiratory infection causes fever, malaise, greenish-yellow productive cough (option 3). Environmental exposure usually causes constrictive symptoms such as wheezing (option 4). **Cognitive Level:** Analysis **Client Need:** Health Promotion and Maintenance **Integrated Process:** Nursing Process: Evaluation **Content Area:** Adult Health: Respiratory **Strategy:** Recognize that the only option that is not a condition causing a physical problem is option 2. Eliminate the options not associated with the changes of aging. **Reference:** D'Amico, D. & Barbarito, C. (2007). *Health & physical assessment in nursing.* Upper Saddle River, NJ: Pearson Education, Inc., p. 367.

6 **Answer: 3** **Rationale:** Second-hand smoke has been linked to respiratory distress and lung cancer (option 3). There is no need to avoid people who are consuming foods to which the client has an allergy. The client will have an allergic reaction only when consuming the food (option 1). Allergy testing is often performed so the client can avoid exposure (option 2). Exercise will not exacerbate allergies (option 4). **Cognitive Level:** Application **Client Need:** Physiological Integrity: Reduction of Risk Potential **Integrated Process:** Nursing Process: Implementation **Content Area:** Adult Health: Respiratory **Strategy:** Recall that continued exposure to allergens may produce anaphylaxis. Smoking

is contraindicated in all circumstances; exercise is usually encouraged. There are very few conditions in which exercise is contraindicated, for example, congenital heart disease. **Reference:** D'Amico, D. & Barbarito, C. (2007). *Health & physical assessment in nursing.* Upper Saddle River, NJ: Pearson Education, Inc., pp. 360–361.

7 **Answer: 3** **Rationale:** A middle-aged adult would have a respiratory rate of 12 to 20 breaths per minute (option 3). An infant would have a more rapid respiratory rate, such as 30 to 40 breaths/minute (option 1). A pregnant female may experience tachypnea and dyspnea due to pressure on the diaphragm (option 2). An older adult client may have tachypnea due to loss of elasticity of the lungs or with lung disease (option 4). **Cognitive Level:** Application **Client Need:** Physiological Integrity: Reduction of Risk Potential **Integrated Process:** Nursing Process: Evaluation **Content Area:** Adult Health: Respiratory **Strategy:** Recall that adults have a respiratory rate of 12 to 20 breaths per minute. Infants have a respiratory rate of about 35 breaths per minute. Due to changes associated with aging and pregnancy these clients may have tachypnea. **Reference:** D'Amico, D. & Barbarito, C. (2007). *Health & physical assessment in nursing.* Upper Saddle River, NJ: Pearson Education, Inc., pp. 360–361.

8 **Answer: 2, 3, 4, 5** **Rationale:** Determining the length of time the client has had the cough is essential to determining its relationship to disease. A description of the cough and mucus production is imperative for the differentiation of disease process. It is important to have information about pain, as a painful cough may indicate underlying lung disease such as lung cancer (options 2, 3, 4, and 5). The nurse would not need to inquire about how long the client believes he or she can tolerate the cough (option 1). **Cognitive Level:** Application **Client Need:** Health Promotion and Maintenance **Integrated Process:** Nursing Process: Assessment **Content Area:** Adult Health: Respiratory **Strategy:** Understanding symptoms will assist in developing a plan of care for the client. Remember that in a client with a cough it is necessary to have information about the cough type, mucus production, pain associated with cough, time of day associated with the cough, and treatments that have provided relief. **Reference:** D'Amico, D. & Barbarito, C. (2007). *Health & physical assessment in nursing.* Upper Saddle River, NJ: Pearson Education, Inc., p. 364.

9 **Answer: 2** **Rationale:** During assessment of the client's lungs, it is essential to evaluate the client's respiratory rate to detect hyperventilation, which could worsen the client's dizziness and increase the risk for falls (option 2). The client may be positioned upright (with orthopnea), on the side, or supine for the assessment depending on comfort level, but the presence of orthopnea is not directly related to risk for falls (option 1). Assessment of apical-radial pulse (option 3) is not a respiratory assessment. Assessment of lung sounds for bibasilar crackles (option 4) is an important assessment but again, this finding does not necessarily contribute to the risk for falls.

Cognitive Level: Application **Client Need:** Safe Effective Care: Safety and Infection Control **Integrated Process:** Nursing Process: Assessment **Content Area:** Adult Health: Respiratory **Strategy:** Note the word *most important* in the question, which tells you that more than one option may be partially or totally correct but that one option is better than all the others. Focus on the critical concept (risk for falls) to select respiratory assessment data that would increase this risk. Eliminate option 3 first because it is a cardiovascular assessment item. Next eliminate option 1 because position of comfort needed with orthopnea is not directly related to risk for falls. While bibasilar crackles (option 4) could lead to decreased oxygenation, this is not a high risk because they are mild (bibasilar). Finally, to help choose option 2 recall that hyperventilation easily leads to dizziness, which can lead to falls. **Reference:** D'Amico, D. & Barbarito, C. (2007). *Health & physical assessment in nursing.* Upper Saddle River, NJ: Pearson Education, Inc., p. 376.

10 Answer: 3 Rationale: In the client with a tumor, dullness would be heard during percussion as it is a solid area (option 1). During percussion in a client experiencing pneumothorax the nurse would elicit hyperresonance (option 2). During percussion for a client experiencing COPD, the nurse would elicit hyperresonance (option 1). Resonance would be elicited during percussion in the client experiencing bronchitis (option 4). **Cognitive Level:** Application **Client Need:** Physiological Integrity: Reduction of Risk Potential **Integrated Process:** Nursing Process: Assessment **Content Area:** Adult Health: Respiratory **Strategy:** Recall that the sound heard during percussion of solid tissue is dullness. Evaluate each option and systematically eliminate each of the incorrect options, since only option 3 represents a health problem that involves solid tissue. **Reference:** D'Amico, D. & Barbarito, C. (2007). *Health & physical assessment in nursing.* Upper Saddle River, NJ: Pearson Education, Inc., pp. 390–391.

References

Bickley, L. (2010). *Bates guide to physical examination and history taking* (10th ed.). Philadelphia: Lippincott Williams & Wilkins.

Bradley, R. (2007). Improving respiratory assessment skills. *Journal for Nurse Practitioners, 3*(4), 276–277.

D'Amico, D. & Barbarito, C. (2007). *Health and physical assessment in nursing.* Upper Saddle River, NJ: Pearson Education, Inc., pp. 348–396.

Jarvis, C. (2008). *Physical examination and health assessment* (5th ed.). St. Louis, MO: Elsevier Saunders.

Moore, T. (2007). Respiratory assessment in adults. *Nursing Standard, 21*(49), 48–56, 58, 60.

Zator Estes, M. (2009). *Health assessment and physical examination* (4th ed.). Clifton Park, NY: Delmar Cengage Learning.

ANSWERS & RATIONALES

7 Gastrointestinal Assessment

Chapter Outline

Health History
Present Health History
Family History

Equipment, Preparation, and
  Positioning
Examination Techniques
Expected Findings

Unexpected Findings
Lifespan Considerations
Documentation

NCLEX-RN® Test Prep

Visit the Companion Website for this book
at www.pearsonhighered.com/hogan to
access additional practice opportunities
and more.

Objectives

➤ Review the anatomy and physiology of the gastrointestinal system.
➤ Conduct a gastrointestinal health history.
➤ Prepare the client for a gastrointestinal assessment.
➤ Utilize the techniques of gastrointestinal assessment.
➤ Describe expected and unexpected findings associated with the
  gastrointestinal system.

Review at a Glance

abdomen a cavity in the body containing the following organs: liver, gallbladder, stomach, spleen, large and small intestines, kidneys, bladder, and reproductive organs

ascites a collection of fluid in the abdominal or peritoneal cavity

borborygmi the presence of increased high-pitched bowel sounds associated with gas or air in the intestines

bruit a vascular blowing sound heard by auscultation with a stethoscope, which is produced when there is an occlusion or stenosis in a blood vessel

dysphagia difficulty in swallowing

gastroenteritis an infection of the gastrointestinal tract causing diarrhea and abdominal discomfort

peritonitis inflammation of the peritoneum

PRETEST

1 When assessing the abdomen, the nurse performs the following examination techniques. In which sequence should the nurse complete the assessment? Place the answers in the correct order using numeric responses.

1. Auscultation
2. Palpation
3. Inspection
4. Percussion

2 When obtaining information about appetite from a client who reports not feeling hungry in the last few weeks, the nurse should ask the client which questions? Select all that apply.

1. "Has your weight changed?"
2. "Can you complete a dietary recall?"
3. "Have you had any changes in your elimination patterns?"
4. "When did you notice your appetite change?"
5. "Are you experiencing any additional symptoms associated with the weight change?"

3 To assess whether a client is having symptoms of abdominal problems, the nurse would ask him or her about which of the following? Select all that apply.

1. Nausea
2. Indigestion
3. Vomiting
4. Fever
5. Dietary intake

4 During an abdominal assessment, an older adult female tells the nurse that she does not regularly include fruits or vegetables in her diet. The nurse should develop a plan of care based upon which of the following nursing diagnoses?

1. Risk for constipation
2. Risk for diarrhea
3. Weight loss related to poor nutrition
4. Risk for chronic pain related to poor nutrition

5 When assessing the client's abdomen the nurse should position the client in which of the following positions?

1. Supine with a pillow under the head
2. Supine with a pillow under the knees and head
3. Sitting with the head upright at a 90-degree angle
4. Standing with feet slightly apart

6 The nurse inspects the client's abdomen and observes a concave shape. The nurse should document this finding using which of the following descriptions?

1. Flat
2. Rounded
3. Scaphoid
4. Protuberant

7 During assessment of the abdomen, the nurse would perform which maneuver to palpate the spleen?

1. Lift the client with the right hand under the rib cage and palpate the right upper quadrant with the left hand
2. Lift the client with the left hand under the rib cage and palpate the left upper quadrant with the right hand
3. Palpate for pulsations by placing a hand below the xiphoid process
4. Palpate for rebound tenderness by pressing into the abdomen with steady pressure while asking if the client is experiencing pain

8 When percussing the liver the nurse would expect to document which of the following findings?

1. Resonance
2. Tympany
3. Dullness
4. Hyperresonance

9 During inspection of the abdomen the nurse notes silvery, shiny stretch marks. The nurse would document this finding as which of the following?

1. Shadows
2. Scars
3. Ascites
4. Striae

10 The nurse finds ascites during assessment of the abdomen. The nurse would conclude that this is most likely associated with which of the following health problems?

1. Overhydration
2. Cirrhosis
3. A mass
4. Trauma

➤ *See pages 137–139 for Answers and Rationales.*

I. HEALTH HISTORY

A. Ask the client to describe his or her appetite; changes in appetite can result from many physical or psychological problems; weight changes may result from either physical or emotional problems; analyze data to determine if weight change is the result of consumption or activity changes; sample questions include the following:
1. "Has your appetite changed? In the last day? In the last month? In the last year?"
2. "What is causing the change in your appetite?"
3. "How are you dealing with the change in appetite?"
4. "Are you experiencing any other symptoms?"
5. "Are you experiencing difficulty swallowing (**dysphagia**)?"

B. Assess weight changes by asking the questions to gather data about food consumption
1. "What is your current weight? Does this represent a change from your usual weight?"
   a. "Over what period of time did the weight change occur?"
   b. "What do you think is causing the weight change?"
2. "Are you experiencing any other symptoms?"
3. "What have you eaten in the last 24 hours?"
4. "How much of each food group are you eating?"
5. "Is this the way you normally eat?"

C. Assess client's bowel habits
1. "Please describe your bowel pattern and the characteristics of your stool."
2. "Have any changes occurred in your stool? If so, what are the changes?"
3. "When did you first notice the change in your bowel habits?"
4. "Do you know what caused the change?"
5. "Have you done anything about the change in your bowel patterns? If so, what?"
6. "Are you using any over-the-counter laxatives or antidiarrheal agents?"

D. If necessary, evaluate whether client is experiencing bloating or increased gas; if so, ask these follow-up questions:
1. "How long have you been experiencing bloating or gas problems?"
2. "Have you changed your diet in a way that may increase gas?"
3. "Have you started taking any medication which may have contributed to bloating or gas?"
4. "Do you use antacids? If so, what do you use and how often? Is this product effective?"
5. "What else, if anything, do you do to reduce the symptoms? Was this effective?"
6. "How much water do you drink per day?"
7. "How much do you exercise?"

E. Evaluate whether the client has any family members with abdominal problems; if so ask these follow-up questions:
1. "What type of abdominal problem does your family member have?"
2. "What family member has the problem?"
3. "How long has your family member had the problem?"
4. "What treatment was prescribed for the problem? How effective was the treatment?"

F. Ask specific questions about disease or infection
1. "Have you ever been diagnosed with a disease affecting the abdomen?"; if so, ask these follow-up questions:
   a. "When were you diagnosed with the problem?"
   b. "What treatment was prescribed for the problem?"

Practice to Pass

A male client who visits the healthcare provider for a physical examination reports to the nurse a 10 pound weight loss over the last month. What type of follow-up questions should the nurse plan to ask?

    c. "Do you do anything else to help manage the problem? If so, what do you do and how effective is it?"

  2. "Have you ever had an abdominal infection?"; if so, ask these follow-up questions:

    a. "What treatment was prescribed?"

    b. "Was the treatment successful?"

    c. "Does the problem reoccur?"; if so ask how often and how it is managed

G. Ask questions about abdominal symptoms

  1. "Do you have any difficulty chewing or swallowing? If so, please describe."

  2. "Do you have dentures or crowns?"

  3. "Do your gums bleed?"

  4. "Do you have indigestion?"; if so, ask these follow-up questions:

    a. "Please describe the frequency and duration of the indigestion."

    b. "What treatments have you used and have they worked?"

    c. "Have you sought treatment for indigestion prior to this visit? If so, what treatment was prescribed and for how long did it work?"

  5. "Do you have nausea or vomiting?"; if so, ask these follow-up questions:

    a. "How long has it been since you started experiencing nausea?"

    b. "How often do you become nauseated? How long does it last?"

    c. "Do you know what is causing the nausea?"

    d. "Can you describe the nausea?"

    e. "Does the nausea occur at different times during the day?"

    f. "Does burning, indigestion, or bloating accompany the nausea?"

    g. "Does vomiting accompany the nausea?"

    h. "Describe the characteristics of the vomitus."

    i. "How much do you vomit?"

    j. "How often does vomiting occur after you experience nausea?"

    k. "Do you have pain with the nausea or vomiting? If so, where is it and what are the characteristics of the pain?"

    l. "Have you sought treatment for the nausea? If so, what was prescribed? Was the treatment successful?"

    m. "If you did not seek treatment, have you used over-the-counter medications for the nausea? If so, what do you use and how often do you use it? Was it effective?"

  6. "Do you experience diarrhea or constipation? If so, please describe."

    a. "Do you know what is causing the diarrhea or constipation? If so, what?"

    b. "What treatment have you sought for the diarrhea or constipation? Is the treatment helping?"

  7. "Are you experiencing rectal itching? If so, please describe."

  8. "Are you experiencing rectal bleeding? If so, please describe."

  9. "What treatment, if any, has been previously prescribed for the rectal itching or bleeding? Was it effective, and if so, how long did it work?"

  10. "Are you having abdominal pain?"; see Table 7-1 for patterns of pain with specific gastrointestinal disorders; if pain is present, ask these follow-up questions:

    a. "Describe the location and characteristics of the pain."

    b. "Does the pain radiate? If so, where?"

    c. "How often do you have pain?"

    d. "What do you believe is causing the pain?

    e. "Does anything relieve the pain? If so, what?"

    f. "Does anything worsen the pain? If so, what?"

H. Ask questions to gather data about problems facing infants or children

  1. Infants

    a. "Is the infant breast or bottle fed?"

    b. "How is the infant tolerating the feeding?"

    c. "How frequently does the infant eat?"

Table 7-1	Pain in Common Abdominal Disorders		
Disorder	**Definition**	**Pain Characteristics**	**Precipitating Factors**
Appendicitis	Acute inflammation of vermiform appendix	Epigastric and periumbilical Localizes to RLQ Sudden onset	Obstruction (fecal stone, adhesions)
Cholecystitis	Acute or chronic inflammation of wall of gallbladder	RUQ, radiates to right scapula Sudden onset	Fatty meals, obstruction of duct in cholelithiasis
Diverticulitis	Inflammation of diverticula (outpouches of mucosa through intestinal wall)	Cramping LLQ Radiates to back	Ingestion of fiber-rich diet, stress
Duodenal Ulcer	Breaks in mucosa of duodenum	Aching, gnawing, epigastric	Stress, use of NSAIDs
Ectopic Pregnancy	Implantation of blastocyte outside of the uterus, generally in the fallopian tube	Fullness in the rectal area Abdominal cramping, unilateral pain	Tubal damage, pelvic infection, hormonal disorders, lifting, bowel movements
Gastritis	Inflammation of mucosal lining of the stomach (acute and chronic)	Epigastric pain	Acute: NSAIDs, alcohol abuse, stress, infection Chronic: *H. pylori* Autoimmune responses
Gastroesophageal Reflux Disorder (GERD)	Backflow of gastric acid to the esophagus	Heartburn, chest pain	Food intake, lying down after meals
Intestinal Obstruction	Blockage of normal movement of bowel contents	Small intestine: aching; large intestine: spasmodic pain Neurogenic: diffuse abdominal discomfort Mechanical: colicky pain associated with distention	Mechanical: physical block from impaction, hernia, volvulus Neurogenic: manipulation of bowel during surgery, peritoneal irritation
Irritable Bowel Syndrome (Spastic Colon)	Problems with GI motility	LLQ accompanied by diarrhea and/or constipation Pain increases after eating and decreases after bowel movement	Stress, intolerated foods, caffeine, lactose intolerance, alcohol, familial linkage
Pancreatitis	Inflammation of the pancreas	Upper abdominal, knifelike, deep epigastric or umbilical area pain	Ductal obstruction, alcohol abuse, use of acetaminophen, infection

Source: D'Amico, D. & Barbarito, C. (2007). *Health & physical assessment in nursing.* Upper Saddle River, NJ: Pearson Education, Inc., p. 543, Table 19.2.

    d. "Have you introduced any new foods in the diet of the infant? If so, what and how was it tolerated?"

    e. "Is the infant colicky? If so, what do you do to relieve the colic?"

    f. "How much water do you give the infant?"

2. Children

    a. "Does the child eat at regular times?"

    b. "What types of foods does the child eat in a typical day?"

    c. "How much does the child eat?"

    d. "Is the child able to feed himself?"

    e. "How often does the child snack? What types of snacks does the child eat?"

    f. "How much water does the child drink?"

    g. "Is the child toilet trained?"

    h. "Does the child bring lunch to school or purchase it at school?"

3. "Does the family eat at least one meal together per day?"

    4. "What kind of food does the family eat?"

    5. "Describe the atmosphere at this meal, such as relaxed, hurried, etc."

I. **Ask questions for the assessment of the older adult**

    1. "Are you incontinent of stool?" (if so, ask client to describe how often and whether treatment has been previously sought)

    2. "Do you have constipation or diarrhea? If so, please describe."

        a. "How often do you have the problem?"

        b. "Do you use over-the-counter remedies? If so, what products do you use and how often do you use them?"

        c. "Are the over-the-counter remedies effective?"

    3. "How many foods containing fiber do you eat per day?"

    4. "Are you able to shop for your own groceries? If not, how to you obtain groceries?"

    5. "Do you have sufficient financial resources to obtain groceries?"

    6. "Do you share your meals with anyone?"

II. PRESENT HEALTH HISTORY

A. **Have the client describe his or her current health status by asking the following questions:**

    1. "How would you describe your current health status?"

    2. "Describe the current health of your digestive tract."

    3. "Are you experiencing any chronic health problems? If yes, please describe."

B. **Have the client describe lifestyle habits contributing to health status by asking the following questions:**

    1. "Are you currently taking any medication? If so, what?"

    2. "Are you taking any over-the-counter medications? If so, what and how often?"

    3. "Do you drink alcohol? If so, what do you drink? How much do you drink and how often? When did you last drink alcohol?"

    4. "Do you smoke? If so, what? How much?"

    5. "Please describe your dietary habits; can you complete a dietary recall?"

C. **Determine current abdominal and gastrointestinal symptoms by asking the following questions:**

    1. "Describe your bowel habits. When was your last bowel movement? Please describe the characteristics of the stool."

    2. "Describe any pain and describe the location and characteristics; what precipitates the pain? What relieves the pain?"

    3. "Please describe any nausea and vomiting; how often does it happen? Describe the characteristics of the vomiting."

    4. "Please describe any indigestion; how often does it happen? When do you experience the indigestion? What precipitates or relieves the indigestion?"

III. FAMILY HISTORY

A. **Family history provides information on any predisposing factors for gastrointestinal or abdominal problems**

B. **Determine significant family history by asking questions such as the following:**

    1. "Is there a family history of gastrointestinal discomfort? If so, please describe."

    2. "Is there a family history of gastric or colon cancer? If so which of your relatives has had gastric or colon cancer?"

    3. "Is there a family history of inflammatory bowel disease? If so, which of your relatives? Is it Crohn's disease or ulcerative colitis?"

IV. EQUIPMENT, PREPARATION, AND POSITIONING

A. **To perform gastrointestinal assessment, gather the following equipment:**

    1. Gown (as client will need to undress)

2. Drape or blanket to cover client
3. Examination gloves
4. Light
5. Stethoscope
6. Skin marker
7. Metric ruler
8. Tissues
9. Tape measure

B. Preparation and positioning

1. Be sure client understands what is going to occur during examination; explain all steps of the procedure and fully answer any client questions

2. Be sure environment is warm and well lit; this will provide optimal comfort for client and visibility for examiner to assess **abdomen** (cavity in the body containing digestive, urinary, and reproductive organs) for color differences, lesions, and movement

3. Locate and confirm that all equipment near examination table is within easy reach of examiner

4. Position client supine with a small pillow under his or her head and knees for comfort and to relax abdominal muscles

5. Place a drape over client's symphysis pubis and legs to preserve his or her dignity (see Figure 7-1)

6. Stand at client's right side, as the liver is on the right side

7. If client is experiencing abdominal pain, the area of pain should be examined last

V. EXAMINATION TECHNIQUES

A. Inspection

1. Inform client of the procedure

2. Encourage client to breathe normally

3. Visually divide abdomen into four quadrants or nine regions (see Figures 7-2 and 7-3)

4. Inspect the abdomen for contour between costal margin and symphysis pubis (see Figure 7-4)

   a. Flat: a straight horizontal plane between costal margin and symphysis pubis

   b. Rounded: abdomen is curved outward between costal margin and symphysis pubis

   c. Scaphoid: abdomen is concave between costal margin and symphysis pubis

   d. Protuberant: abdomen is larger and rounded

5. Inspect and determine position of umbilicus

   a. Centrally located

   b. Inverted

   c. Protruding

Practice to Pass

The clinic nurse needs to complete an abdominal assessment on a client. What equipment does the nurse need to have at hand, and how should the nurse prepare the client?

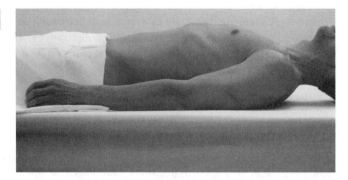

Figure 7-1

Client positioning and draping for abdominal examination

Figure 7-2

Quadrants of the abdomen

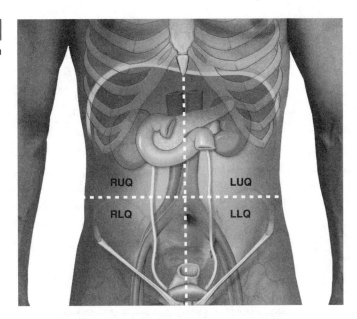

RUQ   **LUQ**

RLQ   **LLQ**

Practice to Pass

The nurse begins to examine a client's abdomen. What should the nurse include when beginning the examination with a visual inspection of the abdomen?

6. Determine skin color

7. Determine texture of skin

8. Inspect abdomen for location and characteristics of lesions, scars, and abdominal markings

9. Inspect for symmetry, bulging, or masses

10. Inspect for pulsations and peristalsis

B. Auscultation

1. Perform auscultation prior to palpation or percussion as they increase peristaltic activity

2. Instruct client about the procedure for assessment of abdomen; ask client to remain still and supine and to breathe normally; tell client that there should be no discomfort

3. Use diaphragm of a stethoscope to auscultate bowel sounds beginning in right lower quadrant and proceeding through quadrants; auscultate each quadrant for at least 60 seconds

4. Use bell of stethoscope to auscultate abdominal vascular sounds

Figure 7-3

Nine regions of the abdomen

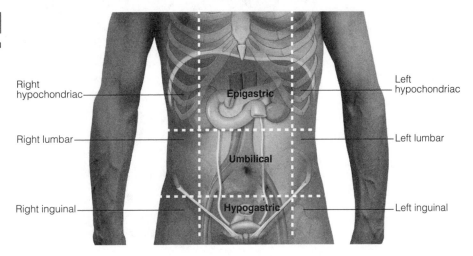

Right hypochondriac

Epigastric

Left hypochondriac

Right lumbar

Left lumbar

Umbilical

Right inguinal

Hypogastric

Left inguinal

Flat. A straight horizontal line is observed from the costal margin to the symphysis pubis.
This contour is common in a thin person.

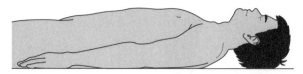

Rounded. Sometimes called a convex abdomen. The horizontal line now curves outward, indicating an increase in abdominal fat or a decrease in muscle tone. This contour is considered a normal variation in the toddler and the pregnant female.

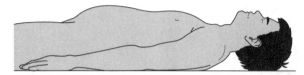

Protuberant. Similar to the rounded abdomen, only greater. This contour is anticipated in pregnancy. It is also seen in the adult with obesity, ascites, and other conditions.

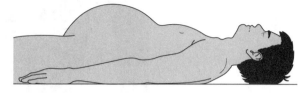

Scaphoid. Sometimes called a concave abdomen.
The horizontal line now curves inward toward the vertebral column, giving the abdomen a sunken appearance. In the adult, this contour is seen in the very thin person.

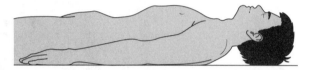

Figure 7-4

Variations in contour of the abdomen

5. Auscultate vascular sounds by first beginning midline below xiphoid process at the aorta and proceeding from side to side over renal, iliac, and femoral areas; auscultate friction rubs by beginning in right lower quadrant and proceeding through quadrants (see Figure 7-5)

6. Auscultate for friction rubs over liver and spleen; friction rubs may produce coarse or grating sounds

C. Percussion

1. Inform client that percussion involves tapping on his or her abdomen by placing the pleximeter, or pointer finger, of nurse's non-dominant hand on abdomen and using a second finger of dominant hand to tap on pleximeter finger to elicit sound

Figure 7-5

Abdominal areas to auscultate for vascular sounds

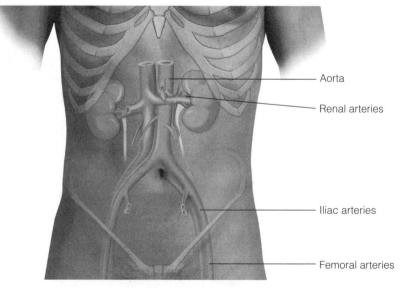

Aorta

Renal arteries

Iliac arteries

Femoral arteries

Figure 7-6

Pattern for percussing
the abdomen

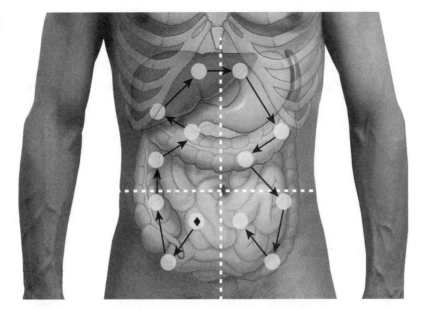

Practice to Pass

The client who reports
abdominal pain needs
to have an abdominal
assessment com-
pleted by the nurse.
After inspecting the
abdomen, what should
the nurse do next?

2. Begin percussion in right lower quadrant and percuss upward to right upper quadrant, left upper quadrant, and finally left lower quadrant (see Figure 7-6)
3. Percuss the liver
   a. Begin percussion at umbilicus in right mid-clavicular line (MCL); percuss upward
      in right MCL toward rib cage; the first percussion sounds heard should be tym-
      pany (see Figure 7-7)

Figure 7-7

Pattern for percussing
the liver

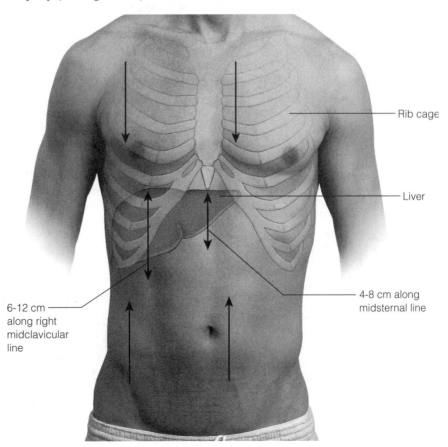

Rib cage

Liver

4-8 cm along
midsternal line

6-12 cm
along right
midclavicular
line

      b. Mark the area, indicating where percussion note changes to dullness; this is the lower border of liver

      c. Next percuss downward in right MCL from the 4th intercostal space; resonance should be heard over lung tissue

      d. Continue percussing until dullness is noted, indicating upper border of liver; mark that spot

      e. Measure distance between these two points, called the liver span

    4. Determine movement of liver during respiration by asking client to take a deep breath and hold it; then percuss upward along midclavicular line; the lower liver border should descend about one inch (see Figure 7-7)

    5. Percuss for dullness over spleen on left side of abdomen posterior to midaxillary line between 6th and 10th intercostal spaces (see Figure 7-8)

    6. Percuss gastric bubble (tympany) between left costal margin and midsternal line below xiphoid process

D. Palpation

    1. Perform palpation to determine organ size and location, muscle rigidity and tenderness, as well as the presence of fluid

    2. Lightly palpate abdomen over four quadrants using dominant hand (see Figure 7-9)

    3. Deeply palpate abdomen by pressing in about two inches

    4. If client is obese use a bimanual technique by placing one hand over other (see Figure 7-10)

    5. Determine size of organs, masses, and any areas of tenderness

    6. Palpate liver by standing on right side of client; place left hand under 11th and 12th ribs; lift rib cage and place right hand into abdomen using an upward and inward motion at intercostal margin (see Figure 7-11)

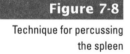

Figure 7-8

Technique for percussing the spleen

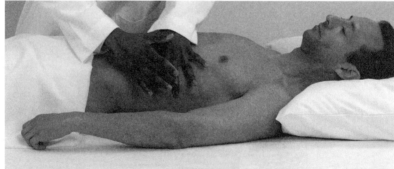

Figure 7-9

Technique for light palpation of the abdomen

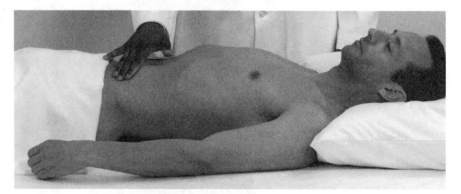

Figure 7-10

Technique for deep palpation of the abdomen

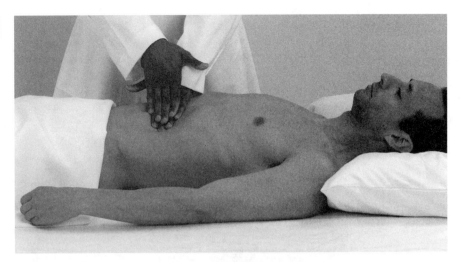

Figure 7-11

Technique for palpating the liver

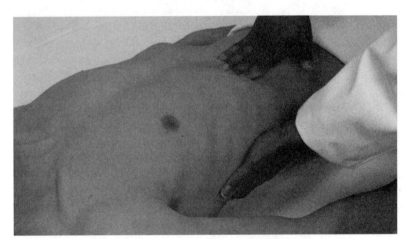

7. Palpate the spleen to determine if there is enlargement by standing at the right side of client; place left hand under lower border of rib cage and elevate rib cage while pressing right hand into left costal margin; ask client to take a deep breath and palpate spleen while diaphragm descends

8. Palpate aorta for pulsations by using fingertips to press into upper abdomen left of midline of xiphoid process; however, do *not* palpate abdomen of a client with a confirmed aortic aneurysm to avoid risk of rupture

9. Palpate for rebound tenderness by depressing hand at a 90-degree angle into the abdominal wall, pressing deeply into abdomen, and then lifting fingers quickly and asking client if he or she has pain (see Figure 7-12)

10. Percuss abdomen for **ascites** (a collection of fluid in abdominal or peritoneal cavity) by positioning client supine; percuss at midline for tympany and progress laterally away from midline until dullness is elicited; mark these areas with a marker

11. Test for psoas sign whenever client is experiencing lower abdominal pain by positioning client supine and placing right hand just above right knee and asking client to raise his or her leg to meet examiner's hand; flexion of hip causes contraction of psoas muscle (see Figure 7-13)

12. Test for Murphy's sign when palpating liver by having client take a deep breath; as diaphragm descends the examiner may feel liver and gallbladder

!

Practice to Pass

The client is suspected of having appendicitis. What should the nurse do to assess for rebound tenderness in this client?

!

!

Figure 7-12

Technique for assessment of rebound tenderness in the abdomen

A. Application of pressure

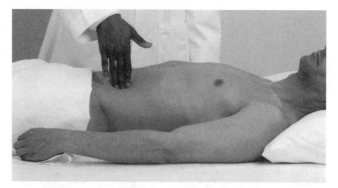

B. Rapid release of pressure

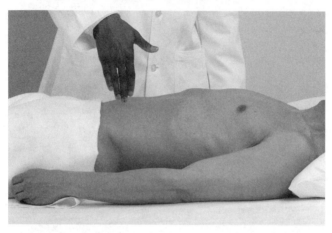

Figure 7-13

Assessing for Psoas sign

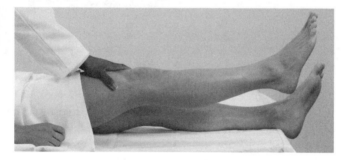

VI. EXPECTED FINDINGS

A. Inspection

1. During inspection of the abdomen, contour should be flat
2. The umbilicus should be inverted or protruding, free of inflammation and drainage
3. Skin color should be same skin tone as rest of body; skin should be smooth, moist, and without blemishes or lesions; macules, moles, and freckles are considered a normal variation
4. Abdomen should be symmetrical without bulges or masses
5. In thin clients, pulsations in aortic area and peristaltic waves may be observable

B. Auscultation

1. Bowel sounds are usually irregular, high-pitched gurgling sounds occurring 5 to 30 times a minute; **borborygmi** (increased high-pitched bowel sounds associated with gas or air in intestines) is a normal finding in clients who have not eaten in hours and may occur up to 320 times per minute
2. During auscultation of abdomen no vascular sounds or friction rubs should be heard

C. Percussion

1. When using assessment technique of percussion, expect to hear tympany over gastric bubble and dullness over liver and spleen and any solid organ
2. Liver span should be between 5 and 10 centimeters (2 to 4 inches) and between 4 and 9 centimeters (1.5 to 3 inches) at midsternal line and approximately 1 inch at lower liver border
3. It is normal to hear splenic dullness between 6th and 10th intercostal spaces

D. Palpation

1. When palpating abdomen it is soft, non-tender, and palpation should not elicit pain
2. Liver is not normally palpable; if palpated it should be smooth, non-tender, and firm
3. Spleen is usually not palpable
4. Normally there should be no aortic pulsations or rebound tenderness
5. Ascites should not be palpable
6. When testing for psoas sign, client should not experience any pain when his or her hip is flexed
7. When testing for Murphy sign, client should not feel pain when liver or gallbladder is palpated

VII. UNEXPECTED FINDINGS

A. Inspection

1. It is abnormal to observe client guarding his or her abdomen; taking several deep breaths may relax abdominal muscles
2. Obesity causes a protuberant abdomen, whereas cachexia may result in a concave abdomen
3. Umbilicus should not have signs of inflammation or infection; a protuberant umbilicus may indicate urinary distention or a hernia, especially in children
4. Skin should be dry and should not have signs of inflammation; if skin is taut and/or glistening it could indicate ascites; striae or stretch marks are silvery, shiny, irregular marks on skin and may result from pregnancy, obesity, or ascites
5. Asymmetry may result from masses, adhesions, or strictures and has a variety of causes
6. Shadows may indicate masses, adhesions, or strictures
7. A bulge may be result of a tumor, cyst, or hernia
8. Pulsations may be abnormal and may indicate an aneurysm
9. Increased peristaltic activity may be result of **gastroenteritis** (an infection of gastrointestinal tract causing diarrhea and abdominal discomfort) or a bowel obstruction

B. Auscultation

1. Gastroenteritis or diarrhea may cause hyperactive bowel sounds
2. Hypoactive bowel sounds may result from abdominal surgery or obstruction
3. If client is experiencing a paralytic ileus, bowel sounds may be absent; absence of bowel sounds should not be determined until abdomen has been auscultated for a full 5 minutes
4. Client should not have a vascular sound; **bruits** are blowing, soft, continuous sounds and are considered abnormal as a bruit results from turbulent blood flow; bruits heard during diastole are usually the result of arterial occlusion
5. Friction rub or grating sound is the result of tissue rubbing together or organs rubbing against peritoneum
6. If client is experiencing a paralytical ileus, suspect an obstruction

C. Percussion

1. Hyperresonance may result from overdistention
2. Dullness in left lower quadrant may indicate stool in bowel

    3. Dullness below costal margin may result from an enlarged liver or spleen

    4. Movement of liver is decreased when client is experiencing a pneumothorax

    5. Dullness over stomach may be result of a heavy meal

D. Palpation

    1. Muscle tightness may produce guarding or abdominal pain

    2. Abdominal pain may be referred

    3. Palpation of a lesion, bulge, mass, or obstruction is considered abnormal

    4. Palpation that elicits pain may indicate gallbladder or liver enlargement

    5. If nodules are palpated over liver it may indicate cirrhosis or metastatic carcinoma

    6. Spleen should not be palpable

    7. Fluid should not be present in abdomen and if present it may indicate cirrhosis or hepatic disease

    8. A positive psoas sign (pain during hip flexion) may indicate peritoneal irritation or **peritonitis** (inflammation of peritoneum)

    9. Sharp abdominal pain (indicating a positive Murphy's sign) occurs with cholecystitis

VIII. LIFESPAN CONSIDERATIONS

A. Infants and children

    1. The abdomen of an infant or child is round

    2. Peristaltic waves may be visible

    3. A toddler has a "potbelly" appearance

B. Pregnant females

    1. As pregnancy progresses, uterus rises to take up an increasing amount of space in abdomen

    2. Height of uterine fundus can be measured at a predictable height in centimeters at specific weeks of gestation (see Figure 7-14)

    3. Compression and displacement of abdominal organs by uterine fundus can lead to constipation, gas, hemorrhoid formation or flares, and frequent voiding

    4. Peristalsis and bowel sounds may decrease because of changing levels of hormones

    5. Common complaints during pregnancy affecting the gastrointestinal tract include heartburn or indigestion, nausea and vomiting, and constipation

    6. Inspection of abdominal skin may reveal stretch marks (striae gravidarum) and a dark line extending midline from umbilicus to symphysis pubis (linea nigra), especially during second half of pregnancy

    7. Abdominal muscles may lose tone because of stretching

C. Older adults

    1. Abdomen may be rounded or protuberant due to adipose tissue and weakened abdominal wall muscle

    2. Muscle structure is softer

    3. Older adult clients may have a loss of teeth, or ill fitting or broken dentures, which may cause gastric problems

    4. Decreased saliva production, digestive enzymes, peristalsis, and gastric activity may lead to constipation, reflux, and other disease processes

    5. Decreased intake of fiber and fluids also contributes to bowel irregularity

    6. Stress may lead to ulcers and inflammatory bowel disease exacerbations

    7. Older adults may have nutritional deficits or may be overweight

IX. DOCUMENTATION

A. Take a health history by obtaining the client's chief complaint and description of problem

B. Document a dietary history

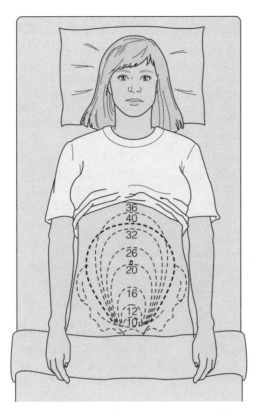

Figure 7-14

Uterine fundal height at various gestational weeks

C. Obtain and interpret vital signs
D. Document weight gain or loss and results of abdominal inspection
E. Document abdominal auscultatory and percussion sounds
F. Document palpation findings last

Case Study

A 50-year-old male truck driver who visits the ambulatory care clinic reports having acid reflux. The client is five feet, ten inches tall and weighs 370 pounds. When the nurse performs a dietary recall, the following diet was consumed in 24 hours:

Breakfast: two frozen breakfast sandwiches and a soda
Midmorning snack: bagel, cream cheese, and coffee
Lunch: Italian cold cut deli sandwich, chips, soda, and macaroni salad
Afternoon snack: cookies
Dinner: macaroni and cheese, meatloaf, crusty bread, and butter
The client reports very little exercise and abdominal pain when lying down.

1. What conclusion should the nurse draw related to the 24-hour dietary recall?

2. What conclusion should the nurse form about the client's diet?

3. In what order should the nurse proceed with assessment techniques when assessing the client's abdomen?

4. Based on the client's reported history what nursing diagnosis will help the nurse develop a plan of care to increase positive health behaviors?

5. What factor contributes to his health problems?

For suggested responses, see page 309

POSTTEST

1 While performing a head-to-toe assessment of a client the nurse hears dullness over the left upper quadrant during percussion. What would be the next assessment the nurse should perform?

1. Inspection of the area
2. Palpation of the area
3. Auscultation of the entire abdomen
4. Inspection of respiratory excursion

2 During a gastrointestinal assessment the client tells the nurse about experiencing chronic flatulence. Which question should the nurse ask the client next?

1. "Are you eating large amounts of broccoli and cauliflower?"
2. "Are you consuming bread products?"
3. "Is fish a staple in your diet?"
4. "Do you consume two quarts of water per day?"

3 The client is vomiting fecal-like material. The nurse would expect to prepare the client for diagnostic testing to evaluate the client for which health problem?

1. Appendicitis
2. Diarrhea
3. Intestinal obstruction
4. A disorder of the throat

4 The adult client presents to the ambulatory care clinic with reports of not being able to chew and swallow easily. The nurse should evaluate the client for which possible contributing factor?

1. Bloating
2. Missing teeth or ill-fitting dentures
3. Gastrointestinal bleeding
4. Pain

5 The nurse is assessing a child and notes a protruding umbilicus. How would the nurse document this finding?

1. A rounded abdomen
2. Ascites
3. A hernia
4. A central striae

6 When assessing the abdomen the nurse would expect to auscultate which sounds?

1. High-pitched gurgling
2. Low-pitched rumbling
3. Bruits
4. Friction rubs

7 When auscultating the abdomen of an adult client, the nurse is unable to hear bowel sounds. For how many minutes should the nurse listen to each quadrant of the abdomen? Provide a numeric answer.

8 While palpating the client's abdomen the nurse notes the client wince in pain and assesses involuntary contraction of the abdominal muscles. The nurse would document which of the following findings?

1. Referred pain
2. Guarding
3. Dullness
4. A gastric bubble

9 The nurse palpates an accumulation of fluid in the abdomen and documents this as ascites. The nurse should also assess the client for which health problems as possible etiological factors? Select all that apply.

1. Chronic obstructive disease
2. Cirrhosis
3. Congestive heart failure
4. Renal failure
5. Appendicitis

10 A client with a history of cholecystitis is admitted to the emergency department with reports of pain. The nurse should assess this pain by palpating in which area on the accompanying diagram?

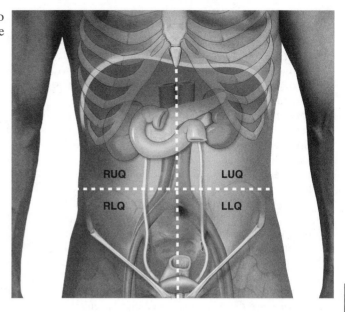

➤ *See pages 139–140 for Answers and Rationales.*

ANSWERS & RATIONALES

Pretest

1 **Answer: 3, 1, 2, 4** **Rationale:** The nurse will use the techniques of assessment in the following order for assessment of the abdomen: inspection, auscultation, palpation, and percussion. Inspection and auscultation are performed first and second so as not to stir abdominal contents through manual manipulation and possibly create inaccurate data. Palpation (light then deep) is performed prior to percussion. **Cognitive Level:** Application **Client Need:** Health Promotion and Maintenance **Integrated Process:** Nursing Process: Assessment **Content Area:** Adult Health: Gastrointestinal **Strategy:** Recall that inspection is completed first. Next recall that bowel sounds can be altered by physical manipulation, which leads you to select auscultation next. Finally recall that the rest of the assessment is conducted in the usual sequence to choose palpation before percussion. **Reference:** D'Amico, D. & Barbarito, C. (2007). *Health & physical assessment in nursing.* Upper Saddle River, NJ: Pearson Education, Inc., p. 528.

2 **Answer: 1, 2, 4, 5** **Rationale:** These questions will elicit information about the client's appetite changes, the client's perceptions of weight changes, and determine factors that may contribute to the weight change. Asking about elimination patterns provides information about the functioning of the intestines in the lower gastrointestinal tract (option 3), but this is not directly related to appetite. **Cognitive Level:** Application **Client Need:** Health Promotion and Maintenance **Integrated Process:** Nursing Process: Assessment **Content Area:** Adult Health: Gastrointestinal **Strategy:** Focus on the critical word in the question, which is *appetite*. Eliminate the option about the lower bowel (elimination) as this question will not provide information about appetite. **Reference:** D'Amico, D. & Barbarito, C. (2007). *Health & physical assessment in nursing.* Upper Saddle River, NJ: Pearson Education, Inc., pp. 520–521.

3 **Answer: 1, 2, 3** **Rationale:** The nurse should ask the client about symptoms of a problem such as nausea, indigestion and vomiting, bloating, dysphagia, diarrhea, or constipation. Fever is a sign of infection, but this is a systemic sign rather than one localized to the gastrointestinal tract (option 4). Asking about dietary intake will provide information about weight, but does not assess an abdominal or gastrointestinal symptom (option 5). **Cognitive Level:** Application **Client Need:** Health Promotion and Maintenance **Integrated Process:** Nursing Process: Assessment **Content Area:** Adult Health: Gastrointestinal

Strategy: The critical words in the question are *symptoms of abdominal problems*. With this in mind, eliminate options that are not symptoms related to the gastrointestinal tract, which include fever (option 4) and dietary intake (option 5). **Reference:** D'Amico, D. & Barbarito, C. (2007). *Health & physical assessment in nursing.* Upper Saddle River, NJ: Pearson Education, Inc., p. 522.

4 Answer: 1 Rationale: The client who consumes a diet low in fruit and vegetables, which provide roughage, is at risk for constipation (option 1). Diarrhea is associated with a high fat diet or a diet high in sugar (option 2). Fruits and vegetables are low calorie foods, so weight loss (option 3) is probably not what this client is experiencing (since the client is not eating those foods). There is no evidence that this client is experiencing pain, either acute or chronic (option 4).
Cognitive Level: Application **Client Need:** Health Promotion and Maintenance **Integrated Process:** Nursing Process: Analysis **Content Area:** Adult Health: Gastrointestinal **Strategy:** First eliminate pain as an option since there is no evidence that the client is in pain. Next eliminate weight loss as the client is probably consuming a high carbohydrate, protein, and fat diet. Choose between the opposite options, which are constipation and diarrhea. Choose constipation over diarrhea because this client consumes no roughage; therefore, the client would have constipation. **Reference:** D'Amico, D. & Barbarito, C. (2007). *Health & physical assessment in nursing.* Upper Saddle River, NJ: Pearson Education, Inc., p. 526.

5 Answer: 2 Rationale: The nurse performing an abdominal assessment should position the client supine with a pillow under the head and under the knees to relax the abdominal muscles (option 2). Placing the client supine with a pillow under the head will not relax the abdominal muscles (option 1). Placing a pillow under the client's head will make the client more comfortable. Sitting and standing will not provide adequate access to the abdominal organs (options 3 and 4).
Cognitive Level: Application **Client Need:** Health Promotion and Maintenance **Integrated Process:** Nursing Process: Assessment **Content Area:** Adult Health: Gastrointestinal **Strategy:** First eliminate options 3 and 4, which do not provide access to the abdomen. Recall that a supine position provides access to the abdomen, but a pillow under the knees will relax the abdomen to choose option 2 over option 1. **Reference:** D'Amico, D. & Barbarito, C. (2007). *Health & physical assessment in nursing.* Upper Saddle River, NJ: Pearson Education, Inc., p. 528.

6 Answer: 3 Rationale: A scaphoid abdomen is an inward concave shape (option 3). A flat abdomen is a straight horizontal plane (option 1). A rounded abdomen is a convex shape (option 2). A protuberant abdomen is a large convex shape (option 4).
Cognitive Level: Comprehension **Client Need:** Health Promotion and Maintenance **Integrated Process:** Nursing Process: Assessment **Content Area:** Adult Health:

Gastrointestinal **Strategy:** Eliminate the flat shaped answer (option 1) as it is not a horizontal plane. Next recognize that rounded and protuberant are convex shapes to eliminate options 2 and 4. Recall that scaphoid is an inward or convex shape to choose option 3 correctly. **Reference:** D'Amico, D. & Barbarito, C. (2007). *Health & physical assessment in nursing.* Upper Saddle River, NJ: Pearson Education, Inc., p. 530.

7 Answer: 2 Rationale: The spleen is located on the left side of the abdomen so the nurse would lift the client under the rib cage with the left hand and palpate the left quadrant with the right hand (option 2). In order to palpate the liver the nurse would lift the client under the rib cage with the right hand and palpate the right quadrant with the left hand (option 1). Palpating the area under the xiphoid process for pulsations is evaluating the client for an aortic aneurysm (option 3). Palpating for rebound tenderness is used to evaluate for peritoneal irritation by pressing into the abdomen with steady pressure and while releasing the pressure asking the client if he or she is experiencing pain (option 4).
Cognitive Level: Application **Client Need:** Health Promotion and Maintenance **Integrated Process:** Nursing Process: Implementation **Content Area:** Adult Health: Gastrointestinal **Strategy:** Recall first that the spleen is located in the left upper quadrant. This helps you to eliminate options 1 (right upper quadrant) and 3 (epigastric area). Next recall that peritoneal irritation is usually reflected in the lower quadrant to eliminate option 4. **Reference:** D'Amico, D. & Barbarito, C. (2007). *Health & physical assessment in nursing.* Upper Saddle River, NJ: Pearson Education, Inc., p. 539.

8 Answer: 3 Rationale: The liver is a dense solid organ and the nurse should expect to document dullness (option 3). Resonance is documented over air filled organs such as the lungs (option 1). Tympany occurs over the stomach's gastric bubble (option 2). Hyperresonance is percussed when there is hyperinflation of the lungs (option 4).
Cognitive Level: Comprehension **Client Need:** Health Promotion and Maintenance **Integrated Process:** Nursing Process: Implementation **Content Area:** Adult Health: Gastrointestinal **Strategy:** Recall first that the lungs are air filled and produce resonance when percussed or hyperresonance when overinflated. This will help you to eliminate options 1 and 4. Next recall that tympany is percussed over the stomach to eliminate option 2. Alternatively, recall that the liver is a solid organ and solid organs produce dullness to choose option 3 over option 2. **Reference:** D'Amico, D. & Barbarito, C. (2007). *Health & physical assessment in nursing.* Upper Saddle River, NJ: Pearson Education, Inc., p. 534.

9 Answer: 4 Rationale: Striae are shiny, silvery stretch marks found on the skin associated with ascites, obesity, and pregnancy (option 4). A shadow would be indicative of a mass (option 1). Scars are the result of surgery or

trauma and are benign (option 2). Ascites is indicative of a liver problem and is associated with fluid accumulation in the abdomen (option 3).
Cognitive Level: Comprehension **Client Need:** Health Promotion and Maintenance **Integrated Process:** Communication and Documentation **Content Area:** Adult Health: Gastrointestinal **Strategy:** First eliminate option 1 recalling that shadows should be palpated as they are associated with masses. Next eliminate option 3 because ascites would be accompanied by abdominal enlargement from fluid accumulation and because ascites is also palpated. Of the remaining two options involving inspection, recognize that option 4 (striae) is the only option describing a stretch mark, while option 2 (scars) is the result of previous trauma or surgery. **Reference:** D'Amico, D. & Barbarito, C. (2007). *Health & physical assessment in nursing.* Upper Saddle River, NJ: Pearson Education, Inc., pp. 530–531.

10 Answer: 2 Rationale: Ascites is associated with cirrhosis, end-stage renal disease, and congestive heart failure (option 2). Overhydration is fluid accumulation but is not associated with fluid accumulation in the abdomen, but rather weight gain due to systemic fluid overload (option 1). A mass is associated with tumor which may be benign or malignant (option 3). Trauma is not associated with ascites (option 4).
Cognitive Level: Analysis **Client Need:** Health Promotion and Maintenance **Integrated Process:** Nursing Process: Evaluation **Content Area:** Adult Health: Gastrointestinal **Strategy:** First recall that ascites is a fluid accumulation in the abdomen. This will help you to eliminate options 3 and 4. Next recall that ascites occurs as a result of congestive heart failure, end-stage renal disease, and cirrhosis to choose correctly. Alternatively, recall that overhydration would lead to systemic fluid overload and edema (not fluid being sequestered in the abdomen). **Reference:** D'Amico, D. & Barbarito, C. (2007). *Health & physical assessment in nursing.* Upper Saddle River, NJ: Pearson Education, Inc., p. 541.

Posttest

1 Answer: 2 Rationale: The order of the abdominal assessment is inspection, auscultation, percussion, and palpation. The respiratory system is not assessed during an abdominal assessment.
Cognitive Level: Application **Client Need:** Health Promotion and Maintenance **Integrated Process:** Nursing Process: Assessment **Content Area:** Adult Health: Gastrointestinal **Strategy:** Eliminate the respiratory option because in the head to toe assessment the respiratory system would be already completed. Recall that inspection and auscultation are completed prior to manipulating the abdomen to prevent stirring the contents of the bowel and creating false bowel sounds. **Reference:** D'Amico, D. & Barbarito, C. (2007). *Health & physical assessment in nursing.* Upper Saddle River, NJ: Pearson Education, Inc., p. 528.

2 Answer: 1 Rationale: Broccoli and cauliflower (in addition to figs and cabbage as examples) will cause bloating and flatulence (option 1). Consuming bread products does not cause gas (option 2). Fish is not associated with gas (option 3). Excessive fluid intake may contribute to a softer stool, whereas inadequate intake is associated with constipation (option 4).
Cognitive Level: Analysis **Client Need:** Health Promotion and Maintenance **Integrated Process:** Nursing Process: Assessment **Content Area:** Adult Health: Gastrointestinal **Strategy:** Eliminate option 4 first because water does not cause gas. Next recall that bread and fish are not associated with flatulence or bloating to eliminate these incorrect options. Alternatively, recall that cruciferous vegetables such as broccoli and cauliflower are gas-forming to choose correctly. **Reference:** D'Amico, D. & Barbarito, C. (2007). *Health & physical assessment in nursing.* Upper Saddle River, NJ: Pearson Education, Inc., p. 521.

3 Answer: 3 Rationale: Intestinal obstruction is associated with fecal-like vomiting (option 3). The client may have vomiting with appendicitis but it should not be fecal-like (option 1). A client with diarrhea should not have fecal-like vomiting (option 2). Throat disorders do not cause fecal-like vomiting (option 4). The client with fecal-like vomiting should be prepared for an x-ray of the abdomen and a CT scan.
Cognitive Level: Analysis **Client Need:** Health Promotion and Maintenance **Integrated Process:** Nursing Process: Assessment **Content Area:** Adult Health: Gastrointestinal **Strategy:** Recall that fecal material is in the intestinal tract to eliminate all other options. **Reference:** D'Amico, D. & Barbarito, C. (2007). *Health & physical assessment in nursing.* Upper Saddle River, NJ: Pearson Education, Inc., p. 523.

4 Answer: 2 Rationale: A client should be evaluated for missing teeth or ill-fitting dentures when complaining of not being able to chew or swallow (option 2). Bloating is associated with abdominal fullness or flatulence (option 1). Gastrointestinal bleeding is associated with blood in the stool (option 3). Pain is associated with cardiac disease, cholecystitis, kidney stones, or diverticulosis (option 4).
Cognitive Level: Application **Client Need:** Health Promotion and Maintenance **Integrated Process:** Nursing Process: Analysis **Content Area:** Adult Health: Gastrointestinal **Strategy:** Note that the client reports difficulty swallowing, which is an upper gastrointestinal problem; whereas bloating, bleeding, and pain are usually found in the lower digestive tract. **Reference:** D'Amico, D. & Barbarito, C. (2007). *Health & physical assessment in nursing.* Upper Saddle River, NJ: Pearson Education, Inc., pp. 523–524.

5 Answer: 3 Rationale: A common finding in children is a protruding umbilicus, which is associated with a hernia (option 3). A rounded abdomen is common in children and is known as a convex abdomen (option 1). Ascites is not common in children and is fluid in the abdomen (option 2). Striae are known as stretch marks and are not commonly found in children (option 4). **Cognitive Level:** Application **Client Need:** Health Promotion and Maintenance **Integrated Process:** Nursing Process: Assessment **Content Area:** Child Health **Strategy:** A rounded abdomen should be eliminated as it is a normal finding. Eliminate ascites as it is associated usually with alcoholism. Eliminate striae as this reflects stretch marks. **Reference:** D'Amico, D. & Barbarito, C. (2007). *Health & physical assessment in nursing.* Upper Saddle River, NJ: Pearson Education, Inc., pp. 530–531.

6 **Answer: 1** **Rationale:** The nurse would expect to auscultate high-pitched gurgling bowel sounds (option 1). Low-pitched sounds are not found during the abdominal assessment (option 2). Bruits are associated with turbulent blood flow (option 3). Friction rubs are associated with organs rubbing together or against the peritoneum, usually caused by inflammation (option 4). **Cognitive Level:** Application **Client Need:** Health Promotion and Maintenance **Integrated Process:** Nursing Process: Assessment **Content Area:** Adult Health: Gastrointestinal **Strategy:** Friction rubs are associated with inflammation of organs, not vascular problems. Bruits are associated with vascular problems of the renal, femoral, or iliac arteries. Low-pitched sounds are not associated with normal bowel sounds. **Reference:** D'Amico, D. & Barbarito, C. (2007). *Health & physical assessment in nursing.* Upper Saddle River, NJ: Pearson Education, Inc., p. 531.

7 **Answer: 5** **Rationale:** Each of the client's abdominal quadrants are auscultated for at least 5 minutes prior to documenting that the client has no or absent bowel sounds. **Cognitive Level:** Application **Client Need:** Health Promotion and Maintenance **Integrated Process:** Nursing Process: Assessment **Content Area:** Adult Health: Gastrointestinal **Strategy:** Specific knowledge is needed to answer this question. This is a critical intervention for the nurse to implement as absent bowel sounds are life-threatening and immediate action is needed. **Reference:** D'Amico, D. & Barbarito, C. (2007). *Health & physical assessment in nursing.* Upper Saddle River, NJ: Pearson Education, Inc., p. 532.

8 **Answer: 2** **Rationale:** Muscle contraction or guarding is involuntary contraction of the abdominal muscles usually indicating peritonitis. The nurse should document this as guarding (option 2). Referred pain is pain that is felt in another area of the body and is not guarding (option 1). Dullness is not palpated but rather per-

cussed (option 3). A gastric bubble is percussed and not palpated (option 4). **Cognitive Level:** Application **Client Need:** Health Promotion and Maintenance **Integrated Process:** Nursing Process: Assessment **Content Area:** Adult Health: Gastrointestinal **Strategy:** Eliminate options 3 and 4, which involve percussion. Recall that pain is a somatic finding. Then recall that guarding is the finding that is founded upon palpation. **Reference:** D'Amico, D. & Barbarito, C. (2007). *Health & physical assessment in nursing.* Upper Saddle River, NJ: Pearson Education, Inc., p. 537.

9 **Answer: 2, 3, 4** **Rationale:** Cirrhosis, congestive heart failure, and renal failure are conditions that may present with the symptom of ascites. Chronic obstructive pulmonary disease produces respiratory symptoms (option 1). Appendicitis does not produce the symptom of fluid accumulation (option 5). **Cognitive Level:** Application **Client Need:** Health Promotion and Maintenance **Integrated Process:** Nursing Process: Assessment **Content Area:** Adult Health: Gastrointestinal **Strategy:** Recall that the disease processes of cirrhosis, congestive heart failure, and renal failure are all associated with fluid accumulation (ascites). Eliminate options that do not involve fluid deposits in the abdomen, which in this question are the respiratory disease option and the appendicitis option. **Reference:** D'Amico, D. & Barbarito, C. (2007). *Health & physical assessment in nursing.* Upper Saddle River, NJ: Pearson Education, Inc., p. 541.

10 **Answer: (The correct answer area is labeled as the right upper quadrant in the original figure.)** **Rationale:** The nurse should palpate and percuss the right upper quadrant as the gallbladder is located in this quadrant. The stomach, spleen, left adrenal gland, and kidney are located in the left upper and lower quadrants. The right lower quadrant contains the colon and sexual organs. The left lower quadrant also contains the sexual organs and the colon. **Cognitive Level:** Application **Client Need:** Health Promotion and Maintenance **Integrated Process:** Nursing Process: Assessment **Content Area:** Adult Health: Gastrointestinal **Strategy:** Be aware that to accurately perform assessment techniques, the location of internal organs must be part of the nurse's knowledge base. Recall that the gallbladder is located in the right upper quadrant to make the correct selection. **Reference:** D'Amico, D. & Barbarito, C. (2007). *Health & physical assessment in nursing.* Upper Saddle River, NJ: Pearson Education, Inc., p. 517.

References

Bickley, L. (2010). *Bates guide to physical examination and history taking* (10th ed.). Philadelphia: Lippincott Williams & Wilkins.

D'Amico, D. & Barbarito, C. (2007). *Health and physical assessment in nursing.* Upper Saddle River, NJ: Pearson Education, Inc., pp. 510–553.

Jarvis, C. (2008). *Physical examination and health assessment* (5th ed.). St. Louis, MO: Elsevier Saunders.

Zator Estes, M. (2009). *Health assessment and physical examination* (4th ed.). Clifton Park, NY: Delmar Cengage Learning.

ANSWERS & RATIONALES

Neurological Assessment

8

Chapter Outline

Health History
Present Health History
Family History

Equipment, Preparation,
and Positioning
Physical Examination
Expected Findings

Unexpected Findings
Lifespan Considerations
Documentation

Objectives

➤ Identify the anatomical structures of the neurological system.
➤ Identify the questions to ascertain information about health history, present history, and family history.
➤ Describe the assessment techniques for assessment of the nervous system.
➤ Describe the expected and unexpected findings in the assessment of the neurological system.
➤ Describe the considerations across the lifespan to be taken into account during assessment of the neurological system.
➤ Describe documentation of the assessment of the neurological system.

 NCLEX-RN® Test Prep

Visit the Companion Website for this book at www.pearsonhighered.com/hogan to access additional practice opportunities and more.

Review at a Glance

anosmia lack of smell as a result of cranial nerve dysfunction
Babinski reflex neurological test of a reflex elicited by stimulating the sole of the foot and observing for fanning of toes, which in clients older than two years of age is considered abnormal
clonus hyperactive reflex indicating upper motor neuron disease; when present there will be alternating flexion and extension

diplopia double vision
dysphagia difficulty swallowing
hypalgesia decreased sensation of pain
hyperalgesia increased sensation of pain
hyperesthesia increased sensation to touch
hypoesthesia decreased sensation to touch

nystagmus involuntary oscillations of the eye
papilledema edema of optic nerve as it enters the retina
tinnitus ringing in the ear associated with cochlear disturbance or dysfunction
vertigo dizziness (often severe) related to alterations of the vestibular apparatus in the ear

PRETEST

1 The husband of a 60-year-old female who hit her head on the dashboard in a car accident is asking, "What is wrong with my wife? She usually has such a gentle spirit. Now she is cursing like I have never heard before." What would be the nurse's best reply?

1. "The behavior is likely to be a result of damage to the frontal lobe from the car accident."
2. "She is just uncomfortable and will stop yelling as soon as we get her pain under control."
3. "I will give her a sedative that will help her to become quiet."
4. "Your wife may have a gentle spirit, but her cursing is really bad right now."

2 While the nurse is performing an admission assessment on a newly admitted client, the client states, "I am very unsteady on my feet." What assessment would the nurse perform to evaluate the client's statement?

1. Test the client's intellectual functioning by asking the client to remember several sequences of numbers
2. Perform assessments to evaluate cerebellar function
3. Assess the client for two point discrimination
4. Test ocular fields to see if there is a visual problem causing unsteadiness

3 The nurse is caring for a client who has been admitted to the neurological unit for evaluation of dizziness and reports of the "room spinning when lying down." The nurse should document this finding as which of the following?

1. Orthostatic hypotension
2. Diplopia
3. Vertigo
4. Bradycardia

4 The nurse is examining an elderly man who is unable to stand with his eyes closed, feet together, and arms at his side. The man leans from side to side during this part of the examination. The nurse would conclude that this is a positive finding for which assessment?

1. Rinne test
2. Weber's test
3. Babinski reflex
4. Romberg test

5 The nurse is testing the client's ability to recognize familiar objects. When the nurse places a coin in the client's hand, the client correctly identifies the object. How would the nurse document this finding?

1. Hyperesthesia
2. Stereognosis
3. Astereognosis
4. Apraxia

6 The nurse is caring for a client who sustained a head injury several days ago. The client is lethargic and tells the nurse that he is on vacation in the islands. Based on these clinical manifestations it is most important that the nurse perform which neurological assessment next?

1. Cranial nerves
2. Deep tendon reflexes
3. Level of consciousness
4. Client's ability to calculate problems

7 The clinical educator on a neurological unit is teaching a new nurse how to elicit deep tendon reflexes. The educator would evaluate the orientee as having appropriate knowledge of a positive triceps reflex when the orientee describes this as which of the following?

1. Fanning of the fingers
2. Rotation of the arm
3. Adduction of the arm
4. Extension of the forearm

8 A nurse on a neurological unit is assessing the memory of a newly admitted 74-year-old client. The client is unable to state his date of birth, social security number, or the names of his wife or children. The nurse concludes that this client is experiencing which of the following?

1. Short-term memory loss
2. Depression
3. Long-term memory loss
4. Emotional problems

9 To evaluate a client for anosmia, the nurse would perform which of the following assessments?

1. Have the client close the eyes and touch his or her nose
2. Have the client close the eyes and identify a familiar smell
3. Ask the client to describe a course of action for a situation
4. Have the client read a Snellen eye chart

10 To evaluate the patellar reflex the nurse would perform the following assessments in what order? Provide a numeric answer.

1. Use distraction
2. Wash hands
3. Palpate the patella
4. Position the client
5. Strike the patella with a reflex hammer

➤ *See pages 160–162 for Answers and Rationales.*

I. HEALTH HISTORY

    A. Nurses must have a thorough knowledge of anatomy and physiology of the neurological system in order to perform an accurate assessment

    B. The neurological system consists of the central nervous system and peripheral nervous system

      1. Central nervous system includes brain and spinal cord

      2. Peripheral nervous system is composed of spinal and peripheral nerves

    C. Brain is encased by meninges and cushioned by cerebrospinal fluid

    D. Brain has four areas, which control all functions in the body: cerebrum, diencephalon, cerebellum, and brain stem (see Figure 8-1)

      1. Cerebrum is responsible for all conscious behavior; it allows client to perceive, remember, and communicate; it is also responsible for involuntary movement; it has four lobes: frontal, parietal, occipital, and temporal (see Table 8-1)

        a. Frontal lobe controls skeletal movement, speech, emotions, and intellectual activities such as the following: intellect, reasoning, judgment, and ability to learn and think abstractly

        b. Parietal lobe is responsible for sensation and somatosensory stimuli such as temperature, pain, and identifying sensations

Figure 8-1

Regions of the brain

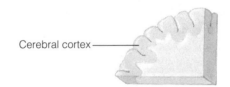

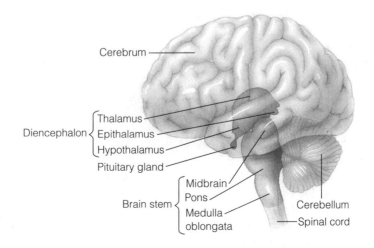

Table 8-1	Structure	Location	Function
Structure, Location, and Function of the Brain	Cerebrum	Top of brain	Responsible for all conscious behavior; perception, communication, involuntary movement, memory
	Cerebral cortex	Outer layer of brain	Responsible for conscious behavior
	Frontal lobe	Front of cerebrum	Responsible for emotions, behavior, intellect, personality, and language
	Temporal lobe	Behind the ear	Responsible for sensations such as hearing, smell, taste, and memory
	Parietal lobe	Back of cerebrum	Responsible for perception and interpretation of pain, temperature, touch, and texture
	Occipital lobe	Back, central	Responsible for perception and visual stimuli
	Thalamus	Diencephalon	Interprets sensory stimuli: warmth, smell, and taste
	Hypothalamus	Coronal section	Controls temperature, heart rate, blood pressure, and sleep
	Cerebellum	Posterior base of brain	Controls muscle movement, strength, coordination, and equilibrium
	Midbrain section of brainstem	Anterior brainstem	Responsible for visual and auditory reflexes, eye movement
	Pons section of brainstem	Between midbrain and medulla	Controls respiratory function, facial and eye movement, and sensation
	Medulla portion of brainstem	Connects brainstem to spinal cord	Controls respiratory and heart rates; blood pressure; and reflexes for coughing, vomiting, swallowing, and sneezing
	Meninges	Brain covering	Protects the brain

Practice to Pass

A client who has experienced a frontal lobe injury would exhibit alterations in which areas of function?

Practice to Pass

The client who is in a motor vehicle accident and develops a fever immediately when entering the Emergency Department is most likely experiencing damage to what area of the brain?

Practice to Pass

What is the function of cerebrospinal fluid (CSF)?

   c. Occipital lobe controls the visual cortex, which permits client to interpret visual stimuli

   d. Temporal lobe allows client to interpret auditory (hearing) and olfactory (smell) stimuli

2. Diencephalon is composed of thalamus, hypothalamus, and epithalamus
   a. Thalamus processes all information in cerebral cortex
   b. Hypothalamus is responsible for blood pressure; heart rate; force of heart contraction; respiratory rate and depth; digestive function; perceptions of pain, fear, rage, and pleasure; body temperature; food intake; water balance; and sleep
   c. Epithalamus controls mood and sleep
3. Cerebellum controls muscle movement, tone and coordination, and equilibrium
4. Brain stem is responsible for autonomic control of respirations, blood pressure; it controls involuntary reflexes such as coughing, hiccuping, sneezing, swallowing, and vomiting

E. Spinal cord is protected by meninges and cerebrospinal fluid; spinal cord transmits impulses to and from brain

F. Reflex activity and the peripheral nervous system involve the cranial nerves and spinal nerves
   1. Reflexes are stimulus response activities; these activities are involuntary and take place at the level of the spinal cord
   2. Reflexes include biceps, triceps, brachioradialis, patellar, Achilles, and plantar

G. Cranial nerves are responsible for a variety of sensory and motor functions (see Table 8-2)

H. Spinal nerves are responsible for sensory and motor activities in various parts of the body; the messages from the spinal nerves are transmitted to the brain via pathways or tracts in the spinal cord (see Table 8-3)

I. To obtain a health history, obtain biographical data
   1. As the client ages, risk increases for some neurological disorders
   2. Ascertain the client's educational level because this will influence questions asked
   3. Ask about geographical locale as certain locations influence risk of certain neurological dysfunction

Table 8-2	Cranial Nerve	Type	Function
Cranial Nerves	I Olfactory	Sensory	Smell
	II Optic	Sensory	Vision
	III Oculomotor	Motor	Opening eye, moving eye in all fields, dilating pupils
	IV Trochlear	Motor	Movement of eye laterally and downward
	V Trigeminal	Mixed	Motor controls muscle of mastication
			Sensory is responsible for facial and eye sensation
	VI Abducens	Motor	Lateral movement of the eye
	VII Facial	Mixed	Motor controls closing eyes, moving mouth and face
			Sensory is responsible for taste on anterior tongue
	VIII Acoustic	Sensory	Hearing and equilibrium
	IX Glossopharyngeal	Mixed	Motor controls swallowing, gag reflex, and salivation
			Sensory is responsible for taste on posterior tongue
	X Vagus	Mixed	Motor controls pharynx and larynx
			Sensory controls sensations in pharynx and larynx
	XI Spinal accessory	Motor	Controls movement of head, neck and shoulders
	XII Hypoglossal	Motor	Tongue movement and swallowing

Practice to Pass

When assessing the gag reflex, the nurse is evaluating the function of which cranial nerve?

4. Ask about occupation as this may cause exposure to substances toxic to nervous system

J. Ask questions about past history to discover risk factors for neurological disorders

1. "Do you have a history of head injury? If so, did you lose consciousness?" (head injury may leave permanent neurological deficits)
2. "Have you had seizures?"
3. "Have you ever had surgery involving the nervous system?"
4. "Have you had treatment for neurological problems?"
5. "Have you had any back or spinal cord injuries?" (may lead to peripheral neurological disease)
6. "Have you had any medical problems such as diabetes, cardiovascular disease or dysrhythmias, cerebrovascular accident, or hypertension?" (these diseases may lead to neuropathy and residual problems)
7. "Have you had any medical problems that may influence your health?" (infections may lead to meningitis)
8. "Have you had any recent immunizations?" (DPT is contraindicated if encephalopathy is present; may suggest that client is in need of Haemophilus influenza type B or meningococcal vaccine)
9. "Are you taking over-the-counter medications? If yes, what?" (medications may adversely affect nervous system)
10. If female, "Are you taking birth control pills or hormone replacement therapy?" (these drugs have been linked to increased risk of stroke and bleeding)

Table 8-3	Tract	Function
Sensory and Motor Tracts of the Spinal Cord	Lateral Spinothalamic	Responsible for pain and temperature
	Anterior Spinothalamic	Responsible for touch
	Posterior Tract	Responsible for pressure, two-point discrimination, vibration, proprioception, and light touch
	Lateral Corticospinal Tract	Controls movement of extremities
	Anterior Corticospinal Tract	Controls voluntary movement
	Corticobulbar Tract	Responsible for cranial nerves
	Rubrospinal Tract	Responsible for coordination of muscle movement
	Reticulospinal Tract	Responsible for posture and movement
	Vestibulospinal Tract	Controls movement

11. "Have you traveled to foreign countries?" (may have contracted virus or parasite)
12. "Have you been in the military?" (may have been exposed to toxins, viruses, or parasites)

II. PRESENT HEALTH HISTORY

A. Ask client general introductory questions such as the following:
1. "What brings you here today? (note whether there is any change in affect or depression if you know the client)
2. "How have you been feeling?"

B. Follow up with specific questions to elicit data about possible neurological problems
1. "Have you had a fever?" (fever may be associated with infection)
2. "Have you had a change in sensation?" (loss of sensation may indicate stroke or neuropathy)
3. "Have you had a change in the function of any of your senses?"
4. "Have you had any headaches? If so, please describe the frequency and location. Are the headaches associated with anything?" (headaches may indicate hypertension or intracranial bleeding)
5. "Have you experienced a head injury? If so what happened? What part of your head did you hit? Did you lose consciousness? If so, for how long?"
6. "Do you ever feel lightheaded or dizzy? If so, when does it occur? How often does it occur? Does it occur with position changes?"
7. "Do you ever feel like the room is spinning? Do you feel like you are spinning? Does this come on suddenly or gradually?"
8. "Have you had a seizure? How long did it last? Does any activity precipitate the seizure? Did your muscles go flaccid or tense up? Are there any physical signs associated with the seizure? What happened after the seizure? Did you sleep? Were you dazed or confused? Before the seizure did you have any physical warning signs?" (some people experience an aura or warning sign prior to the seizure)
9. "Do you have any difficulty speaking or swallowing?" (these symptoms are associated with a stroke)
10. "Have you had visual changes or hearing changes?" (these changes are associated with a stroke)
11. "Do you have any cardiovascular problems?" (cardiovascular disease may increase the risk of a stroke)
12. "Do you have a cardiac dysrhythmia?" (dysrhythmias, especially atrial fibrillation, increase the risk of stroke)
13. "Do you have numbness or tingling in your hands?"
14. "Do you have any weakness in your extremities?" (could indicate a neurological disorder)
15. "Do you experience tremors?" (tremors are involuntary movements and could indicate possible neurological disorder)
16. "Do you have difficulty with your bowel or bladder?" (bladder or bowel problems could be the result of spinal nerve problems, a cerebrovascular accident, or spinal stenosis)
17. "Do you have any problems with coordination?"
18. "Do you have any blood disorders?" (bleeding disorders may increase the risk of stroke)
19. "Do you have thyroid disease?" (thyroid disease may mimic neurological disease because hypothyroidism causes flat affect and weakness)
20. "Do you use proper body mechanics?" (improper body mechanics can lead to either musculoskeletal or neurological dysfunction)

Practice to Pass

What assessment questions should the nurse ask to evaluate a headache?

21. "How many hours of sleep do you get per night?" (sleep deprivation may decrease cerebral function)
22. "Do you smoke?" (smoking may increase risk of cerebrovascular disease)

III. FAMILY HISTORY

A. Family history provides information on any predisposing genetic factors for neurological problems

B. Determine significant family history by asking questions such as the following:
1. "Does anyone in your family have a history of hypertension, cardiovascular disease, stroke, multiple sclerosis, seizures, Alzheimer's disease, cancer, or any neuro-muscular disease?"
2. "Does anyone in your family have a history of psychiatric illness?"
3. "Does anyone in your family have a history of alcoholism?"

IV. EQUIPMENT, POSITIONING, AND PREPARATION

A. Gather the equipment listed below prior to performing examination
1. Stethoscope
2. Blood pressure cuff
3. Gloves
4. Penlight
5. Sterile needle
6. Familiar objects: coin, paperclip, or key
7. Familiar substance to smell: coffee, lemon, or cinnamon
8. Familiar substance to taste: sweet, salt, bitter, and sour substances
9. Test tubes for hot and cold water
10. Reflex hammer
11. Tongue blade
12. Ophthalmoscope
13. Tuning fork

B. Positioning and preparation
1. A full neurological exam is lengthy so it is important to make sure the client is comfortable
2. Throughout the examination ask the client about feelings of fatigue
3. Proper position for a neurological examination is sitting; a chair is more comfortable than the examination table
4. Due to client comfort or client condition, assessment may need to proceed slowly
5. If the client is unsteady, protect him or her from injury

Practice to Pass

In what position is it most appropriate for the nurse to place the client to conduct a neurological examination?

!

V. PHYSICAL EXAMINATION

A. Preliminary assessments
1. Observe client prior to beginning examination
2. Look at client in a systematic manner to relate the clinical manifestation to the neurological dysfunction
3. Upon meeting client, note dress, hygiene, grooming, speech, posture, and body language; if mental status examination is to be performed, do that assessment first (see Chapter 3 for how to conduct a mental status examination)
4. Observe client for symmetry of movement, abnormal movements, and muscle strength
5. Observe if speech is clear or garbled
6. Evaluate hygiene from perspectives of possible physical decline, mental illness, visual deficits, weakness, or cerebral dysfunction

7. Dysarthria, facial asymmetry, or balance difficulties may indicate weakness or cerebellar dysfunction

8. Inappropriate responses to questions or inattention may indicate an underlying cerebral disorder

B. Proceed to obtain vital signs, as neurological system is responsible for control of vital signs

1. Obtain temperature; temperature elevation may indicate infection, inflammatory process, or cerebrovascular accident

2. Monitor blood pressure, as hypertension places client at risk for cerebrovascular accident

3. Evaluate pulse for bradycardia, as it may indicate increased intracranial pressure or could provide information about cardiac irregularity and suggest that client be evaluated for atrial fibrillation

4. Evaluate respiration, as irregular breathing patterns may indicate increased intracranial pressure

C. Assess mental status, including cerebral functioning, cognitive functioning, and communication

1. Cerebral functioning consists of checking arousal and orientation

   a. To check arousal begin by using minimal stimuli such as calling client's name, then (if needed) gently shaking client, and finally using painful stimuli

   b. When calling client's name, speak in a normal tone first and then call client's name louder if needed

   c. Gently touch client, then gently shake client's shoulder

   d. Painful stimuli may include: trapezius squeeze, sternal rub, supraorbital pressure, mandibular pressure, nail bed pressure, and Achilles' tendon squeeze

      1) Trapezius squeeze consists of pinching one to two inches of muscle and gently twisting

      2) To elicit sternal rub, use knuckles of dominant hand and rub

      3) Nail pressure will cause pain when pencil, thumb, or pen is pressed into base of nail

      4) Achilles' tendon pinched between thumb and index finger will elicit pain

      5) Formerly supraorbital pressure and mandibular pressure used to be applied, but these can increase intracranial pressure and, therefore, have fallen out of favor

   e. Assess orientation to determine deteriorating neurological status

      1) Ask client what time it is; if he or she is unable to answer then ask what month or season it is; ask if client knows where he or she is

      2) Being disoriented to person is a sign that constant reorientation is needed and safety is of great concern

2. Evaluate cognitive functioning by assessing level of awareness; this is evaluated by observing behavior, appearance, speech, response to stimuli, memory, and judgment

   a. Evaluate behavior by observing client's actions or obtaining reports from significant others if client is unresponsive

   b. Appearance should reflect cleanliness minimally

   c. Speech should be clear, understandable, and appropriate; client should be able to follow simple directions

   d. Client should be awake, alert, and oriented

   e. Memory should be intact; check recent memory by asking client to state what was eaten for breakfast; assess remote or long-term memory by asking for birth date or major historic event; for remote questions, answers must be verifiable

   f. Evaluate judgment by asking client what would be done in the event of a fire; evaluate whether client's abstract reasoning process is appropriate by asking client to interpret a proverb such as, "A stitch in time saves nine"

▲ *Practice to Pass*

If the client does not respond when the nurse calls his or her name, what should the nurse do next to assess for responsiveness?

g. Evaluate knowledge, vocabulary, and mathematical skills; evaluate general knowledge by asking who current president is; evaluate vocabulary by asking client to define words; assess mathematical skills by asking client to add or subtract money or complete a serial sequence; thought process should be logical and relevant

D. Test cranial nerves (CNs) if there is a deficit

1. Tell client that you will be giving him or her instructions throughout the assessment; inform client that during the examination he or she will close the eyes and you will be touching him or her during parts of the examination

2. To test olfactory nerve (CN I), have client blow nose if obstructed; have client close both eyes and place a familiar scent near one nare, while client occludes other nare; repeat procedure on other side

3. Assess optic nerve (CN II) by having client read a magazine or read from a Snellen eye chart; use an ophthalmoscope to examine fundus of eye; locate optic disc and document shape and color

4. Assess oculomotor (CN III), trochlear (CN IV), and abducens (CN VI) nerves by having client move eyes through cardinal fields of gaze by following an object or finger without moving head; evaluate client's pupillary reaction to light and accommodation; pupils should be assessed for size regularity and equality

   a. Observe direct reaction to light by having client look ahead and shining a penlight in eye and observing for constriction

   b. Observe consensual reaction to light by shining a penlight into one eye and observing other eye for constriction

   c. Observe accommodation by bringing an object close to his or her eyes and observing eyes for constriction

   d. Observe extraocular pupil movement and describe presence of movement in both eyes, type of movement, amplitude (fine, medium, or coarse), frequency (constant or subsides), and plane of movement (horizontal, vertical, or rotary); see Table 8-4 for sample unusual eye movements

5. Test trigeminal nerve (CN V) by having client close eyes and state every time face is touched with a wisp of cotton; evaluate corneal reflex by touching client's eye with a wisp of cotton (client should blink when touched); assess motor function of this nerve by having client clench teeth

6. Evaluate facial nerve (CN VII) by having client smile, frown, show teeth, close eyes, puff cheeks, and raise eyebrows

   a. Assess muscle strength by having client puff cheek and attempt to push air through lips with pressure to cheek

   b. Test anterior aspect of tongue for taste

7. Assess acoustic nerve (CN VIII) to determine adequate hearing and balance

   a. Evaluate hearing by performing Weber test in which a tuning fork is struck and placed on center of head for lateralization of sound

   b. Assess Rinne test by using a tuning fork to compare bone conduction of sound to air conduction; strike tuning fork and place base of fork on mastoid process; ask client to state when sound is no longer heard and note number of seconds; move tines of vibrating tuning fork 1 to 2 centimeters (0.5 inch) in front of external auditory meatus; again ask client to state when sound is no longer heard and record time in seconds

Practice to Pass

What is the most appropriate method to assess the corneal reflex?

Table 8-4	Eye Movement	Characteristics
Eye Movement Characteristics	Pendular movement	Oscillations moving left and right
	Jerk	A quick movement in one direction, slow movement in the opposite direction

Practice to Pass

Is bone conduction longer then air or is air conduction longer than bone?

    c. Use cold-caloric or oculovestibular test to evaluate vestibular aspect of nerve; involves injecting cold water into ear canal and is used when client is unresponsive

    d. To evaluate equilibrium, ask client to stand with eyes closed and feet together and evaluate client's balance

8. Evaluate glossopharyngeal (CN IX) and vagus (CN X) nerves by having client say "ah" and checking gag reflex

    a. Observing client swallow will provide information about motor function of nerves

    b. Evaluate quality of client's voice by listening to client speak

9. Test spinal accessory nerve (CN XI) by having client shrug shoulders; look for symmetry

    a. Have client turn head to right and repeat by turning to left; this evaluates client's sternocleidomastoid muscle

    b. Test sternocleidomastoid muscle by having client turn head to the side while nurse attempts to return head to midline; repeat on other side to test bilaterally

    c. Evaluate trapezius muscle strength by having client raise shoulders and resist while nurse pushes down

10. Evaluate hypoglossal nerve (CN XII) by evaluating tongue

    a. Ask client to protrude (stick out) tongue

    b. Ask client to retract (put tongue back in mouth)

    c. Ask client to move tongue laterally

    d. Ask client to push tongue against cheek while nurse pushes against cheek and then repeats on other side

E. Assess motor function next as musculoskeletal system is innervated by neurological system; motor function is in part related to cerebellar function and is also related to function of motor cortex

    1. Assess client's gait by having client walk across room

        a. Ask client to walk heel to toe while looking straight ahead, not at floor

        b. Ask client to walk on toes and observe balance and coordination

        c. Ask client to walk on heels and observe for balance and coordination

    2. Have client perform Romberg test to assess equilibrium and coordination by standing with feet together, eyes closed, and observe for swaying; protect client from injury

    3. Perform finger to nose test, which is also a test of equilibrium

        a. Have client sit and keep eyes open; extend both arms, touch right finger to nose then return right arm to extended position; repeat with left arm; have client close eyes and repeat

        b. Test coordination by having client close eyes and touch nose then the nurse's finger

    4. Ask client to perform deep knee bend or to hop on one foot to evaluate muscle strength, position sense, and cerebellar function; remember some individuals cannot perform these tests due to age, obesity, or physical dysfunction and musculoskeletal disorders

    5. Assess client's ability to rapidly alternate hands to determine upper motor neuron weakness

        a. Have client sit and place palms face down on lap and alternate position of palms to face up and face down; movement should be smooth and even

        b. Evaluate rapid alternating movement by having client touch finger to thumb

        c. Ask client to lie down and then slide right heel down left shin and repeat with opposite leg

    6. Tests of muscle strength can be considered part of neurological exam, but are conducted as part of examination of musculoskeletal system (see Chapter 9); repeat

neurological checks of a client often include the following elements of
motor function

  a. Ask client to move each extremity to determine ability to perform voluntary
  movement

  b. Ask client to perform hand grasps by squeezing two fingers of examiner's hands and
  note degree of strength and bilateral equality; check upper extremity strength using
  palmar drift method by asking client to extend both arms forward with palms up and
  close eyes for 10 to 20 seconds (arms should stay steady with no downward drift)

  c. Ask client to do straight leg raises (to 90 degrees), one leg at a time, to determine
  lower extremity strength; alternatively, ask client to push one foot at a time
  against resistance of examiner's hand, often stated as "pushing your foot on the
  gas pedal of a car"

  d. For clients with a decreased level of consciousness, motor movement can be elicited
  by noxious stimuli such as pressure, pain, or suctioning; an attempt to push examiner's hand away is considered purposeful and is called *localizing*

F. **Assess sensory function to evaluate client's response to various stimuli; if client responds
to stimuli distally then it is not necessary to assess client's response to stimuli proximally;
client must describe location and stimulus; do not ask client if a pinprick is felt as this may
suggest sensation to client; when testing for sensations do not go rapidly as multiple
sensations may be perceived as one sensation known as summation**

  1. Use a wisp of cotton and have client say when and where touch is felt; assess at ran-
  dom locations

  2. Assess client to discriminate between sharp and dull; using a sterile needle with one
  blunt end, alternate between sharp and dull stimuli over various parts of body; remember to have client state where touch was felt and whether it was sharp or dull

  3. Assess client's ability to discriminate temperature; using tubes filled with hot and
  cold water, alternate between two temperatures, touching various locations around
  body; have client state where touch was and whether it was hot or cold

  4. Assess client's ability to feel vibration by using a tuning fork: striking fork and placing it
  on bony body parts; client should say when and where tuning fork was felt

  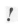 **5.** Evaluate client for stereognosis by having client identify an object placed in hand
  with eyes closed; repeat with a different object in opposite hand

  6. Assess client for graphesthesia to evaluate client's ability to perceive writing on skin;
  have client close eyes and use non-cotton end of cotton tipped applicator to write a
  number or letter on skin; repeat in different locations

  7. Evaluate client for extinction by touching bilaterally with client's eyes closed and asking him or her to state how many sensations there are and where they are felt

  8. Test client for ability to discriminate between two points (two-point discrimination)
  by using non-cotton ends of two cotton-tipped applicators to determine shortest distance between tips that client can feel

  9. Evaluate client for topognosis by having client close eyes and having him or her
  identify part of body touched

  10. Assess client for kinesthesia by having client close eyes while nurse moves a finger or
  big toe up; ask client whether extremity was moved up or down

G. **Assess deep tendon reflexes; have client sit unless his or her physical condition necessitates a
supine position; if client must assume supine position then muscle should be partially extended;
using reflex hammer requires skill—use wrist to elicit reflex, not hand or arm; if reflex not
elicited then client should relax muscle or be distracted so nurse can try again to elicit reflex**

  1. Begin by eliciting bicep's reflex by supporting client's lower arm with nurse's non-
  dominant hand; client's arm needs to be flexed at elbow with palm up; nurse places

thumb of non-dominant hand over bicep tendon and strikes thumb with reflex hammer and muscle should contract

2. Test tricep's reflex by supporting elbow in non-dominant hand and with nurse's dominant hand striking tricep's tendon with reflex hammer; tricep muscle should contract

3. Test brachioradialis reflex by positioning arm on client's lap with elbow flexed and hand resting on lateral side of palm; strike tendon with reflex hammer and observe flexion of arm and supination of hand

4. Assess patellar reflex by locating patella and striking tendon with flat end of reflex hammer; observe for extension of quadriceps muscle

5. Elicit Achilles' tendon reflex by flexing leg at knee and dorsiflexing foot of leg being examined; strike Achilles' tendon with flat end of reflex hammer; should cause plantar flexion of foot

6. Test superficial reflex of abdomen by using handle of reflex hammer or wooden end of cotton-tipped applicator and stroking abdomen

7. In male clients, nurse may elicit cremasteric reflex by stroking inner thigh and observing for elevation of testis on the same (ipsilateral) side

8. Elicit plantar reflex by positioning leg with external rotation of hip and stimulating sole of bottom of foot with stainless steel aspect of hammer and observing for flexion of toes

9. Assess for **Babinski reflex** by using stainless steel end of reflex hammer and stimulating sole of foot from heel to toes and across pad of foot; observe client for fanning of toes

VI. EXPECTED FINDINGS

A. During mental status examination, client should be awake, alert, and oriented

1. Client should have intact memory and appropriate judgment

2. Client should be able to perform simple mathematical calculations and define simple words

3. Abstract thought and reasoning should be logical and relevant; client should be living in reality

4. In order to increase safety the client should have good judgment

B. Cranial nerves should be intact

1. When testing olfactory nerve, client should be able to smell and identify a familiar scent, such as coffee or cinnamon, bilaterally

2. Optic nerve is intact when client is able to read Snellen eye chart or newspaper; optic disk should not be edematous

3. When testing oculomotor, trochlear, or abducens nerve, anticipate that client can elevate or laterally move eye as well as moving eye downward; pupils should directly and consensually react to light; pupils should constrict when tested for accommodation

4. During assessment of CN V, client should feel a touch with a wisp of cotton to his or her face; when cornea is touched with a wisp of cotton, client should blink; motor function of seventh cranial nerve should be checked as well as corneal reflex; when face is touched with a wisp of cotton, client should feel it

5. Expect client to be able to smile, frown, show and clench teeth, close eyes, puff cheeks, and raise eyebrows when checking seventh cranial nerve

6. Client should be able to lateralize sound when checking acoustic nerve; air conduction should be heard longer then bone; when performing the Romberg test, expect client to maintain balance

7. Assessment of glossopharyngeal and vagus nerves should reveal intact gag reflex; uvula should elevate when client says "ah"

8. When evaluating spinal accessory nerve, client should be able to elevate shoulders and resist against nurse when testing for muscle strength

Practice to Pass

What equipment does the nurse need to evaluate a client's vision?

Practice to Pass

When evaluating the client for Bell's palsy, what would the nurse ask the client to do to test CN VII?

Table 8-5	Rating	Interpretation
The Reflex Response Scale	0	No response
	1	Diminished
	2	Normal
	3	Brisk
	4	Hyperactive

9. Hypoglossal nerve assessment reveals that client is able to protrude and retract tongue; client should be able to keep tongue in cheek when nurse pushes on cheek

C. **Motor function of client should be intact to reflect intact cerebellum**
   1. Client should be able to walk across floor effortlessly in a coordinated manner; client should be able to walk heel to toe as well as walking on heels
   2. When evaluating finger to nose test, client should be able to smoothly touch nose with eyes closed easily; rhythmic alternating movement should be smooth and effortless; result should be same for heel to shin test

D. **Sensory function nerves should be intact**
   1. During sensory assessment client should be able to feel every time he or she is touched
   2. Client should be able to differentiate between sharp and dull as well as hot and cold
   3. Vibration should be discernible
   4. During assessment of stereognosis client should be able to identify an object without seeing it
   5. Position of body part should be perceivable at all times
   6. Client should be able to perceive a character drawn on skin with applicator
   7. Two-point discrimination should be within following limits: fingertips 0.3–0.6 cm; hands and feet 1.5–2 cm; lower leg 4 cm
   8. A client should be able to perceive touch bilaterally when a stimulus is applied to a point on both sides of body at one time

E. **Reflex activity is an involuntary activity that is always present in the absence of disease (see Table 8-5)**
   1. Normal response when bicep reflex is elicited is contraction of bicep and flexion of forearm
   2. Expected response to tricep reflex is extension of lower arm with contraction of tricep muscle
   3. During assessment of brachioradialis reflex, expect client to flex lower arm and supinate hand
   4. Patellar reflex produces extension of leg when elicited
   5. During assessment of Achilles' tendon client will flex foot if reflex is intact
   6. Expected adult finding when assessing plantar reflex is to observe curling of toes
   7. When evaluating abdominal reflex abdominal muscle will contract
   8. Cremasteric reflex is tested on males; expected response is that testis will elevate on the same side as the thigh that is stroked (ipsilateral response)
   9. Adult client should not fan toes while being assessed for Babinski reflex

VII. UNEXPECTED FINDINGS

A. **Unexpected findings during evaluation of a client's mental status is a client who has changes ranging from disorientation to unresponsive**
   1. Clients unable to properly groom themselves and care for hygienic needs may be experiencing physical decline or psychiatric illness such as schizophrenia or organic brain syndrome; depression may cause client to have poor posture and body language that does not agree with client's verbal expression

Practice to Pass

True or False—The client can hold a muscle still when the nurse is eliciting a reflex response.

Practice to Pass

Should the nurse assess the Babinski reflex during every assessment?

2. Neurological dysfunction may cause client to have a decreased level of consciousness; examples of dysfunction that cause decreased level of consciousness include cerebrovascular accident, diabetic ketoacidosis, hypoglycemia, and head injury; unresponsive clients may posture (see Figure 8-2 and Table 8-6); spinal cord injury can lead to varying patterns of paralysis (see Table 8-7)

3. Memory, ability to perform mathematical equations, and ability to define vocabulary should remain intact; if client is experiencing decline in intellectual ability or memory, then this may indicate organic brain dysfunction or damage to cerebral cortex

4. If client is unable to think abstractly or does not have a stable mood or emotional status, then client may be experiencing a psychiatric disorder such as depression or schizophrenia; these conditions may manifest a lack of congruence between facial expression and tone of voice with content of conversation

5. Hallucinations, lack of judgment, altered perceptions, and illogical thought may cause clinical manifestations of fever, psychiatric illness, and neurological dysfunction

B. **Abnormal findings associated with cranial nerves include head trauma and intracranial lesions**

1. Client unable to identify familiar smells when olfactory nerve is tested may be experiencing **anosmia** (lack of smell as a result of cranial nerve dysfunction), sinusitis, brain lesion, infection, allergic rhinitis, smoking, cocaine use, or complications of surgical procedure

2. A functional deficiency of the optic nerve may result from neuritis, a brain tumor, or intracranial hemorrhage; optic atrophy will lead to changes in shape and color of disk; swelling of optic disk, known as **papilledema**, signifies intracranial hemorrhage or tumor; if optic nerve is damaged the client may experience **diplopia**, also known as double vision

3. If third, fourth, and sixth cranial nerves are damaged, client may be experiencing myasthenia gravis or brain stem disorder; **nystagmus** is oscillation of eyes, which may be a manifestation of either cerebellar disease or a deficiency in the vestibular system

!

Practice to Pass

What is the medical term for edema of the optic disk?

Figure 8-2	GLASGOW COMA SCALE
Glasgow Coma Scale	**BEST EYE-OPENING RESPONSE** 4 = Spontaneously 3 = To speech 2 = To pain 1 = No response **(Record "C" if eyes closed by swelling)**
	BEST MOTOR RESPONSE to painful stimuli 6 = Obeys verbal command 5 = Localizes pain 4 = Flexion—withdrawal 3 = Flexion—abnormal 2 = Extension—abnormal 1 = No response **(Record best upper limb response)**
	BEST VERBAL RESPONSE 5 = Oriented × 3 4 = Conversation—confused 3 = Speech—inappropriate 2 = Sounds—incomprehensible 1 = No response **(Record "E" if endotracheal tube in place, "T" if tracheostomy tube in place)**

Table 8-6	Posture	Description	Etiology
Abnormal Posturing	Decorticate	Flexion of arms, wrist, and fingers Extension of lower extremities and plantar flexion	Cerebral cortex lesion
	Decerebrate	Upper extremities extended with internal rotation of wrist, palms pronated	Brainstem lesion
	Opisthotonos	Arching of back, heels, and head bent backwards	Meningitis

Table 8-7	Injury	Description
Spinal Injuries	Paraplegia	Complete loss of muscle tone and reflex activity initially below the level of injury in the lower extremities. Reflex activity returns and is usually hyperactive.
	Tetraplegia	Complete loss of muscle tone and reflex activity below the level of injury involves upper and lower extremities.
	Hemiplegia	Incomplete loss of muscle tone due to lesion of brain or spinal cord.

4. During assessment of trigeminal nerve, it is abnormal to have unequal strength bilaterally, asymmetry, or pain when moving face; if client does not have sensation or blink when corneal reflex is assessed, then client may have a lesion on trigeminal nerve

5. Muscle weakness observed upon assessment of cranial nerve VII may be indicative of Bell's palsy, nerve damage, or cerebrovascular accident; most common abnormal findings are sagging of eyelids, loss of nasolabial fold, and asymmetry of cheeks

6. Most common abnormal findings associated with acoustic nerve include **tinnitus** (ringing in ear associated with cochlear disturbance or dysfunction), deafness, and **vertigo** (dizziness, often severe, related to alterations of vestibular apparatus in the ear); if nerve is damaged then client may also experience equilibrium and balance issues

7. Glossopharyngeal and vagus nerve damage may cause client to experience a weak voice, **dysphagia** (difficulty swallowing), and an increased risk of aspiration due to poor gag reflex

8. Damage to spinal accessory nerve may result in muscle atrophy or weakness

9. When hypoglossal nerve is damaged, client will experience muscle atrophy, weakness, or fasciculations; tongue will deviate to side of lesion

C. **Motor system abnormalities are due to dysfunctions of cerebellum**

1. Difficulty with gait could be indicative of alcohol intoxication or a lesion between brain and periphery (see Table 8-8)

2. Abnormal findings associated with cerebellar disease include difficulty with gait; a positive Romberg's test means that body is swaying when eyes are closed; if client is unable to maintain balance when eyes are closed, protect client from falling

3. When testing for rapid alternating movement or coordination, abnormal findings include lack of coordination as evidenced in cerebellar disease

4. When evaluating client's coordination with finger to nose test, the term associated with overestimating examiner's finger is *dysmetria*; when client is reaching for the nurse's finger and deviates to one side it is known as *past pointing*; dysmetria and past pointing are related to cerebellar dysfunction; if heel falls off shin this is also a sign of lack of coordination

D. **Sensory system abnormalities may be due to disrupted integrity of peripheral nerve fibers, sensory tracts, and cortical functioning**

1. Client should be able to determine difference between sharp or dull, and discriminate pain; abnormal findings include increased or decreased sensations of any type (see Table 8-9 for corresponding terms)

2. When assessing for sensation, client should feel vibration; if client is unable to feel vibration it may be due to diabetes, peripheral neuropathy, or alcoholism

Practice to Pass

How would the nurse evaluate for cerebellar disease?

Table 8-8	Common Muscle Description	Etiology	Abnormalities
Motor Function Abnormalities	Atrophy	Small muscle that appears wasted	Disuse, polio, neuropathy, injury, lower motor lesions
	Hypertrophy	Increased muscle size	Exercise
	Paresis	Decreased strength	Lesions
	Pain	Discomfort	Strain, sprain
	Flaccidity	Hypotonicity	Cerebrovascular accident (CVA), muscular dystrophy (MD), spinal cord injury (SCI)
	Spasticity	Increased muscle contraction	SCI
	Rigidity	Resistance to movement	Parkinson's disease
	Cogwheel rigidity	Resistance to movement that eases into a jerk like motion	Parkinson's disease
	Tic	Twitching	Tardive dyskinesia
	Fasciculation	Rapid twitching of resting muscle	Lower motor neuron dysfunction
	Paralysis	Lack of motor function	Trauma, SCI, CVA, MD, diabetes mellitus (DM), multiple sclerosis (MS), myasthenia gravis
	Tremor	Involuntary contractions	Parkinson's disease, MS

Table 8-9	Pain or Sensation Term	Definition
Sensory Function Abnormalities	Hypalgesia	Decreased pain sensation
	Hyperalgesia	Increased pain sensation
	Analgesia	Without pain sensation
	Hypoesthesia	Decreased touch sensation
	Hyperesthesia	Increased touch sensation
	Anesthesia	Without touch sensation

3. Client should have position sense and tactile discrimination; absence of one or both is likely due to a lesion of sensory cortex or posterior column; *akinesthesia* is the term used to describe lack of position sense; *astereognosis* is the term used to describe inability to correctly identify objects with eyes closed
4. Clients should be able to feel two points when testing for two-point discrimination; increase in distance necessary to feel two points indicates there may be a sensory cortex lesion

E. **Reflex abnormalities may indicate dysfunction of cerebral cortex or residual damage from spinal cord injury**
   1. When eliciting reflexes it is abnormal to elicit areflexia, hyporeflexia, or hyperreflexia (see Table 8-10)
   2. Etiology of abnormal reflex activity is spinal cord injury, neuromuscular disease, or lower motor neuron disease (see Tables 8-11 for abnormal reflexes, 8-12 for gait disturbances, 8-13 for neurological infections, and 8-14 for neurological disorders that can affect reflex activity)

Table 8-10	Abnormal Reflex Activity	Definition	Etiology
Types of Abnormal Reflex Activity	Clonus	Jerky muscle contraction	SCI, seizure
	Hyporeflexia	Absence of reflex activity	SCI
	Hyperreflexia	Increased reflex activity	CVA
	Areflexia	No reflex activity	SCI

Table 8-11	Reflex	Assessment	Abnormal Response	Etiology
Abnormal Reflexes	Babinski	Stroke sole of foot with stainless steel end of reflex hammer	Extension of large toe, fanning of last four toes	Spinal injury, infection
	Brudzinski	Flex chin to neck and observe knees and hips	Pain in neck Flexion of hips and knees	Spinal injury or infection
	Kernig	Perform straight leg raise for the client or flex thigh and attempt to straighten	Pain or resistance to straightening Pain down leg	Meningeal irritation

Table 8-12	Gait Disturbances	Description	Etiology
Types of Gait Disturbances	Ataxia	Wide base with slapping of feet and swaying	Multiple sclerosis (MS), cerebellar tumor, alcohol intoxication
	Steppage	foot slapping, lifting knee as though to climb steps	Spinal cord injury (SCI), polio, muscular dystrophy (MD), peripheral neuropathy
	Scissors	Knees are touching during walking, takes great effort to walk	MS, paraparesis (weakness of lower extremities)
	Festinating	Short shuffling steps with stooped posture, turns stiffly while holding body rigidly	Parkinson's disease

Table 8-13	Infection	Description	Etiology
Infections of the Neurological System	Meningitis	Viral or bacterial infection of brain coverings	Gunshot wound, fractured skull, respiratory infection, infection from neurological surgery
	Encephalitis	Inflammation of brain	Sequelae of viral infection, usually childhood viruses (i.e., chickenpox)
	Brain abscess	Accumulation of pus around brain from systemic infection	Gunshot wound, skull fracture
	Myelitis	Infection of the spinal cord	Polio, herpes, measles, gonorrhea

Table 8-14	Disorders	Description	Etiology
Neurological Disorders	Alzheimer's disease	Progressive degenerative disease of brain that results in dementia	Unknown
	Cerebral palsy	Neuromuscular damage due to hypoxia at birth, developmental defect, or infection	Hypoxia, trauma
	Multiple sclerosis	Degeneration of the myelin sheaths	Unknown
	Muscular dystrophy	Progressive weakness of skeletal muscle	Unknown; results in death
	Myasthenia gravis	Chronic weakness with exertion	Unknown
	Parkinson's disease	Degeneration of white matter of cerebellum	Unknown

VIII. LIFESPAN CONSIDERATIONS

A. Infants

1. Infant will be born very alert followed by period of recovery from birth process; baby should have loud, robust cry; if cry is shrill-like then this may signify central nervous system damage

2. Assess infants for motor activity by observing movement; any abnormal muscle movement may be indicative of mental retardation, cerebral palsy, or peripheral neuromuscular dysfunction such as brachial plexus palsy

3. By age six months infant should have head control; an infant who does not have control is considered to have developmental delay; assess head control by placing infant supine and pulling up by wrists while observing for head control; head should be midline; head lag is not normal

4. Evaluate Landau reflex until age 18 months by holding infant prone; newborn will hold head at 45 degrees and flex elbows and knees; after age three months, infant will raise head and arch back; if reflex not present then infant may have mental retardation or motor weakness

5. Sensory assessment not usually performed on infant; infant will respond to pain by crying

6. Assess infant for rooting, Moro, grasp, sucking, Babinski, plantar grasp, stepping, placing, and tonic neck "fencing" reflexes

   a. Assess rooting reflex by stroking face near mouth and infant will turn head to stimuli; reflex lasts three to four months

   b. Elicit Moro reflex by startling infant by making a noise or gently shaking layette while observing infant; infant should look as though it is clinging; arms and legs are extended and abducted; reflex lasts about four months

   c. Grasp is a reflex seen when nurse places finger in hands of infant and infant holds onto nurse's finger; reflex disappears by age four months; absence may indicate brain damage or muscle or nerve damage; if reflex persists longer than four months then infant may have a cerebral lesion

   d. Sucking reflex is seen until one year of age and is evaluated by placing gloved finger near mouth and infant will suck

   e. Babinski reflex is normal until two years of age; assess reflex by stroking sole of foot from heel to toes and observing fanning of toes

   f. Demonstrate stepping reflex by holding infant under arms and placing feet on flat surface; normal response is walking motions and should disappear by the time child is ready to walk; it is abnormal to see crossing of legs

   g. Observe placing reflex by holding infant under arms and placing top of foot on underside of table; child should flex hip and knee to step onto table

   h. To elicit tonic neck "fencing" reflex place baby supine with head turned over a shoulder; arm and leg on same side as turned head will extend whereas opposite extremities will flex

B. Children

1. Children will perceive neurological exam as a game; child will take pride in showing what he or she can do

2. Most of motor system can be assessed by observing child playing; muscular dystrophy may be etiology of abnormal muscle development and strength

3. Coordination and sensation should be intact

4. Deep tendon reflexes are not tested due to lack of relaxation of muscles in children; reflex hammer is not used to elicit reflexes but rather examiner's finger

C. Adults

1. Adults are usually cooperative

2. Assessment may need to be timed to permit client participation without fatiguing the client

D. Older adults

1. Due to normal changes associated with aging, an older client may have slower response time

2. Gait and movement may be more deliberate and it may deviate slightly from a midline path

3. Sensation may be decreased; this may be noted as normal as long as it is bilaterally symmetrical; thus an older adult may need greater stimuli for light touch

4. Deep tendon reflexes may be absent or less brisk due to aging and inability of older adults to relax their muscles; plantar reflex may be absent or difficult to interpret, although a definite extensor response should still be considered abnormal
5. Although cranial nerves may not be tested often, taste and smell may show a declining function

IX. DOCUMENTATION

A. **Adult assessment documentation includes mental status, cranial nerves, motor and sensory functioning, and reflex activity**
B. **Mental status includes appearance, behavior, speech, orientation, recent and remote memory, judgment, and reasoning**
C. **Cranial nerve assessment is documented only when deficit is suspected; pupillary response is usually documented even if no deficits are noted**
D. **Motor and sensory functioning is documented next, with reflex activity documented last**

Case Study

A 40-year-old male client was admitted to the hospital for significant weakness, which has gotten worse over the last year. The client attributed the symptoms to the long working hours required as part of his job (chief executive officer of a health system). When the symptoms first started, the client would resolve with rest so he thought the symptoms were due to fatigue. Recently the client has had vision changes and difficulty urinating. The nurse has performed an assessment and obtained the following data: weakness that has been getting worse, tremors, fatigue, slowed speech, unsteady gait, blurred vision, and numbness.

1. The nurse would develop a plan of care for which priority nursing diagnosis?

2. What nursing interventions are essential for the nurse to identify?

3. In addition to the neurological assessment what other assessments should the nurse complete?

4. What information should the nurse document as subjective?

5. The nurse should conclude that the client would need what diagnostic testing to confirm a medical diagnosis?

For suggested responses, see pages 309–310

POSTTEST

POSTTEST

1 To test the seventh cranial nerve, what is the most appropriate assessment for the nurse to conduct?

1. Direct and consensual pupillary reaction to light
2. Corneal reflex by touching cornea with wisp of cotton
3. Vision by using Snellen eye chart
4. Having the client smile and clench teeth

2 The nurse would use which assessments to evaluate the vestibulocochlear nerve? Select all that apply.

1. Weber test
2. Rinne test
3. Caloric test
4. Romberg test
5. Achilles' reflex test

3 To evaluate topognosis, the nurse would use which procedure when assessing the client?

1. Reposition the client's toe and ask him or her to state what body part was moved and where it was moved
2. Touch the client and ask what body part was touched
3. Use ends of two cotton tipped applicators and touch the client's skin to determine distance between objects that client can feel
4. Ask the client to identify what object was placed in his or her hand

4 The nurse is unable to elicit a patellar reflex. What action should the nurse take next to try to test this reflex?

1. Have client lie on left side
2. Reposition the client
3. Use distraction to facilitate relaxation in the client
4. Take no action; document that the patellar reflex is unable to be elicited

5 The nurse needs to evaluate the client's level of consciousness. What is the most appropriate approach for the nurse to use for this assessment?

1. Ask the client to state his or her name, where he or she is, and what time it is
2. Test the client's memory
3. Use Glasgow Coma Scale
4. Evaluate all cranial nerves

6 The nurse is performing an evaluation of a 20-year-old client's gait and balance. The client is unable to walk heel to toe without swaying. The nurse should further evaluate the client for which problem?

1. Muscle atrophy
2. Alcohol intoxication
3. Paralysis of cranial nerve VII
4. Cranial nerve V dysfunction

7 The client reports an inability to move his or her tongue. What is the most appropriate action for the nurse to take?

1. Test the hypoglossal nerve
2. Evaluate function of the facial nerve
3. Test for sensory function
4. Prepare the client for a computed tomography (CT) scan

8 To examine the oculomotor nerve, the nurse would use which assessment technique?

1. Assess six cardinal fields of gaze
2. Use a Snellen eye chart
3. Touch cornea with a wisp of cotton
4. Touch face with a wisp of cotton

9 The client presents with the inability to move his or her right arm. The nurse should have the client demonstrate the ability to do which of the following?

1. Discern sensation
2. Determine two-point discrimination on face and neck
3. Protrude the tongue
4. Shrug the shoulders and turn the head

10 The nurse has just assessed a client who has a Glasgow Coma Scale score of 7. The nurse should conclude that this client has which status?

1. Awake, alert, and oriented
2. Arousable
3. Unresponsive
4. Coming out of anesthesia

➤ *See pages 162–164 for Answers and Rationales.*

ANSWERS & RATIONALES

Pretest

1 Answer: 1 Rationale: Explaining to the husband that his wife's behavior is the result of damage to the frontal lobe serves two purposes because it provides information and also answers his question (option 1). Option 2 is not truthful, as the behavior is due to the location of the injury in the brain, not pain. Sedatives are usually contraindicated until all baseline assessments are completed so neurological response is not depressed (option 3). Focusing on the cursing is not therapeutic and is inappropriate (option 4). Cognitive Level: Analysis Client Need: Physiological Integrity: Physiological Adaptation Integrated Process: Communication and Documentation Content Area: Adult

Health: Neurological **Strategy:** Recall that the frontal lobe is located in the cerebrum and controls movement, speech, emotions, intellectual activity, learning, judgment, reasoning, and concern for others. **Reference:** D'Amico, D. & Barbarito, C. (2007). *Health & physical assessment in nursing.* Upper Saddle River, NJ: Pearson Education, Inc., p. 732.

2 **Answer: 2** **Rationale:** The cerebellum is the area of the brain that controls balance (option 1). Intellectual functioning is controlled by the frontal lobe. Testing the ability to remember number sequences evaluates memory and not intellect (option 1). Two-point discrimination is used to evaluate sensation (option 3). Visual disorders do not have as much influence on balance as do the auditory, neurological, and musculoskeletal systems (option 4).
Cognitive Level: Analysis **Client Need:** Health Promotion and Maintenance **Integrated Process:** Physiological Integrity: Reduction in Risk Potential **Content Area:** Adult Health: Neurological **Strategy:** Recall that the cerebellum is the area of the brain that controls balance and coordination; therefore, assessments of gross motor function and muscle strength are indicated. **Reference:** D'Amico, D. & Barbarito, C. (2007). *Health & physical assessment in nursing.* Upper Saddle River, NJ: Pearson Education, Inc., pp. 732, 745, 758.

3 **Answer: 3** **Rationale:** Vertigo is a sensation of the room spinning, usually due to vestibular problems (option 3). Orthostatic hypotension is low blood pressure that occurs when a client moves from a sitting or lying position to a standing position (option 1). Diplopia is double vision and has no association with dizziness (option 2). Bradycardia may produce lightheadedness and dizziness but is due to decreased heart rate (option 4).
Cognitive Level: Application **Client Need:** Health Promotion and Maintenance **Integrated Process:** Communication and Documentation **Content Area:** Adult Health: Neurological **Strategy:** Recall that vertigo, dizziness, and lightheadedness are evaluated by the Romberg test and cranial nerve VIII. **Reference:** D'Amico, D. & Barbarito, C. (2007). *Health & physical assessment in nursing.* Upper Saddle River, NJ: Pearson Education, Inc., p. 752.

4 **Answer: 4** **Rationale:** The Romberg test is considered positive when the client is unable to stand with feet together, arms at side, and eyes closed without losing his or her balance (option 4). The Rinne and Weber tests are used to test the eighth cranial nerve (options 1 and 2). A positive Babinski reflex is abnormal in clients over the age of two years (option 3). The Babinski reflex is elicited when the sole of the foot is stimulated and the toes fan.
Cognitive Level: Analysis **Client Need:** Health Promotion and Maintenance **Integrated Process:** Nursing Process: Evaluation **Content Area:** Adult Health: Neurological **Strategy:** Recognize that the Romberg test is always positive when the client is unable to maintain his or her

balance. **Reference:** D'Amico, D. & Barbarito, C. (2007). *Health & physical assessment in nursing.* Upper Saddle River, NJ: Pearson Education, Inc., p. 325.

5 **Answer: 2** **Rationale:** Stereognosis is the ability to correctly identify familiar objects placed in the hand with the eyes closed (option 2). Hyperesthesia is an increased pain sensation (option 1). Astereognosis is the inability to identify familiar objects placed in hands (option 3). Apraxia is the inability to perform a previously known task (option 4).
Cognitive Level: Application **Client Need:** Health Promotion and Maintenance **Integrated Process:** Communication and Documentation **Content Area:** Adult Health: Neurological **Strategy:** Note that astereognosis begins with the letter A and in medical terminology this usually means "without" or "absent." **Reference:** D'Amico, D. & Barbarito, C. (2007). *Health & physical assessment in nursing.* Upper Saddle River, NJ: Pearson Education, Inc., p. 764.

6 **Answer: 3** **Rationale:** The client may be experiencing a decreasing level of consciousness (option 3). Based on this data, the client is not oriented to place. The client should be awake, alert, and oriented. It is not essential that the nurse assess the cranial nerves because this assessment provides data primarily about the senses (option 1). Deep tendon reflexes should be intact unless the spinal cord is injured (option 2). The client does not need the assessment of problem solving ability as the client is not experiencing organic brain disease (option 4).
Cognitive Level: Analysis **Client Need:** Health Promotion and Maintenance **Integrated Process:** Nursing Process: Assessment **Content Area:** Adult Health: Neurological **Strategy:** Recall that if the client is lethargic and not oriented, he or she will not be able to respond to complex activities, so eliminate those options first. The client is experiencing a head injury, not a spinal cord injury, so eliminate that option next. **Reference:** D'Amico, D. & Barbarito, C. (2007). *Health & physical assessment in nursing.* Upper Saddle River, NJ: Pearson Education, Inc., p. 745.

7 **Answer: 4** **Rationale:** The normal response to eliciting the triceps reflex is extension of the arm (option 4). The other options are not responses to a test of the deep tendon reflex.
Cognitive Level: Application **Client Need:** Health Promotion and Maintenance **Integrated Process:** Teaching/Learning **Content Area:** Adult Health: Neurological **Strategy:** Recall that a positive deep tendon tricep reflex is extension of the forearm. Hypoactive reflexes are found when there is a lower motor neuron injury. Upper motor neuron injuries may cause hyperactive reflexes. **Reference:** D'Amico, D. & Barbarito, C. (2007). *Health & physical assessment in nursing.* Upper Saddle River, NJ: Pearson Education, Inc., p. 767.

8 **Answer: 3** **Rationale:** The nurse tests long-term memory loss by asking the client to respond to verifiable questions such as names and ages of family members, birth date, social security number, and work or educational background (option 3). Short-term memory is tested by asking the client to respond to questions about the last three days (option 1). Depression is evaluated by asking the client about feelings and hearing responses such as, "I am depressed" or "It is no use" (option 2). Emotional dysfunction is assessed by evaluating congruence between what the client is saying and the accompanying facial expression and tone of voice (option 4). **Cognitive Level:** Analysis **Client Need:** Health Promotion and Maintenance **Integrated Process:** Nursing Process: Assessment **Content Area:** Adult Health: Neurological **Strategy:** Long-term memory and short-term memory are opposites; so if you have to guess, remember the test taking strategy that when opposites appear in distracters, one of them has an increased likelihood of being the correct response. **Reference:** D'Amico, D. & Barbarito, C. (2007). *Health & physical assessment in nursing.* Upper Saddle River, NJ: Pearson Education, Inc., pp. 745–746.

9 **Answer: 2** **Rationale:** Anosmia is the inability to smell; therefore, having the client identify a familiar smell would be appropriate to test cranial nerve I (option 2). Having the client touch his or her nose with his or her eyes closed is a test of cerebellar function (option 1). Judgment is evaluated by asking the client to describe a course of action for a situation (option 3). The Snellen eye test evaluates cranial nerve II, the optic nerve (option 4). **Cognitive Level:** Application **Client Need:** Health Promotion and Maintenance **Integrated Process:** Nursing Process: Assessment **Content Area:** Adult Health: Neurological **Strategy:** Recall that assessment of the cranial nerves provides the nurse with information about the client's sensory or motor function. The inability to smell (anosmia) and impaired vision are both sensory problems, requiring a choice between those two options. Recall that the other options are not evaluated through the cranial nerves. **Reference:** D'Amico, D. & Barbarito, C. (2007). *Health & physical assessment in nursing.* Upper Saddle River, NJ: Pearson Education, Inc., pp. 745, 748, 759.

10 **Answer: 2, 4, 3, 1, 5** **Rationale:** To evaluate the patellar reflex, the nurse would wash his or her hands, position the client, palpate the patella, use distraction, and strike the patella with the reflex hammer. **Cognitive Level:** Analysis **Client Need:** Health Promotion and Maintenance **Integrated Process:** Nursing Process: Implementation **Content Area:** Adult Health: Neurological **Strategy:** Remember to wash hands first, position the client, perform the assessment, and (although it is not part of this question) document any procedure. **Reference:** D'Amico, D. & Barbarito, C. (2007). *Health & physical assessment in nursing.* Upper Saddle River, NJ: Pearson Education, Inc., pp. 768–769.

Posttest

1 **Answer: 4** **Rationale:** The seventh cranial nerve is the facial nerve and is evaluated by having the client smile, show the teeth, close both eyes and puff out the cheeks, frown, and elevate the eyebrows (option 4). There should be facial symmetry in muscle strength of the facial nerve. Option 1 tests pupillary reflex while option 3 tests vision. Option 2 tests the corneal reflex. **Cognitive Level:** Analysis **Client Need:** Health Promotion and Maintenance **Integrated Process:** Nursing Process: Assessment **Content Area:** Adult Health: Neurological **Strategy:** Recognize that options 1, 2, and 3 are all tests of the eye and option 4 is a test of the facial nerve. This answer is different from the rest; therefore, a test taking strategy would be to pick this answer. **Reference:** D'Amico, D. & Barbarito, C. (2007). *Health & physical assessment in nursing.* Upper Saddle River, NJ: Pearson Education, Inc., pp. 748–750.

2 **Answer: 1, 2, 3, 4** **Rationale:** The Weber test is a test that uses a tuning fork to evaluate if the client is able to determine lateralization of sound. The Rinne test compares bone to air conduction of sound using a tuning fork. The caloric test is an evaluation of the vestibular aspect of the vestibular portion of the nerve. The Romberg assesses equilibrium and coordination. The Achilles' reflex test is an evaluation of eliciting the deep tendon reflex with a hammer and does not evaluate the eighth cranial nerve (option 5). **Cognitive Level:** Application **Client Need:** Health Promotion and Maintenance **Integrated Process:** Nursing Process: Implementation **Content Area:** Adult Health: Neurological **Strategy:** Recognize that the first four options are tests of cranial nerves and the Achilles' reflex test is an evaluation of the deep tendon reflexes. Recall that deep tendon reflexes do not evaluate the eighth cranial nerve. **Reference:** D'Amico, D. & Barbarito, C. (2007). *Health & physical assessment in nursing.* Upper Saddle River, NJ: Pearson Education, Inc., p. 752.

3 **Answer: 2** **Rationale:** Topognosis is the ability of the client to identify an area of the body that has been touched (option 2). Repositioning the client's toe and asking the client to state what body part was moved and where it was moved is a test of position sense (option 1). Dermatome testing is two point discrimination to determine the distance between two points (option 3). Asking the client to identify what object was placed in his or her hand is a test of stereognosis (option 4). **Cognitive Level:** Application **Client Need:** Health Promotion and Maintenance **Integrated Process:** Nursing Process: Assessment **Content Area:** Adult Health: Neurological **Strategy:** Recall that testing for topognosis is a method to evaluate sensory or cortical disease. The client is asked to identify an area of the body that has been touched. The client should also be asked to point to what area of the body has been touched. **Reference:** D'Amico, D. &

Barbarito, C. (2007). *Health & physical assessment in nursing*. Upper Saddle River, NJ: Pearson Education, Inc., pp. 764–766.

4 **Answer: 3** **Rationale:** The use of distraction helps to facilitate eliciting the reflex (option 3). Repositioning the client or having the client lie on his or her left side will not facilitate obtaining the reflex (options 1 and 2). Documenting that the reflex is not able to be elicited is not appropriate until distraction is used or the Achilles' reflex is elicited (option 4). If the client has a reflex that is distal to the one that is not able to be obtained then the reflex pathways would be intact.
Cognitive Level: Application **Client Need:** Health Promotion and Maintenance **Integrated Process:** Nursing Process: Implementation **Content Area:** Adult Health: Neurological **Strategy:** Recall that relaxation is often needed to obtain reflex activity. The nurse may use any form of distraction. **Reference:** D'Amico, D. & Barbarito, C. (2007). *Health & physical assessment in nursing*. Upper Saddle River, NJ: Pearson Education, Inc., pp. 768–769.

5 **Answer: 3** **Rationale:** The Glasgow Coma Scale is used to evaluate the client's level of consciousness (option 3). The scale evaluates best eye opening, motor function, and verbal response. Having the client state his or her name, location, and time is a test of orientation (option 1). Testing the client's memory will provide information on organic brain disorders (option 2). Testing cranial nerves will provide information on sensory and motor function (option 4).
Cognitive Level: Application **Client Need:** Health Promotion and Maintenance **Integrated Process:** Nursing Process: Implementation **Content Area:** Adult Health: Neurological **Strategy:** The Glasgow Coma Scale provides information on the level of consciousness. The highest score the patient can obtain is 15 and the lowest is 3. A score of 7 or less indicates a coma state. The options involving memory or cranial nerves do not have any relation to the level of consciousness and can be eliminated.
Reference: D'Amico, D. & Barbarito, C. (2007). *Health & physical assessment in nursing*. Upper Saddle River, NJ: Pearson Education, Inc., p. 773.

6 **Answer: 2** **Rationale:** The client who is unable to walk heel to toe may be experiencing alcohol intoxication, motor neuron weakness, or muscle weakness (option 2). A client experiencing muscle atrophy would have decreased strength (option 1). Facial paralysis would be the result of paralysis of the seventh cranial nerve (option 3). Cranial nerve V dysfunction is impairment of the trigeminal nerve (option 4).
Cognitive Level: Analysis **Client Need:** Health Promotion and Maintenance **Integrated Process:** Nursing Process: Evaluation **Content Area:** Adult Health: Neurological **Strategy:** Motor function is evaluated by assessing gait and balance, the Romberg test, finger to nose test, rapid alternating action, and heel to shin test. **Reference:** D'Amico, D. & Barbarito, C. (2007). *Health & physical*

assessment in nursing. Upper Saddle River, NJ: Pearson Education, Inc., pp. 757–761.

7 **Answer: 1** **Rationale:** Movement of the tongue is controlled by the hypoglossal or cranial nerve XII (option 1). The facial nerve is assessed by puffing the cheek, raising the eyebrow, or clenching teeth (option 2). Sensory assessment does not provide information on motor function (option 3). A CT scan does not provide information on tongue movement (option 4).
Cognitive Level: Application **Client Need:** Health Promotion and Maintenance **Integrated Process:** Nursing Process: Assessment **Content Area:** Adult Health: Neurological **Strategy:** The assessment of the hypoglossal nerve would provide information on tongue movement. The client would be asked to stick out his or her tongue and to use the tongue to push against the inside of the cheek bilaterally to test for tongue strength. **Reference:** D'Amico, D. & Barbarito, C. (2007). *Health & physical assessment in nursing*. Upper Saddle River, NJ: Pearson Education, Inc., p. 756.

8 **Answer: 1** **Rationale:** The oculomotor nerve is evaluated by having the client move his or her eyes through the six cardinal fields of gaze (option 1). The Snellen eye chart tests vision (option 2). Touching the cornea and face with a wisp of cotton evaluates blink reflex and function of the trigeminal nerve (options 3 and 4).
Cognitive Level: Analysis **Client Need:** Health Promotion and Maintenance **Integrated Process:** Nursing Process: Implementation **Content Area:** Adult Health: Neurological **Strategy:** Recall that to evaluate the oculomotor nerve, the nurse would test the six cardinal fields by having the client move his or her eyes through all motions (up, down, and laterally). **Reference:** D'Amico, D. & Barbarito, C. (2007). *Health & physical assessment in nursing*. Upper Saddle River, NJ: Pearson Education, Inc., p. 748.

9 **Answer: 4** **Rationale:** The client should demonstrate the ability to shrug shoulders and turn his or her head (option 4). The inability to move the arm is a motor problem and not sensory (options 1 and 2). Protruding the tongue is a test of cranial nerve XII (option 3).
Cognitive Level: Analysis **Client Need:** Health Promotion and Maintenance **Integrated Process:** Nursing Process: Evaluation **Content Area:** Adult Health: Neurological **Strategy:** Recall that motor function of the arm and shoulder is evaluated by testing cranial nerve XII. The client should be able to shrug the shoulder, raise the arm, and turn the head. **Reference:** D'Amico, D. & Barbarito, C. (2007). *Health & physical assessment in nursing*. Upper Saddle River, NJ: Pearson Education, Inc., p. 756.

10 **Answer: 3** **Rationale:** The Glasgow Coma Scale measures best eye opening, best verbal, and best motor response. The minimum score that the client can obtain is a 3 and the maximal score is a 15. A score of 7 would indicate that the client is unresponsive (option 3). A higher score indicates that the client is awake, alert, and oriented (option 1). A client who is arousable (option 2) describes only the best eye opening part of the scale. The Glasgow Coma Scale does not reflect anesthesia recovery (option 4).

Cognitive Level: Analysis **Client Need:** Health Promotion and Maintenance **Integrated Process:** Nursing Process: Analysis **Content Area:** Adult Health: Neurological

Strategy: Recall that the Glasgow Coma Scale is an indicator of level of consciousness. The higher the score the more alert the client; a lower score indicates that the client is more unresponsive. **Reference:** D'Amico, D. & Barbarito, C. (2007). *Health & physical assessment in nursing.* Upper Saddle River, NJ: Pearson Education, Inc., p. 773.

References

Bickley, L. (2010). *Bates guide to physical examination and history taking* (10th ed.). Philadelphia: Lippincott Williams & Wilkins.

D'Amico, D. & Barbarito, C. (2007). *Health and physical assessment in nursing.* Upper Saddle River, NJ: Pearson Education, Inc., pp. 348–396.

Jarvis, C. (2008). *Physical examination and health assessment* (5th ed.). St. Louis, MO: Elsevier Saunders.

Zator-Estes, M. (2009). *Health assessment and physical examination* (4th ed.). Clifton Park, NY: Delmar Cengage Learning.

ANSWERS & RATIONALES

Musculoskeletal Assessment

9

Chapter Outline

Health History
Present Health History
Family History

Equipment, Preparation, and
  Positioning
Examination Techniques
Expected Findings

Unexpected Findings
Lifespan Considerations
Documentation

Objectives

➤ Discuss the assessment questions used during an assessment of
the musculoskeletal system.
➤ Describe the positioning and preparation of the client undergoing
assessment of the musculoskeletal system.
➤ Identify the techniques used during an assessment of the
musculoskeletal system.
➤ Describe normal and abnormal findings obtained from assessment
of the musculoskeletal system.
➤ Describe the variations found during a musculoskeletal system
assessment across the lifespan.

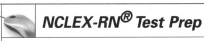

NCLEX-RN® Test Prep

Visit the Companion Website for this book
at www.pearsonhighered.com/hogan to
access additional practice opportunities
and more.

Review at a Glance

abduction moving a limb away from
the midline of the body
adduction moving a limb toward the
midline of the body
ballottement a technique to detect
fluid or floating body structures by displacing body fluid and palpating the
return impact on the body structure
dorsiflexion upward flexion of the
ankle so the superior aspect of the foot
moves toward the shin
eversion moving the sole of the foot
outward at the ankle
extension straightening a limb at
a joint

flexion bending a limb at a joint
fracture a partial or complete break
in a bone's continuity caused most often
by trauma
inversion moving the sole of the foot
inward at the ankle
joint a point in the body where two or
more bones meet
kyphosis an exaggerated thoracic dorsal curve that causes asymmetry between
the two sides of the posterior thorax
ligaments bands of flexible tissue
that attach bone to bone
lordosis an exaggerated lumbar
curve that compensates for conditions

such as pregnancy, obesity, or other
skeletal changes
opposition movement that involves
touching the thumb of a hand to any of
the fingertips of the same hand
plantar flexion movement (extension)
of the ankle by pointing the toes downward
rotation turning of a bone around its
own long axis
scoliosis lateral curvature of the spine
subluxation partial dislocation of
a joint
tendons tough fibrous bands that
attach either muscle to bone or muscle
to muscle

PRETEST

1 The nurse is obtaining a health assessment on a client who reports leg pain and inability to perform activities of daily living (ADLs). The nurse would ask which questions to obtain information about the client's ability to carry out ADLs? Select all that apply.

1. "Can you tell me how the pain is affecting your life?"
2. "Do you know what is causing the problem?"
3. "Does anyone in your family have any musculoskeletal problems?"
4. "Can you describe how your activity level has changed?"
5. "Can you tell me about your hobbies?"

2 To determine alleviating factors for symptoms of a musculoskeletal injury, it is essential that the nurse ask the client which question?

1. "When were you injured?"
2. "How were you injured?"
3. "Have you been able to carry out your regular activities?"
4. "Have you used over-the-counter medications?"

3 When performing an assessment of the client presenting with a musculoskeletal problem, which action should the nurse take first?

1. Palpate the area that is the source of the problem
2. Inspect the area of pain or inflammation
3. Assess range of motion to determine the extent of the area involved
4. Palpate the area to determine the presence of pulses and edema

4 What action would the nurse take to examine the temporomandibular joint?

1. Have the client open and close the mouth while palpating the joint in front of the tragus
2. Assess the function of cranial nerve II
3. Have the client shrug the shoulders and observe for symmetry
4. Have the client lift the arms and observe for symmetry

5 When testing range of motion of a client's shoulder, the nurse hears a grating sound. The nurse should document which of the following assessment findings?

1. Clicking
2. Crepitus
3. A strain
4. A sprain

6 The client reports shoulder pain without palpation or movement. The nurse should evaluate this client further for which health problem?

1. A strain
2. A sprain
3. A cardiac problem
4. A rotator cuff tear

7 The nurse has assessed the client's shoulder strength and finds that the client has full resistance and range of motion. The nurse should document this finding with which of the following ratings?

1. Normal (5)
2. Good (4)
3. Fair (3)
4. Poor (2)

8 To use a goniometer to measure a client's range of motion in the elbow, the nurse should take which action?

1. Place the joint in extension and then flex the joint as far as possible and measure
2. Place the joint in a neutral position, flex the joint as far as possible and measure, and then fully extend the joint as far as possible and measure
3. Flex the joint as far as possible and measure
4. Extend the joint as far as possible and measure

9 The nurse palpates a round, fluid-filled cyst on the dorsum of the wrist. The nurse interprets this finding as consistent which of the following?

1. Carpal tunnel syndrome
2. A ganglion
3. Rheumatoid arthritis
4. Crepitus

10 The nurse is assessing the client's knee for ballottement. After having the client lie supine with the leg in extension, the nurse should take which action?

1. Grasp the tibia and push fluid in the suprapatellar bursa to move between the tibia and patella
2. Grasp the tibia and push fluid in the suprapatellar bursa to move between the femur and patella
3. Grasp the tibia and push fluid in the suprapatellar bursa to move between the tibia and femur
4. Grasp the thigh above the knee and push fluid in the suprapatellar bursa to move between the femur and patella

➤ *See pages 185–187 for Answers and Rationales.*

I. HEALTH HISTORY

A. Obtain a description of client's general mobility

1. Today
2. Two months ago
3. Two years ago

B. Determine client's ability to carry out activities of daily living (ADLs) by asking about the following:

1. "Can you describe any changes in your activity level?"
2. "Do you have an idea about what is causing these changes?"
3. "What have you done about these changes until now?"
4. "How long have these changes been present?"
5. "Have you discussed these changes with a healthcare professional?"
6. "Do your joint/muscle/bone disorders put limits on your ability to do any of the following?
   a. Bathe self (get in or out of tub, turn on faucets)
   b. Toilet self (urinate or move bowels, get on or off toilet, wipe or cleanse self)
   c. Dress self (manipulate buttons and zippers, fasten openings behind neck, pull clothes over head, pull up pants or socks, tie shoes, get shoes that fit)
   d. Groom self (brush teeth, comb or brush hair, shave, apply makeup)
   e. Eat (prepare meals, pour liquids, cut up food, bring food to mouth, drink)
   f. Move purposefully in environment (walk, walk up or down stairs, get in or out of bed, get out of house)
   g. Communicate (talk, use phone, write)

C. Because some conditions predispose to musculoskeletal problems, determine presence of the following chronic health problems as well as their progression, treatments, and effects on ADLs

1. Diabetes mellitus
2. Hypothyroidism
3. Sickle cell anemia
4. Lupus erythematosus
5. Rheumatoid arthritis

D. Determine personal history of illness, infection, or injury to musculoskeletal system

1. Musculoskeletal illnesses or infections
   a. "When was the illness or infection diagnosed?"
   b. "What treatment was prescribed and how helpful was it?"
   c. "What other things did you do to help with the problem?"
   d. "Did the problem resolve (acute) or is it still present (chronic)?"
   e. "How are you managing the problem now (for chronic problems)?"

Table 9-1	Term for Injury	Definition
Terms for Musculoskeletal Trauma	Joint dislocation	Displacement of bone away from its normal position in a joint
	Muscle strain	Partial tear of a muscle caused by muscle overstretching or overuse
	Muscle sprain	Stretching or tearing of the capsule or ligament of a joint because of forced movement to the joint beyond the normal range of motion
	Bone fracture	Partial or complete break in the continuity of a bone

2. Musculoskeletal injuries
   a. "Have you ever had any **fractures** (break in continuity of a bone)? If so, can you tell me about when they occurred, the cause, their location, treatment, and any present problems with daily activities?"
   b. "Have you ever had any penetrating wounds, such as from a nail, sharp object, knife, or gunshot? If so, can you describe them?"
   c. Have you had other types of trauma to muscles or bone, such as joint dislocations or muscle strains or sprains?" (see Table 9-1)

II. PRESENT HEALTH HISTORY

Practice to Pass

A client visits the healthcare provider because of a problem with the left knee. What symptoms of common knee problems should the nurse assess for?

A. **Assess for current common symptoms of musculoskeletal problems**
   1. **Joints** (points in body where two or more bones meet)
      a. Pain
      b. Stiffness
      c. Swelling, heat, redness
      d. Limitation of movement
   2. Muscles
      a. Pain
      b. Cramping
      c. Weakness
   3. Bones
      a. Pain
      b. Deformity
      c. Trauma (fractures, sprains, dislocations)

B. **For each symptom, ask about the following:**
   1. Location
      a. "Where is it located?"
      b. "Is it on one side (unilateral) or both sides (bilateral)?"
   2. Quality
      a. "What does it feel like?" (Answers will often include aching, stiff, sharp, dull, or shooting)
      b. "Is it constant or intermittent?"
   3. Severity: "How strong is the symptom?" (often used for pain; use a rating scale of 1 to 10)
   4. Onset: "When did it start?"
   5. Timing
      a. "What time of day does it occur?"
      b. "How often does it occur?"
      c. "How long does it last?"
   6. Aggravating and alleviating factors
      a. "Is the symptom aggravated by movement, rest, specific position, or weather?"
      b. "Is the symptom relieved by rest, application of heat or cold, medications (prescribed or over-the-counter? If so, how often are these needed/used?"

III. FAMILY HISTORY

A. Determine family history of musculoskeletal problems, which may recur in other family members

B. Assess for the above by asking the following:

1. "What is the disease or health problem?"
2. "Who in the family has this problem?"
3. "When was this problem diagnosed?"
4. "What treatments have been used?"
5. "How effective have the treatments been?"

IV. EQUIPMENT, PREPARATION, AND POSITIONING

A. Equipment

1. Tape measure
2. Goniometer, to measure joint angles
3. Skin marking pen

B. Preparation and positioning

1. Make client comfortable, provide examination gown, and drape for full visualization of body part
2. Depending on the area being examined, client may be in a sitting or standing position
3. Joints: support the joint being examined at rest
4. Muscles: need to be in a position that allows them to be soft and relaxed for accurate assessment
5. Inflamed areas: use gentle movement and firm support, as well as gentle return to a relaxed state, to avoid causing pain and/or muscle spasm

Practice to Pass

The nurse is preparing to do a musculoskeletal exam on a client. What equipment does the nurse need and how should the client be prepared for the exam?

V. EXAMINATION TECHNIQUES

A. General information

1. Techniques include inspection, palpation, range of motion (ROM), and muscle testing; recall types of movements that are normal for each joint while conducting examination (see Table 9-2)
2. Inspect for overall appearance, posture, and position of client
3. Observe for deformities, inflammation, and immobility; inflammation and/or accompanying pain (acute problems) must be assessed first if present

B. Facial area

1. Inspect temporomandibular joints (TMJs) on both sides of face
2. Palpate TMJs (Figure 9-1)
   a. Place finger pads of index and middle fingers in front of tragus of ear
   b. Ask client to open and close his or her mouth while palpating TMJs
3. Palpate jaw muscles by asking client to clench teeth while palpating masseter and temporalis muscles
4. Test ROM of TMJs
   a. Ask client to open his or her mouth widely to determine that it opens with ease
   b. Next ask client to push out lower jaw (with mouth slightly open), move lower jaw side to side, and finally close mouth
   c. Repeat actions in *a.* and *b.* against opposing force or resistance to test for muscle strength and motor function of cranial nerve V, the trigeminal nerve

C. Shoulders

1. Inspection: with client facing examiner, compare shape and size of shoulders, clavicles, and scapula

Table 9-2 Joint Movement

Type of Movement

Gliding movements are the simplest type of joint movements. One flat bone surface glides or slips over another similar surface. The bones are merely displaced in relation to one another.

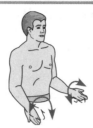
The terms **supination** and **pronation** refer only to the movements of the radius around the ulna. Movement of the forearm so that the palm faces anteriorly or superiorly is called *supination*. In *pronation*, the palm moves to face posteriorly or inferiorly.

Flexion is a bending movement that decreases the angle of the joint and brings the articulating bones closer together. **Extension** increases the angle between the articulating bones. (**Hyperextension** is a bending of a joint beyond 180 degrees.)

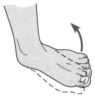
The terms **inversion** and **eversion** refer to movements of the foot. In *inversion,* the sole of the foot is turned medially. In *eversion,* the sole faces laterally.

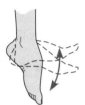
Flexion of the ankle so that the superior aspect of the foot approaches the shin is called **dorsiflexion**. Extension of the ankle (pointing the toes) is called **plantar flexion**.

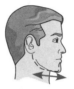
Protraction is a nonangular anterior movement in a transverse plane. **Retraction** is a nonangular posterior movement in a transverse plane.

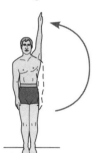
Abduction is movement of a limb away from the midline or median plane of the body, along the frontal plane. When the term is used to describe movement of the fingers or toes, it means spreading them apart. **Adduction** is the movement of a limb toward the body midline. Bringing the fingers close together is adduction.

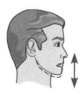
Elevation is a lifting or moving superiorly along a frontal plane. When the elevated part is moved downward to its original position, the movement is called **depression**. Shrugging the shoulders and chewing are examples of alternating elevation and depression.

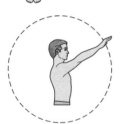
Circumduction is the movement in which the limb describes a cone in space: while the distal end of the limb moves in a circle, the joint itself moves only slightly in the joint cavity.

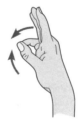
Oppostion *of the thumb* is only allowed at the saddle joint between metacarpal 1 and the carpals. It is the movement of touching the thumb to the tips of the other fingers of the same hand.

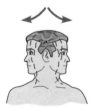
Rotation is the turning movement of a bone around its own long axis. Rotation may occur toward the body midline or away from it.

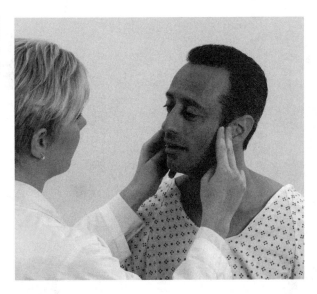

Figure 9-1

Palpation of the temporomandibular joints

2. Palpation of shoulders and surrounding areas
   a. Palpate at sternoclavicular joint and move laterally along clavicle joint to acromioclavicular joint
   b. Palpate downward into subacromial area and greater tubercle of humerus
3. Test range of motion of shoulders using both arms at same time
   a. Have client shrug shoulders by flexing them forward and upward
   b. With elbows extended, have client raise arms forward and upward in an arc
   c. Have client return arms to sides, and with elbows extended, move arms as far backward as possible
   d. Check internal **rotation** (turning of a bone around its own long axis) by placing back of client's hands as close as possible to scapulae (Figure 9-2A)
   e. Check external rotation by asking client to clasp his or her hands behind his or her head (Figure 9-2B)
   f. Ask client to swing his or her arms out to the sides in arcs, touching palms together above head
   g. Ask client to swing each arm toward body midline with elbows extended
4. Test shoulder muscle strength
   a. Repeat assessments in number 3 while providing opposing force (resistance)
   b. Rate muscle strength using the appropriate number in Table 9-3

D. Elbows
1. In turn, support each arm and inspect lateral and medial aspects of elbow
2. Palpate lateral and medial aspects of olecranon process using thumb and middle fingers to palpate grooves on either side of the olecranon process

Table 9-3

Muscle Strength Ratings

Rating	Description of Function	Classification
5	Full range of motion against gravity with full resistance	Normal
4	Full range of motion against gravity with moderate resistance	Good
3	Full range of motion with gravity	Fair
2	Full range of motion without gravity (passive motion)	Poor
1	Palpable muscle contraction but no movement	Trace
0	No muscle contraction	Zero

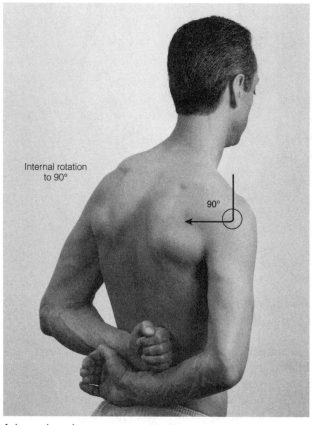

Internal rotation
to 90°

90°

A. Internal rotation

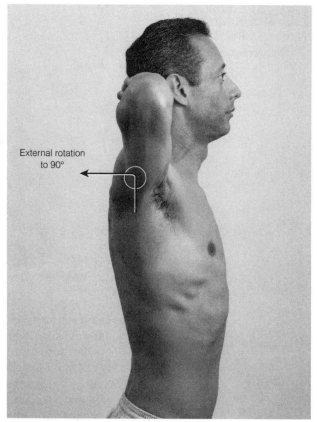

External rotation
to 90°

B. External rotation

Figure 9-2

Testing shoulder range of motion

3. Check range of motion of each elbow by instructing client to do the following:
   a. Bend elbow by bringing forearm forward and touching fingers to shoulder
   b. Straighten elbow
   c. To measure elbow range of motion using a goniometer, place joint in a neutral position, then flex joint as far as possible and measure angle with goniometer; repeat measurement after extending joint as far as possible and compare readings to expected findings (Figure 9-3)
   d. Hold arm straight out and turn palm upward facing ceiling, then downward facing floor
4. Test muscle strength
   a. Stabilize client's elbow with examiner's nondominant hand while holding wrist in dominant hand
   b. Ask client to flex and then extend elbow against resistance

E. **Wrists and hands**
   1. Inspect size, shape, symmetry, and color of wrists and dorsum of hands
   2. Inspect palms of hands
   3. Palpate wrists and hands for temperature and texture
   4. Palpate each joint of wrists and hands, keeping client's wrist straight, and noting temperature of hand at same time
      a. Move thumbs from side to side gently but firmly over dorsum of hand, with fingers resting under area being palpated
      b. To palpate interphalangeal joints, pinch them gently between thumb and index finger

Figure 9-3

Measuring joint range of
motion using a goniometer

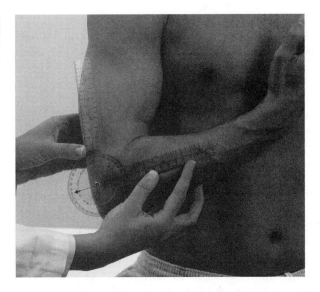

Figure 9-3

Measuring joint range of
motion using a goniometer

5. Test each wrist's range of motion by asking client to do each of the following:
   a. Straighten hand
   b. Using wrist as a pivot point, bring fingers backward as far as possible and then bend wrist downward as far as possible
   c. Turn palms down; move hand laterally toward fifth finger and then medially toward thumb; ensure that movement is from wrist and not elbow
   d. If carpal tunnel syndrome is suspected, test for Phelan's sign by having client bend his or her wrists downward and pressing backs of the hands together to cause **flexion** (bending a limb at a joint) of 90 degrees (Figure 9-4)
6. Test range of motion of hands and fingers by asking client to do the following:
   a. Make a tight fist with each hand with fingers folded into palm and thumb across knuckles (thumb flexion)
   b. Open fist and stretch fingers (**extension**, straightening a limb at a joint)
   c. Point fingers downward toward forearm, then back as far as able
   d. Spread fingers far apart and then together; move thumb toward ulnar side of hand and then away from hand to extent possible
   e. Touch thumb to tip of each finger and to base of little finger
7. Test muscle strength of each wrist
   a. Place client's arm on table with palm facing upward
   b. Stabilize forearm with one hand while holding client's hand with the other
   c. Ask client to flex his or her wrist while opposing resistance is applied

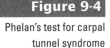

Figure 9-4

Phelan's test for carpal
tunnel syndrome

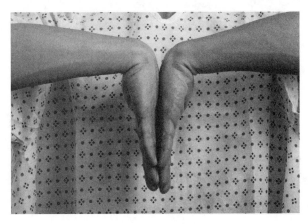

8. Test muscle strength of fingers
   a. Ask client to spread fingers and then try to force fingers together
   b. Ask client to touch little finger with thumb while examiner places resistance on thumb to prevent movement

F. Hips
   1. Inspect position of each hip with client lying supine
   2. Palpate each hip joint and upper thighs
   3. Test range of motion in hips by asking client to do the following:
   a. Raise each leg up from examining table or bed (while keeping the knee straight) one at a time, and return leg to its original position (Figure 9-5)
   b. Raise each leg, one at a time, with knee flexed toward chest as far as it will go
   c. Move foot away from midline as knee moves toward midline (internal hip rotation)
   d. Move foot toward midline as knee moves away from midline (external hip rotation)
   e. Move leg away from midline then as far as possible toward midline; **abduction** is the term used when a body part is moved away from body midline, and **adduction** is when a body part is moved toward body midline
   f. After client turns onto abdomen (or is sidelying), ask him or her to extend knees and then raise each leg backward and upward as far as possible; this may be assessed later during spine assessment with client standing
   4. Test muscle strength of hips by doing the following:
   a. Assist client back to a supine position
   b. Press examiner's hands on client's thighs and ask client to raise his or her hip
   c. Place hands outside client's knees and ask client to spread both legs against resistance
   d. Place hands between client's knees, and ask client to bring legs together against resistance

G. Knees
   1. Inspect knees with client in a sitting position

Figure 9-5

Hip flexion with straight leg raising

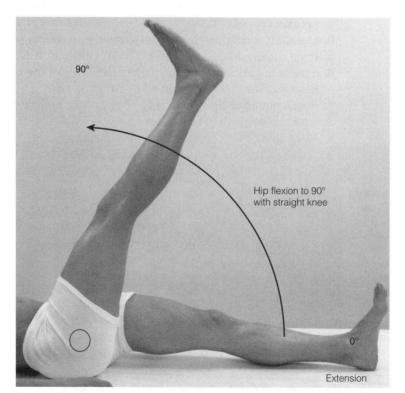

90°

Hip flexion to 90° with straight knee

0°

Extension

2. Inspect quadriceps muscle in anterior thigh for symmetry
3. Use thumb, index, and middle fingers to palpate about 10 cm above patella and then palpate downward to evaluate each area
4. Palpate tibiofemoral joint
   a. With client's knee in flexed position, use thumbs to palpate deeply along each side of tibia toward outer aspects of knee
   b. Next palpate along lateral collateral ligament
5. Test for bulge sign to detect presence of small amounts (4–8 mL) of fluid in supra-patellar bursa
   a. With client in supine position, first use firm pressure to stroke medial aspect of knee upward several times, displacing fluid
   b. Then apply pressure to lateral side of knee while observing medial side (Figure 9-6)
6. Perform **ballottement**
   a. This is used to detect large amounts of fluid or floating body structures by displacing body fluid and then palpating return impact on body structure
   b. Use fingers of left hand to quickly push patella downward against femur and note any movement (Figure 9-7)
7. Test range of motion of each knee by having client bend each knee against chest (flexion) as far as possible
8. Test for muscle strength by having client flex each knee while examiner applies opposing force; then have client extend each knee again
9. Inspect knee while client is standing; ask client to stand erect or hold onto back of chair if unsteady; then ask client to walk at a comfortable pace with a relaxed gait

H. Ankles and feet
1. Inspect ankles and feet while client is sitting, standing, and walking
2. Palpate ankles by grasping heels with fingers of both hands while palpating anterior and lateral aspects of ankle with thumbs
3. Palpate length of calcaneal (Achilles) tendon at posterior ankle
4. Palpate metatarsophalangeal joints just below ball of foot
5. Palpate deeply each metatarsophalangeal joint
6. Test range of motion of each ankle and foot by asking client to do the following:
   a. Point foot toward nose (**dorsiflexion**) and then toward floor (**plantar flexion**)
   b. Turn sole of the foot outward at ankle (**eversion**) and then inward (**inversion**)
   c. Curl toes downward (plantar flexion)
   d. Spread toes as far as possible (abduction) and then bring toes together (adduction)

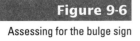

Figure 9-6

Assessing for the bulge sign

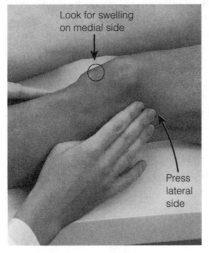

Look for swelling on medial side

Press lateral side

Figure 9-7

Assessing for ballottement

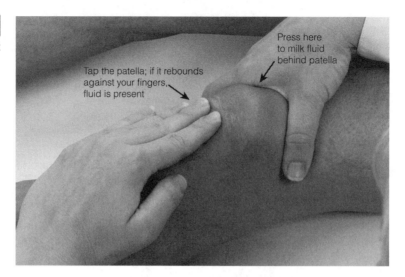

Tap the patella; if it rebounds against your fingers, fluid is present

Press here to milk fluid behind patella

7. Test muscle strength of ankle by asking client to dorsiflex and plantar flex against resistance
8. Test muscle strength of foot by asking client to flex and extend toes against resistance
9. Palpate each interphalangeal joint, also noting temperature of extremity

I. Spine

1. Inspect position and alignment of spine from all sides by walking around client's body with client in a standing position
   a. Observe for concave curve in cervical and lumbar areas, and convex curve in thoracic area
   b. Imagine a vertical line falling from level of thoracic vertebra 1 (T1) to gluteal cleft to confirm that spine is straight (Figure 9-8)
   c. Imagine a horizontal line across top of scapulae and observe whether they are level and symmetrical
   d. Check that heights of iliac crests and gluteal folds are level and symmetrical using a horizontal imaginary line
   e. Finally ask client to bend forward and assess alignment of vertebrae
2. Palpate each vertebral process with thumb
3. Palpate bilateral neck and back muscles
4. Assess range of motion of cervical spine by asking client to do the following:
   a. Touch chest with chin (flexion)
   b. Look upward toward ceiling (hyperextension)
   c. Try to touch each shoulder with ear on the same side, keeping shoulder level (lateral bending or lateral flexion)
   d. Turn head to face each shoulder to greatest extent possible (rotation)
5. Assess range of motion of thoracic and lumbar spine
   a. Sit or stand behind client, who is also standing; stabilize pelvis with examiner's hands and ask client to bend sideways to right and left; note degree of flexion
   b. Ask client to bend forward and touch toes (flexion) and observe whether concavity disappears with this movement and back then has a single C-shaped convexity
   c. Ask client to bend backward as far as comfortable to measure hyperextension
   d. Ask client to twist shoulders to left and right to measure rotation

Practice to Pass

The nurse is conducting a musculoskeletal assessment. What observations should the nurse expect in a healthy client during inspection and palpation of the hips?

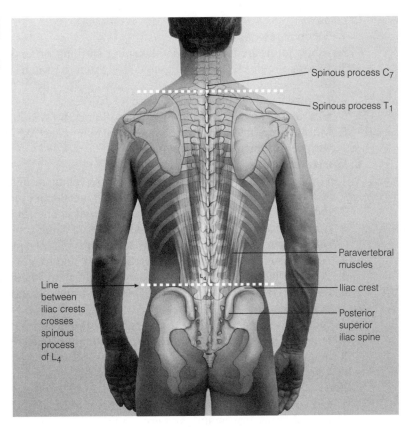

Figure 9-8

Determining posterior spine landmarks for assessment

Spinous process C7

Spinous process T1

Paravertebral muscles

Line between iliac crests crosses spinous process of L4

Iliac crest

Posterior superior iliac spine

VI. EXPECTED FINDINGS

A. Facial area

1. TMJs are symmetrical and without pain or swelling
2. During palpation, examiner's fingers should glide into shallow depression of TMJs
3. Motion of mandible is smooth
4. TMJ may click audibly and palpably as mouth opens and is a normal finding
5. Masseter and temporalis muscles are symmetrical, firm, and nontender
6. ROM of TMJ: mouth opens as much as 3–6 cm between upper and lower incisors, jaw protrudes and retracts with ease, jaw moves side to side 1–2 cm without deviation or dislocation, and mouth closes completely without pain or discomfort

B. Shoulders

1. Shoulders, clavicles, and scapulae are symmetrical and similar in size anteriorly and posteriorly
2. Shoulders and surrounding areas are firm and nontender; scapulae are level
3. Shoulders have forward flexion of 180 degrees and backward extension of up to 50 degrees
4. Internal rotation and external rotation should both be 90 degrees
5. Shoulder adduction is 180 degrees and abduction is as much as 50 degrees
6. Full resistance during shoulder shrug indicates adequate spinal accessory nerve (CN XI) function

C. Elbows
1. Elbows are symmetrical
2. Elbow joints are free of pain, thickening, swelling, or tenderness
3. Elbows can flex to 160 degrees and straighten to form a straight line with upper arm (0 degrees)
4. Elbows can supinate and pronate to 90 degrees
5. Elbows can go through full range of motion without difficulty or discomfort
6. Muscle strength during flexion and extension of each elbow is equal and is normal with or without applied resistance

D. Wrists and hands
1. Wrists and hands are symmetrical without swelling or deformity; ends of ulna or radius may protrude further in some individuals than others
2. Palm has a rounded protuberance over thenar eminence (proximal to thumb)
3. Color and temperature of wrists and hands are similar to rest of body (pink and warm); skin is smooth but may be rougher around interphalangeal joints
4. All wrist and hand joints are firm, nontender, and free of swelling
5. Wrist should hyperextend to 70 degrees and flex to 90 degrees
6. Ulnar deviation should be up to 55 degrees, while radial deviation should be up to 20 degrees
7. Client has no pain, numbness, or tingling with Phelan's sign
8. Fingers flex to 90 degrees and hyperextend up to 30 degrees
9. Fingers abduct to 20 degrees and adduct fully (to touch)
10. There is full resistance to wrist flexion and full muscle strength of fingers

E. Hips
1. Legs are slightly apart and toes should point toward ceiling in a lying position
2. Hip joints are firm, stable, and nontender
3. Hip flexion with straight knee should reach 90 degrees, and with flexed knee should reach 120 degrees
4. Internal hip rotation should reach 40 degrees and external hip rotation should reach 45 degrees
5. Abduction should reach 45 degrees and adduction should reach 30 degrees
6. Hips should hyperextend to 15 degrees

F. Knees
1. Patella is centrally located in each knee and normal depressions along each side of patella are sharp and distinct
2. Skin color is similar to surrounding areas
3. Quadriceps muscles are symmetrical
4. Quadriceps muscle and surrounding soft tissue are firm and nontender; suprapatellar bursa is often not palpable
5. Tibiofemoral joint is firm and nontender
6. No fluid is present normally with testing of bulge sign
7. Patella sits firmly over femur, with little or no movement with patellar pressure
8. Knee flexion is of normal strength and equal, even against resistance
9. Knees are in alignment with thighs and ankles when standing
10. Client can walk with a relaxed gait

G. Ankles and feet
1. Color and temperature of ankles and feet are similar to rest of body
2. Ankles and feet are symmetrical with no broken skin; feet are in alignment with long axis of lower leg; client's weight falls on middle of foot and no swelling is present
3. Ankle joints are firm, stable, and nontender
4. Calcaneal tendon is free of pain, tenderness, and nodules

5. Metatarsophalangeal joints are firm and nontender
6. Dorsiflexion reaches 20 degrees, while plantar flexion reaches 45 degrees
7. Ankle eversion is to 20 degrees while inversion is to 30 degrees
8. Client can perform dorsiflexion and plantar flexion, and toe flexion and extension against resistance

H. Spine

1. Cervical and lumbar curves are concave on inspection, and thoracic curve is convex
2. Spine is straight and heights of scapulae, iliac crests, and gluteal folds are level
3. Vertebral processes are aligned and uniform in size; they are firm, stable, and nontender
4. Neck muscles are fully developed, symmetrical, smooth, firm, and nontender
5. Client is able to complete flexion, hyperextension, lateral bending, and rotation of cervical spine
6. Right and left lateral flexion of lumbar spine should reach 35 degrees
7. With forward bending to touch toes, lumbar concavity disappears and single C-shaped curvature appears
8. Thoracic and lumber hyperextension by bending backwards should reach 30 degrees
9. Rotation of thoracic and lumbar spine by twisting shoulders to left and right should reach 30 degrees

VII. UNEXPECTED FINDINGS

A. Facial area

1. An enlarged or swollen TMJ appears as a rounded protuberance
2. Pain or discomfort in TMJ area, swelling, limited movement, or crackling sounds require further evaluation for TMJ syndrome or dental or neurological problems
3. Swelling and tenderness of masseter and temporalis muscles may indicate arthritis or myofascial pain syndrome

B. Shoulders

1. Swelling, deformity, atrophy, and misalignment of shoulders (especially when combined with limited motion, pain, and/or crepitus) suggest degenerative joint disease, trauma (strain or sprain), or inflammatory conditions (such as rheumatoid arthritis, bursitis, or tendonitis)
2. Shoulder pain without palpation or movement may result from insufficient circulation to myocardium, and is called referred pain; this finding requires medical assistance if client exhibits other corresponding symptoms such as chest pain or indigestion, or other cardiovascular changes
3. Shoulder discomfort during ROM may result from conditions that increase intraabdominal pressure, such as hiatal hernia or gastrointestinal disease
4. When increased or decreased ROM is noted, use a goniometer to measure the angle precisely
   a. Place joint in a neutral position and then flex joint as far as possible and measure angle with goniometer
   b. Repeat measurement after extending joint as far as possible
5. A torn rotator cuff may be present if client cannot perform abduction without lifting or shrugging affected shoulder; it is also accompanied by pain, tenderness, and muscle atrophy

C. Elbows

1. Pain, deformity, swelling, or malalignment needs further evaluation
2. **Subluxation** (partial dislocation of a joint) is accompanied by deformity and misalignment of forearm
3. Elbow grooves feel soft and spongy with inflammation, and surrounding tissue may be reddened, warm to hot, and painful

Practice to Pass

A client seeks health care for facial pain in front of the ear. The client says he has a friend who had TMJ syndrome, and worries that he has it too. What assessment findings would lead the nurse to conclude that this client may indeed have TMJ syndrome?

4. Inflammatory conditions may include arthritis, bursitis, and lateral epicondylitis (tennis elbow) or medial epicondylitis (pitcher's or golfer's elbow)

5. Pain occurs during attempts to extend wrist against resistance with lateral epicondylitis and during attempts to flex wrist against resistance with medial epicondylitis

D. Wrists and hands

1. Redness, tenderness, swelling, or deformity in joints warrants further evaluation and may indicate rheumatoid arthritis, especially if accompanied by ulnar deviation of proximal phalanges

2. Carpal tunnel syndrome occurs when inflamed wrist tissues cause pressure on median nerve, which innervates hand; it may be accompanied by thenar atrophy, which could also occur to some extent with aging

3. A ganglion is an often painless, round, fluid-filled mass that arises from tendon sheaths or dorsum of wrist or hand; if it is more prevalent with wrist flexion, it does not interfere with ROM or joint function

4. Cool extremity temperature may indicate impaired vascular supply, which in turn may reduce muscle strength

5. About 80% of those with carpal tunnel syndrome experience Phelan's sign; which is wrist pain and tingling and numbness that can radiate to the arm, shoulder, neck or chest within 60 seconds

6. If carpal tunnel syndrome is suspected, follow-up testing of Tinel's sign (percussing lightly over median nerve) will result in numbness, tingling, and pain along the median nerve; the client will also have weakness when attempting **opposition** of thumb (movement involving touching thumb of a hand to fingertips of same hand)

7. A client with Dupuytrens's contracture will be unable to extend fourth and fifth fingers; this is a painless inherited disorder that causes severe flexion in affected fingers

E. Hips

1. Classic signs of a fractured femur are external rotation of lower leg and foot and a shortened leg on affected side

2. A fractured femur should be suspected if hip joint is unstable and deformed

3. Inflammatory or degenerative disorders of hip may cause pain, tenderness, swelling, deformity, crepitus, and limited motion (especially internal rotation)

4. A herniated disk can produce back and leg pain along course of sciatic nerve during straight leg raising

F. Knees

1. Swelling and signs of fluid in knee or surrounding structures requires additional evaluation for inflammation, trauma, or degenerative joint disease

2. Atrophy of quadriceps muscles accompanies disuse or chronic disorders

3. Pain, swelling, thickening or heat in knee noted during knee palpation indicates inflammation of bursa (bursitis), while painless swelling is more common in degenerative joint disease

4. Pain and tenderness (inflammation) in tibiofemoral joint may indicate degenerative joint disease, synovitis, or torn meniscus; bony ridges or prominences on outer aspect of joint compatible with osteoarthritis

5. Medial side of knee bulges during bulge test if abnormal amount of fluid is present in joint

6. Patella "floats" over femur during ballottement with abnormal fluid levels, and a palpable click is felt when patella is snapped against femur when fluid is present

7. Abnormal knee alignments include *genu varum* (bowlegs), *genu valgum* (knock knees), or *genu recurvatum* (excessive hyperextension of knees with weight bearing because of weak quadriceps muscles

G. Ankles and feet

1. Gouty arthritis may be present if great toe is swollen, hot, red, and very painful
2. *Hallux valgus* (bunion) shows a great toe that deviates laterally from midline, crowding other toes; this is caused by an enlarged and inflamed metatarsophalangeal joint and bursa
3. *Hammertoe* is a flexion of the interphalangeal joint of toe and hyperextension of metatarsophalangeal joint; it may be accompanied by a callus or corn on surface of flexed joint
4. *Pes planus* (flatfoot) occurs when arch of foot is flattened and may come in contact with floor; may only be noticeable when client is standing and bearing weight on foot
5. Degenerative joint disease is accompanied by pain or discomfort on palpation and movement of affected joints, as well as limited range of motion, and signs of inflammation may be present or absent
6. Tendonitis or bursitis may be present if there is pain and tenderness along a tendon; small nodules occur at times with rheumatoid arthritis
7. Inflammation of a joint may be accompanied by pain, swelling, or tenderness
8. Cooler temperature of lower extremities that is significant may indicate vascular insufficiency, which in turn can lead to musculoskeletal abnormalities from tissue malnutrition

H. Spine

1. Thoracic surgery, such as lung removal, can cause a lack of symmetry of scapulae
2. **Kyphosis** is an exaggerated thoracic dorsal curve that results in asymmetry between sides of posterior thorax
3. **Lordosis** is an exaggerated lumbar curve that often appears in compensation for pregnancy, obesity, or other skeletal changes
4. A flattened lumbar curve, or less concave lumbar curve, often occurs when lumbar muscles are in spasm
5. A list, a leaning to left or right, (plumb line drawn from T1 does not fall between gluteal cleft) may occur with paravertebral muscle spasm or herniated intervertebral disk
6. **Scoliosis**, a spinal curvature to right or left, can lead to an exaggerated thoracic convexity on affected side; because body compensates, a plumb line dropped from T1 falls between the gluteal cleft; because unequal leg length may contribute to scoliosis, legs should be measured with client supine from anterior superior iliac spine to medial malleolus (crossing tape measure at medial side of knee)
7. Compression fractures (especially at T8 and L3) may occur in older adults, and should be considered if client has back pain and tenderness and restricted back movements
8. Muscle spasms are palpated as hardened or knotlike formations; they may be accompanied by pain and restricted movement in affected area, which tends to occur more often in TMJ area or as a *spasmodic torticollis*, in which neck muscle spasms cause head to be pulled to one side
9. Limited ROM, crepitation, or pain with movement in spinal area warrants further evaluation
   a. A sharp pain in lower back that radiates down leg and/or occurs with straight leg raising test may indicate a herniated disk
   b. With a positive straight leg raising test, client has pain when his or her leg is raised (with knee extended) and may be worsened with subsequent dorsiflexion of foot on affected side while leg is still raised

VIII. LIFESPAN CONSIDERATIONS

A. Infants and children

1. Musculoskeletal anomalies in newborn caused by fetal positioning and delivery include *tibial torsion*, a curving apart of tibias, and *metatarsus adductus*, in which forefoot tends to turn inward; these are normally self-correcting with growth and the start of walking

2. Newborns tend to have flat feet, with arches gradually developing during preschool years

3. The presence of hair, cyst, or mass on newborn's spine may indicate spina bifida and requires further evaluation

4. The clavicle(s) may be fractured during birth and go unnoticed, so palpation at each infant office visit is needed to detect lumps or irregularities from callus formation, and also observe range of motion of arm on affected side

5. Infants are assessed at birth and at every office visit until 1 year of age for congenital hip dislocation; place infant supine, flex infant's knees while keeping femurs aligned, and compare height of knees; uneven leg length demonstrated by uneven knee height is called Allis' sign

6. Infants have normal shoulder strength if infant remains upright between nurse's hands while hands are positioned beneath infant's axillae

7. Infants tend to have *genu varum (*bowlegs) before learning to walk, which reverses gradually once walking has begun

8. By age 4 many children have *genu valgum* (knock knees), and this resolves on its own usually by late childhood or early adolescence

9. Bone growth is rapid during infancy, continues at a more steady pace during childhood, and occurs rapidly again at adolescence (growth spurt); long bones increase in length and width

10. Because **ligaments** (bands of flexible tissue that attach bone to bone) are stronger than bones in children, injuries to long bones and joints tend to produce fractures rather than sprains

11. The nurse may use normal play activities, such as jumping, hopping, skipping, and climbing, as ways to assess range of motion and muscle strength

12. Generalized muscle weakness in children may be noted if child places hands on knees and pushes trunk up to rise (Gower's sign) from a sitting position

13. Screening for scoliosis should be done at each office visit during childhood

14. A child's gait changes over time; it is broad-based before age 3 and gradually narrows

15. Arm range of motion is assessed at each visit to screen for subluxation of head of radius, which may occur if adults dangle children from their hands or forcibly remove their clothing

16. Sports activity should be assessed at each visit to determine need for special assessments or to conduct preventive teaching, such as use of helmets or other safety equipment

B. Pregnant females

1. Change in hormones during pregnancy causes cartilage in pelvis to soften, which increases mobility of sacroiliac, sacrococcygeal, and symphysis pubis joints

2. Center of gravity shifts forward during pregnancy, and client shifts weight farther back on lower extremities, causing strain on lower back and lower back pain that is common in late pregnancy

3. Waddling gait develops as pregnancy progresses because of enlarged abdomen and relaxed mobility in joints

4. These pregnancy-induced changes in posture and gait reverse shortly after pregnancy ends

C. Older adults

1. Older adults have bone changes including decreased calcium absorption and reduced osteoblast production
2. The rate of bone resorption is faster than new bone growth, leading to decreased bone density typical of osteoporosis over time, especially in vertebrae and long bones
3. Medications taken for chronic illness, such as glucocorticoids, thyroid hormones, anticonvulsants and others, may have a negative effect on bone density
4. Bone mass and strength may also be reduced by insufficient intake of calcium and vitamin D, or in those who are housebound or immobile
5. Shortening of vertebral column from thinning intervertebral discs leads to a decrease in height, which is compounded by osteoporosis
6. Kyphosis tends to occur with increasing age
7. Slight flexion of hips and knees may be noted when client is standing, and this changes the center of gravity and places client at increased risk for falls
8. Size and quantity of muscle fibers decreases with aging, while amount of connective tissue fibers increases, making muscles fibrous or stringy; **tendons** (tough fibrous bands that attach either muscle to bone or muscle to muscle) also become less elastic, all of which cause progressive decrease in reaction time, speed of movement, agility, and endurance
9. Joint degeneration leads to thickening and decreased viscosity of synovial fluid, fragmentation of connective tissue, and scarring and calcification in joint capsules
10. Joint cartilage becomes frayed, thin, and cracked, leading to erosion of underlying bone, with less shock absorbency of joints and decreased flexibility and range of motion (osteoarthritis)
11. Heberden's nodes also occur with osteoarthritis, and are hard, often painless bony enlargements in distal interphalangeal joints
12. Age-related changes in gait for both males and females include slower walking with an increased need for support while moving
    a. Older adult males tend to walk with head and trunk in a flexed position, with short high steps, a wide gait, and smaller arm swing
    b. Older adult females tend to have a bowlegged stance caused by reduced muscle control, which alters normal angle of hip and increases susceptibility to falls and fractures
13. The general decreased reaction time and speed of performance of tasks in older adulthood can increase risks to safety, especially if unexpected environmental factors interfere (such as loose carpeting, throw rugs, objects on floor, wet surfaces)
14. A well-balanced diet and regular exercise are helpful in slowing progression of musculoskeletal changes of aging
15. Musculoskeletal assessment in older adults is similar in nature to that of other adults, but may need to be conducted more slowly, and careful attention must be paid to not causing pain, discomfort, or joint damage while testing range of motion

IX. DOCUMENTATION

A. Document normal findings found on inspection and palpation for temporomandibular joint of face, shoulders, elbows, wrists and hands, hips, knees, ankles and feet, and spine
B. Document range of motion in joints noted previously and also muscle strength of various muscle groups
C. Document and follow up on manifestations such as pain or tenderness, crepitation, pain with movement, limited range of motion, or other abnormal findings

Case Study

A 72-year-old client has come to the healthcare provider's office for a yearly examination. The nurse is conducting the initial health assessment and is ready to begin the musculoskeletal portion of the examination.

1. What questions should the nurse ask the client to detect common symptoms of bone and joint problems?

2. How should the nurse position the client to begin the examination?

3. What are the four items that should be assessed for each joint during the examination?

4. What are the musculoskeletal age-related changes that are likely in this client?

5. What general recommendations would the nurse make to the client to promote musculoskeletal health and reduce safety risks?

For suggested responses, see page 310

POSTTEST

1 To detect a small amount of fluid in the supra patellar bursa the nurse should perform which action to elicit the bulge sign?

1. Place the client supine and stroke the medial aspect of the knee, applying pressure to the lateral aspect of the knee and observing the medial aspect for fluid
2. Place the client supine and stroke the lateral aspect of the knee and observe the lateral aspect for fluid
3. Squeeze the thigh with fingers and thumb and observe fluid in the suprapatellar bursa move between the patella and femur
4. Squeeze the quadriceps muscle and palpate the bursa

2 When assessing the range of motion of a client's ankle the nurse would place the client through which movements? Select all that apply.

1. Dorsiflexion
2. Hyperextension
3. Plantar flexion
4. Inversion
5. Eversion

3 The nurse is examining the spine of a client who is experiencing an extreme curvature of the lumbar area. How should the nurse document this finding?

1. Kyphosis
2. Scoliosis
3. Lordosis
4. A list

4 When examining cervical range of motion on a client the nurse should ask the client to perform which type of movement? Select all that apply.

1. Touch chin to chest
2. Look toward the ceiling
3. Touch the right ear to the right shoulder
4. Bend at the waist
5. Touch the left ear to the left shoulder

5 The nurse is examining an elderly client and notes an exaggerated curvature of the thoracic spine. The nurse should document this finding as which of the following?

1. Scoliosis
2. Kyphosis
3. Lordosis
4. Tendonitis

6 The client has a history of gouty arthritis and reports pain and swelling of the elbow. The nurse concludes that these manifestations are consistent with which disorder?

1. Osteoarthritis
2. Olecranon bursitis
3. Rheumatoid arthritis
4. Ulnar deviation

7 The nurse is teaching the client about manifestations of gout. The nurse evaluates that the client understands the instruction when the client states which of the following as symptoms of gout?

1. Synovial effusion and pain in small toe
2. Inflammation and pain of the bursa
3. Tophi, erythema, pain, and edema
4. Adducted great toe and pain

8 The nurse assesses the range of motion of an ankle by moving the ankle through which types of movements? Select all that apply.

1. Plantar flexion
2. Dorsiflexion
3. Inversion
4. Eversion
5. Rotation

9 What questions should the nurse include in the assessment of a 50-year-old postmenopausal woman's musculoskeletal system?

1. "How many times have you fallen?"
2. "Do you use any walking aids?"
3. "Do you take calcium supplements?"
4. "Do you play sports?"

10 To test cranial nerve V, the nurse would have the client engage in which activity?

1. Open and close the mouth, push out the lower jaw, and move it side to side
2. Smile and then return the face to a normal position
3. Read a magazine held at fourteen inches from the face
4. Shrug the shoulders and then allow them to relax to normal position

➤ *See pages 187–189 for Answers and Rationales.*

ANSWERS & RATIONALES

Pretest

1 **Answers: 1, 4** **Rationale:** During musculoskeletal assessment, it is important to determine how problems interfere with ADLs. Because pain may limit movement and activity, the nurse would ask open-ended questions, such as how the pain is affecting the client's life (option 1). Asking how the client's activity level has changed (option 4) will also yield data about limitations that affect ADLs. Although it is helpful to ask the client if he or she knows the cause of the problem as part of the interview (option 2), this will not provide information about reduced ability to perform ADLs. Inquiring about family history is an important part of the interview (option 3); however, this also will not provide information about ADLs. Hobbies (option 5) are useful as recreational activities and could possibly yield data about injury; however, hobbies are not part of ADLs, so it is not needed when determining ADL status. **Cognitive Level:** Application **Client Need:** Health Promotion and Maintenance **Integrated Process:** Nursing Process: Assessment **Content Area:** Adult Health: Musculoskeletal

Strategy: Note that the focus of the question is on ADLs. Eliminate the option to describe hobbies (option 5) as it is not a general question related to pain or problems with the musculoskeletal system. Hobbies may provide information about potential risk for injury. Next eliminate options that determine the etiology of a musculoskeletal problem (option 2) or family history (option 3) as they do not address ADLs. **Reference:** D'Amico, D. & Barbarito, C. (2007). *Health & physical assessment in nursing*. Upper Saddle River, NJ: Pearson Education, Inc., p. 684.

2 **Answer: 4** **Rationale:** The questions to elicit information about what relieves (alleviates) the client's symptoms or pain include "What over-the-counter medications do you use?" "What home remedies have you used?" "How often do you need to use the over-the-counter remedies?" Asking the client when the injury occurred (option 1) will indicate to the nurse whether ice or heat is needed for the injury. Asking how the client was injured (option 2) provides information about the mechanism of injury. Asking whether the client has been able to carry out regular activities (option 3) provides information about the severity of the injury. **Cognitive Level:** Application **Client Need:** Health Promotion and Maintenance **Integrated Process:** Nursing Process: Assessment **Content Area:** Adult Health: Musculoskeletal **Strategy:** The critical words in the question are *relieves symptoms* and *injury*. Note that only option 4 provides information about relief of pain or symptoms that would occur with an injury. Eliminate all of the remaining distracters after noting that they investigate the actual injury (options 1 and 2) or effects of the injury (option 3). **Reference:** D'Amico, D. & Barbarito, C. (2007). *Health & physical assessment in nursing.* Upper Saddle River, NJ: Pearson Education, Inc., p. 685.

3 Answer: 2 Rationale: The area of pain or inflammation is always addressed first and inspection is the physical assessment skill that is also performed first. Palpation (options 1 and 4) is performed after inspection. The area is not put through range of motion exercises (option 3) until after the area is assessed to prevent discomfort or further injury. **Cognitive Level:** Application **Client Need:** Health Promotion and Maintenance **Integrated Process:** Nursing Process: Assessment **Content Area:** Adult Health: Musculoskeletal **Strategy:** Eliminate option 3 first because range of motion is assessed last to reduce the risk of inflicting further injury. Note that two options reflect palpation, so options 1 and 4 are eliminated next. To choose option 2 as the correct option, recall that inspection is always performed prior to palpation. **Reference:** D'Amico, D. & Barbarito, C. (2007). *Health & physical assessment in nursing.* Upper Saddle River, NJ: Pearson Education, Inc., p. 689.

4 Answer: 1 Rationale: The temporomandibular joint is assessed by placing the fingers in front of the tragus in front of the ear and having the client open and close the mouth (option 1). Cranial nerve II (option 2) is the optic nerve and has no facial innervations. Shrugging the shoulder (option 3) evaluates the spinal accessory nerve as does lifting the arms (option 4). **Cognitive Level:** Application **Client Need:** Health Promotion and Maintenance **Integrated Process:** Nursing Process: Assessment **Content Area:** Adult Health: Musculoskeletal **Strategy:** Eliminate option 2 first as cranial nerve II is the optic nerve and refers to vision. To eliminate options 3 and 4 note that shrugging the shoulders and lifting the arms are similar and that these actions evaluate the spinal accessory nerve. **Reference:** D'Amico, D. & Barbarito, C. (2007). *Health & physical assessment in nursing.* Upper Saddle River, NJ: Pearson Education, Inc., pp. 690–691.

5 Answer: 2 Rationale: Crepitus is a grating sound produced when a joint is placed through range of motion exercises. A strain (option 3) is an overstretching of a muscle, while a sprain (option 4) involves ligaments. Clicking (option 1) is a sound produced when a joint is opened and closed. The sound is produced by putting the joint through range of motion exercises.

Cognitive Level: Application **Client Need:** Health Promotion and Maintenance **Integrated Process:** Communication and Documentation **Content Area:** Adult Health: Musculoskeletal **Strategy:** Eliminate options 1 and 4 first because each of these is a medical diagnosis. Eliminate option 3 as this sound cannot occur because the shoulder does not open or close and this action is needed to produce a clicking sound. **Reference:** D'Amico, D. & Barbarito, C. (2007). *Health & physical assessment in nursing.* Upper Saddle River, NJ: Pearson Education, Inc., pp. 691–692.

6 Answer: 3 Rationale: Cardiac problems such as angina pectoris or even myocardial infarction can produce referred pain in the shoulder that is unrelated to shoulder movement. A strain (option 1) and a sprain (option 2) produce pain upon movement. A rotator cuff tear (option 4) can only be evaluated when the extremity is moved. **Cognitive Level:** Application **Client Need:** Health Promotion and Maintenance **Integrated Process:** Nursing Process: Assessment **Content Area:** Adult Health: Musculoskeletal **Strategy:** Eliminate options 1 and 2 first after recalling that the pain of a sprain or strain is reproducible with palpation or movement. Similarly, eliminate option 4 after recalling that a rotator cuff tear produces pain with movement as well. Alternatively, select option 3, noting that angina pectoris of cardiac origin can produce heaviness or substernal pain that may radiate to the arms, shoulder, or jaw. **Reference:** D'Amico, D. & Barbarito, C. (2007). *Health & physical assessment in nursing.* Upper Saddle River, NJ: Pearson Education, Inc., p. 692.

7 Answer: 1 Rationale: Full range of motion with full resistance is considered normal. A rating of good (option 2) is full range of motion with moderate resistance. A rating of fair (option 3) indicates full range of motion with gravity. A rating of poor (option 4) is full range of motion without gravity. **Cognitive Level:** Application **Client Need:** Health Promotion and Maintenance **Integrated Process:** Communication and Documentation **Content Area:** Adult Health: Musculoskeletal **Strategy:** The critical words in the question are *full resistance and range of motion.* Note that these are normal findings and choose option 1, which has maximal functioning. **Reference:** D'Amico, D. & Barbarito, C. (2007). *Health & physical assessment in nursing.* Upper Saddle River, NJ: Pearson Education, Inc., p. 695.

8 Answer: 2 Rationale: A goniometer measures the full range of motion of a joint. To obtain this measurement, the nurse should place the joint in neutral position, then flex the joint as far as possible and measure, and finally fully extend the joint and measure. In option 1, the client is not in neutral position and this procedure does not measure extension. Note that it is easier for a client to flex than to extend, which is why flexion measurements are taken first. Option 3 describes the procedure for taking a flexion measurement and omits extension. Option 4 does not measure the degree of flexion.

Cognitive Level: Application **Client Need:** Health Promotion and Maintenance **Integrated Process:** Nursing Process: Assessment **Content Area:** Adult Health: Musculoskeletal **Strategy:** The critical words in the question are *range of motion.* Recall that assessment of full range of motion requires that the joint be flexed and extended. Eliminate options 3 and 4 because option 4 does not measure flexion and although option 3 is the procedure for measuring flexion, it does not include extension. Next recall that flexion begins with the letter "f" and is done first (as it is usually easier to flex an extremity than to extend it), so choose option 2 over 1. **Reference:** D'Amico, D. & Barbarito, C. (2007). *Health & physical assessment in nursing.* Upper Saddle River, NJ: Pearson Education, Inc., p. 696.

9 **Answer: 2** A ganglion is a round, fluid-filled cyst that is the result of stress to the tendon sheath. Carpal tunnel syndrome (option 1) is inflammation of wrist tissue that results in nerve damage. Rheumatoid arthritis (option 3) is an inflammatory condition that causes pain and swelling. Crepitus (option 4) is a grating sensation in the extremity.
Cognitive Level: Analysis **Client Need:** Health Promotion and Maintenance **Integrated Process:** Nursing Process: Assessment **Content Area:** Adult Health: Musculoskeletal **Strategy:** Eliminate crepitus (option 4) first as it is an assessment finding and not a conclusion about a health problem. Eliminate options 1 and 3 next as these are inflammatory processes that do not result in a cyst. **Reference:** D'Amico, D. & Barbarito, C. (2007). *Health & physical assessment in nursing.* Upper Saddle River, NJ: Pearson Education, Inc., p. 699.

10 **Answer: 4** **Rationale:** To detect fluid in the suprapatellar bursa, grasp the thigh above the knee with the fingers and thumb, and then observe the suprapatellar bursa for movement between the patella and the femur. Option 1 is incorrect as pushing on the tibia will not make fluid move to an observable position. Option 2, squeezing the tibia, will not make the fluid move in an observable position because ballottement is a test to observe fluid between the patella and the femur. Option 3, pushing on the tibia, will not cause fluid to move into the space between the patella and the femur.
Cognitive Level: Application **Client Need:** Health Promotion and Maintenance **Integrated Process:** Nursing Process: Assessment **Content Area:** Adult Health: Musculoskeletal **Strategy:** Eliminate options with squeezing the tibia between fingers and thumb, as this type of movement will not push fluid between the patella and femur. **Reference:** D'Amico, D. & Barbarito, C. (2007). *Health & physical assessment in nursing.* Upper Saddle River, NJ: Pearson Education, Inc., p. 707.

Posttest

1 **Answer: 1** **Rationale:** The nurse should assess the suprapatellar bursa for small amounts of fluid by stroking the medial aspect of the knee and applying pressure to the lateral aspect of the knee and observing the medial aspect. This is known as the bulge test (option 1). Option 2 is incorrect as it instructs to observe the lateral aspect of the knee; the bulge test is observing the medial aspect. Option 3, squeezing the thigh with the fingers and thumb and observing the suprapatellar bursa move between the patella and femur, is the ballottement test. Option 4 is incorrect because when palpating the quadriceps muscle the bursa should not be palpable.
Cognitive Level: Application **Client Need:** Health Promotion and Maintenance **Integrated Process:** Nursing Process: Assessment **Content Area:** Adult Health: Musculoskeletal **Strategy:** The bulge test is a test for small amounts of fluid. The term *bulge* implies out of the sides, so eliminate options 3 and 4. Most disorders of the knee cause medial edema and not lateral edema. **Reference:** D'Amico, D. & Barbarito, C. (2007). *Health & physical assessment in nursing.* Upper Saddle River, NJ: Pearson Education, Inc., p. 707.

2 **Answers: 1, 3, 4, 5** **Rationale:** Dorsiflexion (option 1) is pointing the toes toward the nose; they should reach 20 degrees on the goniometer. Plantar flexion (option 3) is pointing the toes toward the floor; they should measure 45 degrees on the goniometer. Inversion (option 4) is pointing the toes inward; the goniometer should measures 30 degrees. Eversion (option 5) is pointing the toes outward; they should measure 20 degrees on the goniometer. Hyperextension (option 2) cannot be performed on an articulating joint.
Cognitive Level: Application **Client Need:** Health Promotion and Maintenance **Integrated Process:** Nursing Process: Assessment **Content Area:** Adult Health: Musculoskeletal **Strategy:** According to test-taking strategies, narrow the choices to opposites. Dorsiflexion and plantar flexion are opposites and inversion and eversion are opposites. **Reference:** D'Amico, D. & Barbarito, C. (2007). *Health & physical assessment in nursing.* Upper Saddle River, NJ: Pearson Education, Inc., p. 710.

3 **Answer: 3** **Rationale:** Lordosis is an exaggerated curvature of the spine. Kyphosis (option 1) is an extreme curvature of the thoracic curvature. Scoliosis (option 2) is a lateral curvature of the spine. A list (option 4) is a right or left lean of the spine due to paravertebral muscle spasms.
Cognitive Level: Application **Client Need:** Health Promotion and Maintenance **Integrated Process:** Nursing Process: Assessment **Content Area:** Adult Health: Musculoskeletal **Strategy:** First eliminate list (option 4) as it is caused by muscle spasm. Recall that kyphosis (option 1) is a thoracic curvature and scoliosis (option 2) is a lateral curvature to eliminate them next. Select lordosis (option 3) because it occurs in the lumbar region and both lordosis and lumbar begin with the letter "l." **Reference:** D'Amico, D. & Barbarito, C. (2007). *Health & physical assessment in nursing.* Upper Saddle River, NJ: Pearson Education, Inc., p. 711.

4 **Answers: 1, 2, 3, 5** **Rationale:** Touching the chin to the shoulder (option 1) measures flexion. Looking toward the ceiling (option 2) measures hyperextension. Option 3, touching the right ear to the right shoulder, evaluates lateral flexion. Option 5, touching the left ear to the left shoulder, evaluates lateral flexion. Bending at the waist (option 4) does not evaluate cervical range of motion as the waist is in the thoracic-lumbar area of the spine. **Cognitive Level:** Application **Client Need:** Health Promotion and Maintenance **Integrated Process:** Nursing Process: Assessment **Content Area:** Adult Health: Musculoskeletal **Strategy:** Read each option carefully and visualize the area of the spine involved. Eliminate option 4 because bending at the waist measures flexibility of the thoracic-lumbar area instead of the cervical area. **Reference:** D'Amico, D. & Barbarito, C. (2007). *Health & physical assessment in nursing.* Upper Saddle River, NJ: Pearson Education, Inc., p. 713.

5 **Answer: 2** **Rationale:** Kyphosis is an exaggerated convex curvature of the spine that occurs because of a congenital abnormality, fractures, arthritic conditions, or sexually transmitted diseases. Scoliosis (option 1) is a lateral curvature of the spine. Lordosis (option 3) is an exaggerated curvature of the lumbar spine due to obesity or pregnancy. Tendonitis (option 4) is inflammation due to overuse of the extremity and tendon. **Cognitive Level:** Application **Client Need:** Health Promotion and Maintenance **Integrated Process:** Communication and Documentation **Content Area:** Adult Health: Musculoskeletal **Strategy:** Eliminate option 4 first because tendonitis is an inflammatory condition. Recall that scoliosis is an S-shaped lateral curvature to eliminate option 1 next. Eliminate option 3 after recalling that lordosis is a lumbar curvature and that both begin with "l." Alternatively, recall that kyphosis is the exaggerated convex curvature of the thoracic area to choose option 2. **Reference:** D'Amico, D. & Barbarito, C. (2007). *Health & physical assessment in nursing.* Upper Saddle River, NJ: Pearson Education, Inc., p. 717.

6 **Answer: 2** **Rationale:** Olecranon bursitis is an inflammation and swelling of the elbow. Osteoarthritis (option 1) produces Bouchard and Heberden nodes in the distal phalanges. Rheumatoid arthritis (option 3) has fusiform swelling of the joints. Ulnar deviation (option 4) is lateral deviation of the interphalangeal joints. **Cognitive Level:** Application **Client Need:** Health Promotion and Maintenance **Integrated Process:** Nursing Process: Assessment **Content Area:** Adult Health Physical Assessment: Musculoskeletal **Strategy:** Recall that options 1 and 3 are similar in that they are forms of arthritis and that option 4 is a clinical manifestation of rheumatoid arthritis. Next recall that bursitis is an inflammatory condition to choose that over the other options. **Reference:** D'Amico, D. & Barbarito, C. (2007). *Health & physical assessment in nursing.* Upper Saddle River, NJ: Pearson Education, Inc., pp. 718–720.

7 **Answer: 3** **Rationale:** Gout is an alteration of purine metabolism that produces tophi, erthyema, pain, and edema. Synovitis (option 1) produces an effusion and distention of the synovium. An inflamed bursa (option 2) is the result of bursitis. An adducted great toe (option 4) is the result of a hallux vagus. **Cognitive Level:** Application **Client Need:** Health Promotion and Maintenance **Integrated Process:** Nursing Process: Assessment **Content Area:** Adult Health: Musculoskeletal **Strategy:** Recall that when there are multiple parts to an option, all of the parts must be correct for the option to be correct. First eliminate option 4 because an adducted toe is not a result of inflammation. Next recall that synovitis (option 1) and bursitis (option 2) are similar in that they are inflammatory conditions and can therefore be eliminated. To reach a final conclusion, recall that gout produces a red, swollen edematous joint with nodes and thus choose option 3 as correct. **Reference:** D'Amico, D. & Barbarito, C. (2007). *Health & physical assessment in nursing.* Upper Saddle River, NJ: Pearson Education, Inc., p. 722.

8 **Answers: 1, 2, 3, 4** **Rationale:** Plantar flexion (option 1) is the ability to flex the ankle by pointing the toes downward. Dorsiflexion (option 2) is the ability to flex the ankle by pointing the toes upward. Inversion (option 3) is the ability of the client to point the foot inward, while eversion (option 4) is the ability to move the foot outward. Rotation (option 5) is movement of a bone on an axis. **Cognitive Level:** Application **Client Need:** Health Promotion and Maintenance **Integrated Process:** Nursing Process: Assessment **Content Area:** Adult Health: Musculoskeletal **Strategy:** First recall that the ankle is a joint. Eliminate option 5 because the ankle is not on a long axis bone. Choose each of the other options because a joint is capable of inversion, eversion, plantar flexion, and dorsiflexion. **Reference:** D'Amico, D. & Barbarito, C. (2007). *Health & physical assessment in nursing.* Upper Saddle River, NJ: Pearson Education, Inc., pp. 674–675.

9 **Answer: 3** **Rationale:** Postmenopausal women should be asked about whether they take calcium supplements to reduce the risk of osteoporosis. A 50-year-old should not be at risk for falls since falls occur most often in older adulthood (option1). Most 50-year-olds do not walk with canes or walkers (option 2). Asking about playing sports (option 4) is usually a question asked of children. **Client Need:** Health Promotion and Maintenance **Integrated Process:** Nursing Process: Assessment **Content Area:** Adult Health: Musculoskeletal **Strategy:** Note the age of the client in the question and first conclude that the core issue of the question may focus on asking an age-appropriate question. With this in mind, eliminate option 2 first because a 50-year-old should not need a walking aid and option 1 because clients in middle adulthood are not at great risk for falls. Finally, recall that most 50-year-old women do not play sports to eliminate option 4. **Reference:** D'Amico, D. & Barbarito, C. (2007). *Health & physical assessment in nursing.* Upper Saddle River, NJ: Pearson Education, Inc., pp. 686–687.

10 **Answer: 1** **Rationale:** To evaluate cranial nerve (CN) V, the trigeminal nerve, the mouth is opened and closed and the jaw is pushed in and out and moved side to side. Smiling (option 2) evaluates CN VII, the facial nerve. Reading (option 3) evaluates near vision and tests the CN II. Shrugging the shoulders evaluates CN XI, the spinal accessory nerve. **Client Need:** Health Promotion and Maintenance **Integrated Process:** Nursing Process: Assessment **Content Area:** Adult Health: Musculoskeletal **Strategy:** Recall that smiling evaluates the CN VII to eliminate option 2 first. Reading a magazine evaluates CN II, so option 3 can be eliminated because this is not a test of motor function. Next recall that shrugging the shoulders evaluates CN XI to eliminate option 4. Alternatively, recall that CN V involves evaluating the motor function of the mouth and jaw to choose option 1. **Reference:** D'Amico, D. & Barbarito, C. (2007). *Health & physical assessment in nursing.* Upper Saddle River, NJ: Pearson Education, Inc., p. 691.

References

Bickley, L. (2010). *Bates guide to physical examination and history taking* (10th ed.). Philadelphia: Lippincott Williams & Wilkins.

D'Amico, D. & Barbarito, C. (2007). *Health & physical assessment in nursing.* Upper Saddle River, NJ: Pearson Education, Inc., pp. 263–303.

Jarvis, C. (2008). *Physical examination and health assessment* (5th ed.). St. Louis, MO: Elsevier Saunders.

Zator Estes, M. (2009). *Health assessment and physical examination* (4th ed.). Clifton Park, NY: Delmar Cengage Learning.

Breasts and Axillae Assessment *10*

Chapter Outline

Health History
Present Health History
Family History

Equipment, Preparation, and
 Positioning
Examination Techniques
Expected Findings

Unexpected Findings
Lifespan Considerations
Documentation

NCLEX-RN® Test Prep

Visit the Companion Website for this book
at www.pearsonhighered.com/hogan to
access additional practice opportunities
and more.

Objectives

➤ Discuss the assessment questions used during an assessment of
  the breasts.
➤ Describe the positioning and preparation of the client undergoing
  assessment of the breasts and axillae.
➤ Identify the techniques used during an assessment of the breasts
  and axillae.
➤ Describe normal and abnormal findings of an examination of the
  breasts and axillae.
➤ Describe the variations found during the assessment of the breasts
  and axillae across the lifespan.

Review at a Glance

areola a darker area that surrounds
the nipple of the breast and contains
sebaceous Montgomery glands
fibroadenoma a noncancerous
mass occurring most commonly during
early adolescence or young adulthood,
although it can occur occasionally in
post-menopausal females

galactorrhea lactation not associated with childbearing or breastfeeding,
most commonly occuring with some
endocrine disorders, medications such
as antihypertensives or antidepressants,
or with excessive nipple stimulation
mastalgia pain in the breast, most
commonly associated with the menstrual cycle

nipple a protuberant area of the
breast that contains the milk duct; there
are 15–20 lactiferous ducts (arranged
cylindrically) around the tip of the nipple
peau d'orange a term used to
describe breast tissue that appears like
the skin of the orange; may indicate
inflammatory breast cancer

PRETEST

1 The nurse is teaching the client about breast self-examination. The client asks, "Are there any areas of the breast where cancer is more likely to occur?" What is the nurse's best response?

1. In the nipple area
2. In the inferior aspect
3. Near the sternal border
4. In the upper outer quadrant

2 The client presents to the emergency room with pain, redness, warmth and swelling in the left breast. The nurse will further evaluate this client for which health problem?

1. Infection
2. Lesions
3. Everted nipples
4. Cystic breast disease

3 The mother of a 16-year-old female calls the clinic information hotline. The mother is screaming and crying on the phone as she tells the nurse that her daughter found a lump in her breast. What is the nurse's best initial action?

1. Tell the mother that teenage girls do not often get breast cancer
2. Instruct the mother to go to the emergency department
3. Offer the mother support and provide concerned listening to decrease anxiety
4. Tell the mother that if she does not have breast cancer then her daughter is not likely to have it

4 A 50-year-old male client with a history of cardio-vascular disease tells the nurse, "It seems like my breasts are getting bigger as I get older." What is the nurse's best response?

1. "Please tell me what medications you are taking, because some medications cause breast enlargement."
2. "Have you increased your caloric intake during the last 6 months?"
3. "As we age our metabolic needs decrease and if we still consume the same number of calories, our weight increases."
4. "This is probably because the healthcare provider ordered female hormones as adjunct treatment for your heart disease."

5 When assessing the breasts in female clients, the nurse performs the assessment using which assessment techniques?

1. Inspecting and palpating the breast
2. Palpating and percussing the breast
3. Inspecting and percussing the breast
4. Inspecting and auscultating the breast

6 A 20-year-old female asks the nurse, "Why do my breasts feel bumpy a few days during the month?" What is the nurse's best response to the client?

1. "There is a good chance that you have breast cancer and you should be evaluated further."
2. "Breast nodules are a result of monthly hormonal changes."
3. "Breast nodules increase during times of stress. Have you been under unusual stress lately?"
4. "Is there a possibility you can be pregnant?"

7 The nurse is teaching a pregnant, third-trimester client about what to expect during delivery when the woman states, "I think I have a breast infection. I have yellow discharge coming from my breasts." What would be the nurse's initial action?

1. Obtain a culture and sensitivity of the discharge and then notify the healthcare provider
2. Obtain a healthcare provider order for a broad spectrum antibiotic since the client is in the third trimester of pregnancy
3. State that this discharge is called colostrum, which is a precursor to milk, and is normal during pregnancy
4. Prepare the client for a breast assessment for further evaluation of this finding

8 When performing a breast assessment on a client, the nurse finds a brown spot below the right breast. It has a nipple located in the center. The nurse should document this finding using which description?

1. Right breast mole
2. Suspicious lesion needing further evaluation
3. Lymphatic tissue requiring further evaluation
4. Benign supernumerary nipple

9 A woman who gave birth one month ago is in the emergency department with a red, warm, swollen, and tender left breast. The client has a temperature of 100 degrees Fahrenheit and reports fatigue and chills. Based on these findings the nurse should prepare to initiate a plan of care for which nursing diagnosis?

1. Self-care deficit related to breast cancer
2. Pain related to infected lymph nodes
3. Impaired tissue integrity related to mastitis
4. Self-care deficit related to influenza

10 When teaching a multicultural group of women over 40 years of age about breast cancer the nurse should include which statement?

1. All women are at equal risk for breast cancer
2. All women should perform yearly self-breast examinations
3. Mammography should be performed every 3 years
4. Caucasian women are at greatest risk for developing breast cancer

➤ *See pages 201–202 for Answers and Rationales.*

I. HEALTH HISTORY

    A. Consists of a group of questions to provide data about problems

    B. Includes biographical data, ethnic background, and questions about general health

        1. Biographical data, such as age, is important to determine since breast cancer risk increases with age

        2. Information about a client's ethnic background is useful because ethnic background influences risk of developing a disease and progression of that disease

           a. Caucasian clients have an increased risk of cancer after age 40

           b. African-American clients under age 40 have an increased risk of breast cancer

           c. Non-white clients are more likely than whites overall to lack access to care, which increases risk of more advanced health problems when they are finally detected

        3. Ask if client has a history of breast lumps; **fibroadenomas** are noncancerous masses that occur in young adults

        4. Ask when client began to menstruate; early menstruation (prior to age 12) increases risk of breast cancer

        5. Ask about breast injury or trauma, as sports injuries in teens could be an issue; lumps may result from deep tissue bruising

        6. Ask if client has ever had breast surgery

           a. "Was it a mastectomy or lumpectomy?"

           b. "Was it a breast reduction?"

           c. "Was there breast augmentation?"

        7. Ask if client has ever had a breast problem

        8. Ask client when was last mammogram

        9. Ask if client has ever been diagnosed with cancer

      10. Ask client if he or she takes any medications

           a. Medications may increase risk of cancer

           b. Some medications, such as cardiac glycosides and female hormones, may cause gynecomastia in men (see Table 10-1)

> **Practice to Pass**
>
> Why is it important to determine the age of onset of menstruation?

Table 10-1	Drug Classification	Effect
Medications Affecting Breast Health	Androgen	Females: Decreased breast size
		Males: Gynecomastia
	Antipsychotics	Females: Galactorrhea, mastalgia
		Males: Gynecomastia
	Cardiac glycosides	Females: Mastalgia
		Males: Gynecomastia
	Estrogen	Females: Breast enlargement, tenderness
		Males: Gynecomastia, tenderness
	Oral contraceptives	Females: tenderness, enlargement
	Tricyclic antidepressants	Females: Galactorrhea
		Males: Gynecomastia

II. PRESENT HEALTH HISTORY

A. Ask client about any pain or discomfort in breasts
  1. "Where is the pain?"
  2. "Do you feel burning or a pulling?"
  3. "Is a localized spot tender?"
  4. "Is the pain associated with activity?"
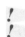
    a. Mastalgia (pain in breast tissue) may be associated with trauma, inflammation, or infection
    b. Cyclic pain may be associated with menstruation or oral contraceptive disease
    c. Pain may be due to a cyst or fibrocystic disease

B. Ask client about any changes in *nipples*
  1. "Is there any discharge from the nipples?"
    a. "When did it first occur?"
    b. "Please describe discharge."
    c. "Does it have an odor?"

    d. Galactorrhea, or lactation not associated with childbirth, may be a side effect of medications
    e. Blood-tinged discharge may be related to malignancy
  2. Ask client about nipple changes; nipples may be inverted or everted

C. Ask client about any changes observed in breast tissue
  1. Ask client about presence of a rash on breast; if seen ask the following:
    a. "Where did the rash start?" (a skin rash that is scaly and red at the nipple may indicate Paget's disease, a malignancy)
    b. "How long ago did the rash start?"

Practice to Pass

The nurse notes during physical assessment that a client has dimpling of the skin on the breast. What conclusion might the nurse draw from this data?

  2. Ask client about any swelling and whether swelling is associated with any conditions
    a. Conditions such as menses can cause swelling
    b. Pregnancy and breastfeeding may contribute to swelling
  3. Ask client about any redness or dimpling of breasts
    a. Dimpling is associated with malignancy
    b. Redness is indicative of mastitis
  4. Ask client if changes in breast size, shape, or contour have been noted; if so, this may be a symptom of breast disease

D. Ask client specific questions that elicit data about an increased risk for cancer
  1. Ask client about any shortness of breath; breast cancer often causes metastasis to lung
  2. Ask client about any abdominal discomfort; the liver is often a site for metastasis from breast cancer

Box 10-1	Female	Obesity
Breast Cancer Risk Factors	Increasing age	Increased alcohol intake
	Immediate relative with breast cancer	Nulliparity, pregnancy after age 30, or lack of breastfeeding
	Menstruation prior to age 12 years	
	Caucasian race	Use of oral contraceptives or hormone replacement therapy
	Sedentary lifestyle	

!
3. Ask client if oral contraceptives were ever taken; this is linked to breast cancer (see Box 10-1)
4. Ask client about hormone replacement therapy; this has been linked to increased risk of breast cancer

Practice to Pass

What factors have been related to breast cancer?

E. **Ask female client if she has ever been pregnant**
  1. If so, at what age did pregnancy occur?
  2. Has client ever experienced infertility?
  3. Being pregnant over age 30, infertility, and never being pregnant have been linked to breast cancer
F. **Ask client about breastfeeding; this has been demonstrated to reduce risk of breast cancer**
G. **Ask client about measures used to promote breast health**
  1. Ask client about monthly performance of breast self-examination

!
  2. Ask client if the health-care provider performs complete breast examinations; every 3 years, breasts should be examined by a healthcare provider
H. **Ask client about lifestyle and habits that influence breast health**
  1. Ask whether client eats high fat or sodium foods; diets high in fat or sodium aggravate fibrocystic breast disease
  2. Ask client about exercise; lack of exercise is associated with increased cancer risk
  3. Ask client about use of alcohol; this has also been linked to cancer (see Box 10-1 for a summary of breast cancer risk factors)

Practice to Pass

During the assessment of family history the nurse should confirm a family history of breast cancer in what relatives?

  4. Ask whether client conducts a breast self-examination (BSE)
    a. Inquire about frequency (monthly at same time of month, such as 5 days after onset of menses, or same day of month in postmenopausal women)
    b. Realize that in Latina and many immigrant cultures, BSE may not be well accepted because looking at or touching oneself is prohibited, so this requires support and additional education by nurse
    c. Use opportunity to review and reinforce knowledge of BSE technique during the actual physical examination

III. FAMILY HISTORY

A. **Ask client about family history of breast cancer**
  1. Women with relatives (mother, sisters, or aunts) who had breast cancer have an increased risk
  2. Breast cancer may be genetically linked, with presence of BRCA1 or BRCA2 gene
B. **Ask client about family history of any type of cancer**

IV. EQUIPMENT, PREPARATION, AND POSITIONING

A. **Equipment**
  1. Small pillow to elevate shoulder
  2. Mirror to permit client to observe breast
  3. Ruler for measuring lesion
  4. Gloves to prevent disease transmission to client or nurse

5. Specimen slide to prepare specimen for examination
6. Culture swab to obtain culture of discharge

B. Preparation: client will need to disrobe from waist up
1. Use a gown that has an opening in front, and expose one breast at a time
2. If a gown that opens in back must be used, lift gown to expose only one breast at a time
3. Clients are often embarrassed to undergo a breast examination; thus it is important to demonstrate professionalism and be conscious of privacy and exposure (such as covering breast not being examined)

C. Positioning: breast assessment will be completed in multiple positions
1. Use of a sitting position or standing while leaning forward facilitates exam for large-breasted women
2. Raising hands over head or placing them on hips assists in detecting dimpling or contour of breasts
3. A supine position permits breast tissue to be evenly distributed over chest wall and will be used when doing breast palpation

V. EXAMINATION TECHNIQUES

A. Inspection
1. Assess symmetry of size, shape, condition of skin, nipples, and venous patterns (see Figure 10-1)
   a. Position the client sitting with hands over head
   b. When the client lifts the arms, the breasts should move symmetrically
   c. Client should place hands on hips and push hands together to contract pectoralis muscle
   d. Large-breasted women should lean forward in sitting and standing positions and perform these maneuvers
2. Assess nipples for inversion or eversion and presence or absence of discharge
3. The **areola** (a darker area that surrounds nipple of breast) should have an even color without redness or lesions
4. Assess area around breast and chest wall for presence of a supernumerary nipple; this finding is benign and appears as a mole but with examination can be determined to be a nipple

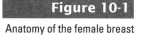

Figure 10-1

Anatomy of the female breast

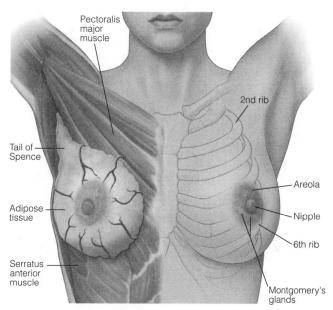

5. Evaluate condition of skin of breast and assess for edema and overall appearance
6. While client is sitting assess axillae for bulging nodes or discoloration; lift client's arm so muscles are relaxed

B. Palpation

1. Have client lie supine with a small pillow or towel roll under shoulder of side being examined; place client's arm over head to displace breast tissue evenly
2. Palpate breast for lumps, masses, or thickening of skin
3. Use light, medium, and deep palpation to feel masses, using a slightly rotary motion to press breast tissue against chest wall
4. Palpate from clavicle to seventh rib to midaxillary line on each side, using one of the following methods:
   a. Concentric circles (most commonly used method): imagine breast as the face of a clock; start at outer aspect of breast at 12 o'clock and move through the numbers, and then move two fingerbreadths inward and repeat procedure until reaching nipple (see Figure 10-2A)
   b. Vertical strip method begins with palpation at sternal edge, moving up and down until reaching midaxillary line
   c. Pie method examines a wedge of breast at a time, moving around breast
   d. Back and forth technique begins at bottom of breast in midclavicular line and moves upward and outward as shown in Figure 10-2B
   e. Large breasted women may need bimanual palpation technique, which is supporting inferior aspect of breast with nondominant hand and using dominant hand to palpate anterior aspect against supporting hand
5. Palpation is performed bilaterally; be sure to palpate breast to tail of Spence (upper outer quadrant) carefully, as upper outer quadrant is a common site for masses
6. Palpate nipple by using index finger and thumb to apply pressure; repeat around entire nipple

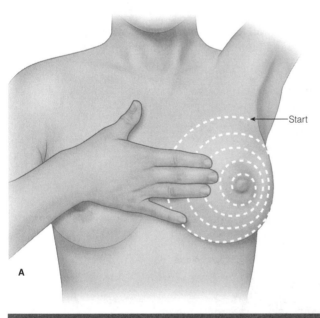
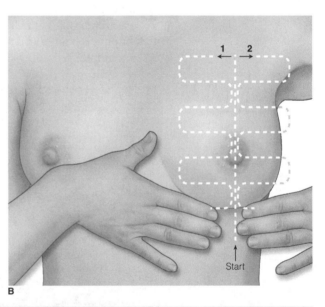

Start

1 2

Start

A

B

Figure 10-2

Alternative patterns for palpation. A. Concentric circles. B. Back and forth technique.

Figure 10-3

Lymph nodes of the breast

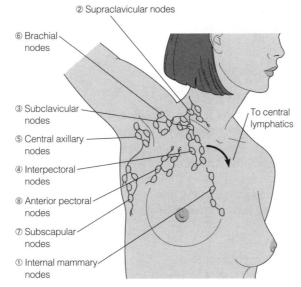

② Supraclavicular nodes

⑥ Brachial nodes

③ Subclavicular nodes

⑤ Central axillary nodes

④ Interpectoral nodes

⑧ Anterior pectoral nodes

⑦ Subscapular nodes

① Internal mammary nodes

To central lymphatics

7. Palpate axillae using fingertips with client sitting; palpate in all directions using light, medium, and deep palpation
   a. Palpate left axilla with right hand while supporting client's left arm so client's muscles are relaxed
   b. Palpate anterior border of axilla (for anterior or subpectoral lymph nodes), central area along rib cage (central axillary nodes), posterior border (subscapular nodes), and along inner aspect of upper arm (lateral nodes); remaining nodes are palpated while conducting palpation of breast tissue (see Figure 10-3)
   c. Repeat procedure on opposite arm
8. Palpation may be enhanced by a friction-free examination
   a. Assessment technique may be performed by using a warm, soapy lather so nurse's hands glide over breasts; provide a damp washcloth to remove soapy lather after exam
   b. Powder may be used during assessment to enable nurse's hands to glide over breasts; apply powder to gloves, not directly to client's skin, and face away from client while applying powder to prevent client aspiration of powder
   c. After exam, give client a cloth to remove any excess powder, which could be an irritant or remain on client's clothing

VI. EXPECTED FINDINGS
A. Inspection
1. Breast should be conical and symmetrical; however, not all women have breasts of equal size, because hand dominance can affect breast size
2. Skin tone and texture should be smooth and even
3. Breasts should be free of lesions, redness, edema, dimpling, or retractions
4. Nipples should be everted, pointing in same direction, with no discharge or lesions
5. Axillae should have no lesions or rashes
B. Palpation
1. Breasts should be soft, non-tender, and elastic with absence of masses
2. Premenopausal women should have firm breasts
3. Postmenopausal women may have breasts that feel cordlike

    4. Nipples should be elastic, nontender, and without discharge

    5. Lymph nodes should not be palpable

VII. UNEXPECTED FINDINGS

A. Inspection (see Table 10-2)

1. Asymmetrical breasts, lesions, dimpling, or retractions may be signs of breast cancer
2. Edema and **peau d'orange** (dimpled orange skin appearance) may be a sign of lymphatic blockage, which can occur with breast cancer
3. Redness may signify infection or carcinoma of breast
4. Nipple changes or nipples with lesions may indicate a metastatic process
5. Rashes may indicate an infection
6. Paget's disease is characterized by a malignant lesion of nipple with discharge and scaly erosion
7. Fibrocystic breast disease is characterized by one or more cysts that are thicker, nodular, mobile tender areas
8. Mastitis is characterized by breast tenderness, redness and warmth that occurs approximately one month after delivery
9. Interductal papilloma is accompanied by serous or serosanguineous discharge in one breast that may cause the client pain

B. Palpation

1. Enlarged, tender axillary lymph nodes may indicate infection of breast, arm, or hand
2. Hard, fixed lymph nodes that are usually painless may indicate cancer or lymphoma
3. Hard, fixed masses (usually not painful) with irregular borders in breast may indicate cancer

VIII. LIFESPAN CONSIDERATIONS

A. Infants

1. In either sex, a newborn's breast may be enlarged due to estrogen crossing placenta
2. There may be clear or white discharge from nipples that disappears within a few weeks after birth
3. Nipples should be symmetrical and flat

Table 10-2	Abnormal Breast Findings
Finding	**Description**
Fibrosis	Asymmetrical breast distortion due to malignant or nonmalignant tumor in breast; is nonmobile
Fibrocystic breast	Tender breast, swelling, mastalgia, nodule development, lumps, and discharge
Fibroadenoma	Single mass that is solid, nontender, firm but elastic, and moveable
Cancer	Nontender, hard, dense irregularly bordered mass may infiltrate nodes; dimpling, retraction, elevation, and discharge common
Mastitis	Pain; breast tenderness; warm, red breast with axillary node enlargement occurring about one month after delivery
Interductal papilloma	Serous or serosanguineous discharge unilaterally occurring toward end of menopause
Mammary ectasia	Nipple discharge and retraction with pain usually occurring in early menopause with enlarged lymph nodes
Peau d'orange	Skin of breast that has become thick, hard, and immobile and has an orange peel appearance; caused by interference with lymphatic drainage in breast cancer
Supernumerary nipple	Congenital benign finding in which there is an additional areola with a nipple

  B. **Female children**
   1. Breast tissue development begins in the prepubertal period
   2. Nipples should be symmetrical with no discharge
  C. **Adolescence**
   1. Female breasts may be symmetrical during development
   2. Breasts should be firm, without lesions or masses
  D. **Pregnant/lactating female**
   1. Breasts and nipples become enlarged
   2. Breasts develop a blue vascular pattern
   3. Breasts may develop striae (stretch marks)
   4. Nipples and areola become darker and larger
   5. Montgomery glands enlarge
   6. Discharge known as colostrum (precursor to milk) may be expressed from nipples during early pregnancy; it is yellow in color and rich in antibodies
   7. In lactating woman, milk production begins and breasts become enlarged, shiny, and firm to hard in texture
   8. During lactation, breasts may become sore or tender
   9. In lactating woman, if nipples and/or surrounding breast tissue becomes red and cracked, nipples should be kept dry and exposed to air
  E. **Older adults**
   1. Breasts lose elasticity of subcutaneous tissue and skin turgor and become pendulous and flat
   2. Nipples may invert or retract
   3. Tissue may feel cordlike and thickening may be present
  F. **Males**
   1. Breast tissue should feel like a thin disc under skin
   2. Males with gynecomastia (enlarged breasts) should not have masses
   3. Breasts should have no lumps or swelling
   4. Areolae should be flat and nipples should be flat and be free of discharge

IX. DOCUMENTATION

  A. **Document presence of lumps, swelling or edema, pain, redness, discharge, skin dimpling or retractions, skin discoloration or peau d'orange, skin texture, rashes, or cracked nipples (especially in lactating women)**
  B. **Document any findings during palpation such as lesions, nodules, changes in skin texture and consistency, or discharge**

Case Study

A 50-year-old female is in the nurse practitioner's office for an annual pelvic and breast examination. The client tells the nurse that "she felt a lump" in her left breast.

1. What questions should the nurse ask the client?

2. In what position(s) should the nurse place the client to perform the breast examination?

3. The nurse is having a difficult time palpating the breast due the client's dry skin. What technique can be employed to assist in the assessment?

4. What other clinical manifestations should the nurse assess for with the client?

5. What findings should the nurse document?

For suggested responses, see page 310

POSTTEST

1 When assessing the breasts of a 60-year-old woman, the nurse palpates the breasts and notes breast tissue that is pendulous with loss of elasticity. What action would the nurse take at this time?

1. Document this as a normal finding
2. Have a physician evaluate the client for underlying pathology
3. Prepare the client for mammography as this indicates fibrocystic breast disease
4. Assess the client for Paget's disease

2 The nurse performing a breast examination on a woman finds a crusty, scaly lesion on the right breast at the nipple. Based on this finding the nurse concludes that the client may have which health problem?

1. Fibrocystic breast disease
2. Mastitis
3. Paget's disease
4. Interductal papilloma

3 The nurse is teaching the client to perform breast self-examination (BSE). The nurse should teach the client to perform the steps of the examination in what order? Place the steps of the procedure in numerical order.

1. Palpate the axilla
2. Palpate the breast from the center outward using the finger pads
3. Inspect the axilla
4. Inspect the breast
5. Palpate the nipple

4 When teaching the pregnant woman about her breasts, the nurse would evaluate that the client understands the instruction when the client makes which statement?

1. "I will stop performing monthly breast exams until after the baby is born."
2. "Colostrum is present in the breasts until about one week after delivery."
3. "Colostrum is present in the breasts somewhere around the fourth month of pregnancy."
4. "Colostrum is not present in the breasts until one week postpartum."

5 The nurse is examining the breasts of a 15-year-old girl. The client asks the nurse why her right breast is larger than the left. What is the nurse's best answer?

1. "There may be a cancerous mass in the right breast so we will order a mammography."
2. "Hormonal changes throughout the month may increase the size of a breast during the month."
3. "One breast may grow faster than the other during adolescence."
4. "Try not to worry about it. We will keep an eye on it."

6 The nurse is assessing the breasts of an obese female. What is the most appropriate technique for the nurse to use to examine the breast?

1. Use a circular technique, starting from the nipple outward
2. Use any technique that permits the examiner to assess the breast
3. Position the client prone with breasts hanging over the examination table
4. Use the bimanual technique

7 The nurse is instructing a 47-year-old female client about mammography. The nurse should include which instruction?

1. Obtain a mammogram every year
2. Perform a breast self-examination (BSE) prior to having a mammogram
3. Obtain a mammogram when the client is menstruating
4. Schedule mammography at the same time as a pelvic examination

8 When documenting the findings of a breast examination on a pregnant female the nurse should expect to document which observation?

1. Nipple retraction
2. Mobile mammary ducts
3. Blue vascular pattern over breasts
4. Mobile nodule in each breast by the fourth month

9 The nurse working in a women's health clinic is teaching a female client about breast lesions. The nurse would explain that which characteristics are associated with a benign lesion? Select all that apply.

1. Soft
2. Mobile
3. Tenderness
4. Regular borders
5. Well-defined

10 Before assessing a female client's breasts for dimpling the nurse will position the client in which best position?

1. Supine
2. Sitting with hands over the head
3. Sitting with hands on the hips
4. Lateral

➤ *See pages 203–204 for Answers and Rationales.*

ANSWERS & RATIONALES

Pretest

1 **Answer: 4** **Rationale:** The incidence of breast cancer is highest in the upper outer quadrant of the breasts, including the tail of Spence. If the mass is in the tail of Spence, it must then be distinguished from enlarged lymph nodes. Breast cancer is not commonly detected in the nipple area (option 1), the inferior portion of the breasts (option 2), or near the sternal border of the breasts (option 3).
Cognitive Level: Application **Client Need:** Health Promotion and Maintenance **Integrated Process:** Teaching/Learning **Content Area:** Adult Health: Reproductive **Strategy:** Recall that the outer quadrant contains the tail of Spence and the lymph nodes, and therefore is the most common site for breast cancer. **Reference:** D'Amico, D. & Barbarito, C. (2007). *Health & physical assessment in nursing.* Upper Saddle River, NJ: Pearson Education, Inc., p. 412.

2 **Answer: 1** **Rationale:** The client who presents with a breast infection will have the following clinical manifestations: redness, swelling, edema, fever, pain, enlarged nodes surrounding the breast, and possibly discharge. Lesions (option 2) are manifested by the presence of a mass. Everted nipples (option 3) may be either a normal finding or may be present with cancer, not infection. Cystic breast disease (option 4) is manifested by thickening or the presence of mobile tender nodular area(s) in the breast.
Cognitive Level: Application **Client Need:** Health Promotion and Maintenance **Integrated Process:** Nursing Process: Assessment **Content Area:** Adult Health: Reproductive **Strategy:** Recall that classic signs of infection, regardless of location, are pain, redness, and swelling. With this in mind, you can systematically eliminate each of the incorrect responses easily. Recall specifically that infection of the breast usually manifests as pain; warmth; and red, cracked, tender breast with enlarged nodes.
Reference: D'Amico, D. & Barbarito, C. (2007). *Health & physical assessment in nursing.* Upper Saddle River, NJ: Pearson Education, Inc., p. 415.

3 **Answer: 3** **Rationale:** This mother is clearly upset. Since a lump is not an airway or circulatory issue the nurse can offer emotional support and permit the mother to verbalize anxiety. Most breast lesions found in teenagers are cancerous and it is inappropriate to state it is not cancerous without evaluation (option 1). The lump does not require a trip to the emergency room but should be evaluated in a gynecologist's office and mammography suite (option 2). Even though breast cancer has a familial tendency it is inappropriate to tell the mother her daughter does not have cancer (option 4).
Cognitive Level: Analysis **Client Need:** Psychosocial Integrity **Integrated Process:** Caring **Content Area:** Adult Health: Reproductive **Strategy:** Note that the client in this question is the mother of the adolescent. Because the client is clearly upset, therapeutic communication principles should be employed. This is the only distracter that is therapeutic and permits the mother to verbalize feelings. **Reference:** D'Amico, D. & Barbarito, C. (2007). *Health & physical assessment in nursing.* Upper Saddle River, NJ: Pearson Education, Inc., p. 401.

4 **Answer: 1** **Rationale:** Cardiac glycosides such as digoxin (Lanoxin) can cause gynecomastia in males. Increased caloric intake and sedentary lifestyle cause weight gain but not necessarily enlarged breasts (options 2 and 3). Female hormones would not be ordered for cardiovascular disease (option 4).
Cognitive Level: Application **Client Need:** Nursing Process: Analysis **Integrated Process:** Communication and Documentation **Content Area:** Adult Health: Reproductive **Strategy:** First note that the client in the question is male and the core issue of the question is enlarged breasts, so the focus is on gynecomastia. Next note that options 2 and 3 are similar, so eliminate them both. Finally choose option 1 over option 4 as this is the true statement. Cardiac glycosides have a side effect of gynecomastia, which is enlarged breasts in males. **Reference:** D'Amico, D. & Barbarito, C. (2007). *Health & physical assessment in nursing.* Upper Saddle River, NJ: Pearson Education, Inc., p. 419.

POSTTEST

ANSWERS & RATIONALES

5 **Answer: 1** **Rationale:** The first step for a breast examination is inspection of the breasts and then axillae; the second step is palpation of the breast and then the axillae. Percussion and auscultation are not performed during the breast examination.
Cognitive Level: Knowledge **Client Need:** Health Promotion and Maintenance **Integrated Process:** Nursing Process: Assessment **Content Area:** Adult Health: Reproductive **Strategy:** Remember that when there are multiple parts to an option, all parts must be correct in order for the option to be correct. To easily eliminate each of the incorrect options, recall that percussion and auscultation have no use in examination of the breasts. **Reference:** D'Amico, D. & Barbarito, C. (2007). *Health & physical assessment in nursing.* Upper Saddle River, NJ: Pearson Education, Inc., pp. 408–415.

6 **Answer: 2** **Rationale:** Cyclic hormonal changes may cause cyclic breast nodules. Breast cancer may be associated with palpable masses but would be present continuously, not for a few days each month (option 1). Stress should not cause breast nodules (option 3). Pregnancy may cause breast tenderness but not cyclic nodules (option 4).
Cognitive Level: Analysis **Client Need:** Health Promotion and Maintenance **Integrated Process:** Communication and Documentation **Content Area:** Adult Health: Reproductive **Strategy:** The critical words in the question are *nodular* and *a few days during the month*. Eliminate option 1 first because breast cancer would not have intermittent findings. Eliminate option 4 next because pregnancy may cause breast tenderness and enlargement but not nodules. Recall that monthly hormonal changes may cause cyclic breast nodularity to choose option 2 over option 3. **Reference:** D'Amico, D. & Barbarito, C. (2007). *Health & physical assessment in nursing.* Upper Saddle River, NJ: Pearson Education, Inc., p. 404.

7 **Answer: 3** **Rationale:** After about the fourth month, colostrum may be released from the breasts. It is a thin, yellow liquid that is a precursor to milk. It is not necessary to obtain a culture and sensitivity or start the client on antibiotics (options 1 and 2). A breast assessment is not necessary (option 4) as this is a normal finding and requires client education.
Cognitive Level: Application **Client Need:** Health Promotion and Maintenance **Integrated Process:** Nursing Process: Implementation **Content Area:** Adult Health: Reproductive **Strategy:** Note that options 1 and 2 both imply there is an infection, and because they are similar they must be eliminated. Note also that the correct option involves teaching, a cognitive intervention, whereas the other distracters are physical interventions, so choose option 3 over 4. Recall that teaching about normal developments during pregnancy is therapeutic and appropriate and permits the mother to verbalize feelings. **Reference:** D'Amico, D. & Barbarito, C. (2007). *Health & physical assessment in nursing.* Upper Saddle River, NJ: Pearson Education, Inc., p. 402.

8 **Answer: 4** **Rationale:** A supernumerary nipple has the appearance of a mole but is benign. It is not an actual mole (option 1). It is not a suspicious lesion and does not need further evaluation (option 2). It is not lymphatic tissue (option 3).
Cognitive Level: Application **Client Need:** Health Promotion and Maintenance **Integrated Process:** Nursing Process: Assessment **Content Area:** Adult Health: Reproductive **Strategy:** Specific knowledge is needed to answer this question. The critical words in the question are *brown spot* and *nipple located in the center.* Associate these words with the term *supernumerary nipple* in the correct option. Recall next that this finding is not significant and does not require further evaluation. **Reference:** D'Amico, D. & Barbarito, C. (2007). *Health & physical assessment in nursing.* Upper Saddle River, NJ: Pearson Education, Inc., p. 400.

9 **Answer: 3** **Rationale:** Mastitis is an infection in the breast that manifests as a red, warm, swollen breast with accompanying fever. The signs of breast cancer include presence of a mass and possible skin changes and/or pain (option 1). Infected lymph nodes would manifest as fever, enlarged node or mass (option 2). Influenza would present as a respiratory infection (option 4).
Cognitive Level: Analysis **Client Need:** Health Promotion and Maintenance **Integrated Process:** Nursing Process: Assessment **Content Area:** Adult Health: Reproductive **Strategy:** The critical words in the question are *gave birth one month ago.* With this in mind, evaluate each of the options for a possible postpartum complication. Eliminate options 1 and 4 first since breast cancer and influenza are not postpartum complications. Next choose option 3 over option 2 because it is a better match for the client's symptoms. Recall that mastitis most commonly occurs one month after delivery and manifests as a reddened, swollen, warm breast with fever. **Reference:** D'Amico, D. & Barbarito, C. (2007). *Health & physical assessment in nursing.* Upper Saddle River, NJ: Pearson Education, Inc., p. 868.

10 **Answer: 4** **Rationale:** Caucasian women over age 40 have the greatest risk for breast cancer, especially if they carry the BRCA 1 or 2 genes. African-American females under age 40 have a greater risk than their peers. All women do not have equal risk (option 1). Breast self-examinations should be performed monthly (option 2) and mammography should be performed yearly (option 3).
Cognitive Level: Application **Client Need:** Health Promotion and Maintenance **Integrated Process:** Teaching/Learning **Content Area:** Adult Health: Reproductive **Strategy:** First eliminate options 2 and 3 because of incorrect timeframes. Then recall that, as with most disease processes, the risk of developing breast cancer varies with genetic predisposition, so eliminate option 1. **Reference:** D'Amico, D. & Barbarito, C. (2007). *Health & physical assessment in nursing.* Upper Saddle River, NJ: Pearson Education, Inc., p. 403.

Posttest

1 **Answer: 1** **Rationale:** Pendulous breast tissue is a normal change that occurs with age (option 1). The physician does not need to evaluate this client as this is a benign finding (option 2). Fibrocystic breast disease presents as a nodular, soft, movable lesion (option 3). Paget's disease is a malignancy that starts as a scaly, crusty lesion on the nipple (option 4).
Cognitive Level: Analysis **Client Need:** Health Promotion and Maintenance **Integrated Process:** Communication and Documentation **Content Area:** Adult Health: Reproductive **Strategy:** Recall that as people age breast tissue is replaced with adipose fibrous tissue. Elderly people lose muscle mass, causing breasts to become pendulous. **Reference:** D'Amico, D. & Barbarito, C. (2007). *Health & physical assessment in nursing.* Upper Saddle River, NJ: Pearson Education, Inc., p. 402.

2 **Answer: 3** **Rationale:** Paget's disease is a malignant lesion of the nipple with discharge and scaly erosion (option 3). Fibrocystic breast disease manifests as a thicker, nodular, mobile tender area (option 1). Mastitis is characterized by breast tenderness, redness and warmth that occurs approximately one month after delivery (option 2). Interductal papilloma is a serous or serosanguineous discharge in one breast that may cause the client pain (option 4).
Cognitive Level: Analysis **Client Need:** Physiological Integrity: Physiological Adaptation **Integrated Process:** Nursing Process: Assessment **Content Area:** Adult Health: Reproductive **Strategy:** First eliminate mastitis as it ends in *-itis* and therefore is an infection. Next recall that interductal papilloma is a blocked duct to eliminate option 4. Finally, recall that fibrocystic breast disease is a thickened nodular area in the breast that may be tender to eliminate option 1. Alternatively, recall that Paget's disease is a malignant disorder that begins with a scaly erosion of the nipple to choose option 3 **Reference:** D'Amico, D. & Barbarito, C. (2007). *Health & physical assessment in nursing.* Upper Saddle River, NJ: Pearson Education, Inc., p. 410.

3 **Answer: 4, 3, 2, 1, 5** **Rationale:** The client should be taught to inspect the breast then the axilla by looking in a mirror with arms elevated and the hands on hips. After inspection the client should be taught to palpate the breast, axilla, and nipple using the fingerpads systematically. This procedure should be performed monthly and can be done in the shower or in front of a mirror. The client needs to be taught to report any usual findings to the healthcare provider.
Cognitive Level: Analysis **Client Need:** Health Promotion and Maintenance **Integrated Process:** Nursing Process: Implementation **Content Area:** Adult Health: Reproductive **Strategy:** To correctly answer this question, remember that inspection is always completed first and the sequencing is breast tissue, then axilla, and finally nipple. **Reference:** D'Amico, D. & Barbarito, C. (2007). *Health & physical assessment in nursing.* Upper Saddle River, NJ: Pearson Education, Inc., pp. 408–416.

4 **Answer: 3** **Rationale:** After the fourth month of pregnancy, a thick yellow precursor to milk (colostrum) is present in the breasts (option 3). Colostrum is full of antibodies to protect the newborn after delivery. Monthly breast examinations should be performed to detect lesions (option 1). Colostrum is in the breasts during pregnancy, after delivery, and until milk production is established, usually within the first few days postpartum (options 2 and 4).
Cognitive Level: Analysis **Client Need:** Health Promotion and Maintenance **Integrated Process:** Nursing Process: Implementation **Content Area:** Adult Health: Reproductive **Strategy:** You can eliminate the first option because it does not promote health. Eliminate options 2 and 4 as they are both postpartum answers, while option 3 is during pregnancy. **Reference:** D'Amico, D. & Barbarito, C. (2007). *Health & physical assessment in nursing.* Upper Saddle River, NJ: Pearson Education, Inc., p. 402.

5 **Answer: 3** **Rationale:** One breast may grow faster than the other throughout the period of adolescence (option 3). If the nurse felt a mass in the breast then the nurse would refer the client to a physician for further evaluation (option 1). Hormonal changes may cause breast tenderness throughout the month (option 2). It is inappropriate to tell a client not to worry as it negates his or her feelings (option 4).
Cognitive Level: Analysis **Client Need:** Health Promotion and Maintenance **Integrated Process:** Teaching/Learning **Content Area:** Adult Health: Reproductive **Strategy:** Eliminate option 4 first, realizing that it is not a therapeutic communication. Nurses should encourage open lines of communication to allow clients to express their feelings. Next eliminate option 1 because nurses do not order diagnostic tests. Choose correctly between the two remaining options either by recalling that breast growth may be uneven during adolescence or by noting that the phrase *throughout the month* in option 2 is strangely worded. **Reference:** D'Amico, D. & Barbarito, C. (2007). *Health & physical assessment in nursing.* Upper Saddle River, NJ: Pearson Education, Inc., p. 401.

6 **Answer: 4** **Rationale:** The bimanual technique is used to support the breast and permit the breast to be compressed between the hands (option 4). The breasts may be examined using a vertical, circular, or bimanual technique as long as the technique is systematic, but the bimanual technique in large-breasted women facilitates assessment (options 1 and 2). For inspection, the client should be positioned sitting and standing, hands over head and hands on hips; for palpation the client should be in the supine position for proper examination of the breasts (option 3).
Cognitive Level: Application **Client Need:** Health Promotion and Maintenance **Integrated Process:** Nursing Process: Implementation **Content Area:** Adult Health: Reproductive **Strategy:** Recall that the bimanual technique facilitates assessment of large breasts. Breasts should be inspected with the client sitting and standing with hands over head

and on hips and palpated when the client is supine.
Reference: D'Amico, D. & Barbarito, C. (2007). *Health & physical assessment in nursing*. Upper Saddle River, NJ: Pearson Education, Inc., p. 414.

7 **Answer: 1** **Rationale:** Mammography should be performed yearly for the women in this age range (option 1). The client should perform a BSE during the fourth to seventh day of the menstrual cycle (option 2). During menses the breasts may be tender (option 3). It is not necessary to perform the mammogram at the same time as the pelvic examination (option 4).
Cognitive Level: Application **Client Need:** Health Promotion and Maintenance **Integrated Process:** Teaching/Learning **Content Area:** Adult Health: Reproductive **Strategy:** Recall that mammography should be performed yearly after age 40 to quickly eliminate each of the incorrect options. **Reference:** D'Amico, D. & Barbarito, C. (2007). *Health & physical assessment in nursing*. Upper Saddle River, NJ: Pearson Education, Inc., p. 405.

8 **Answer: 3** **Rationale:** During pregnancy the woman often develops a vascular pattern over the breasts (option 3). Nipple retraction is associated with breast cancer (option 1). Mammary ducts are not mobile (option 2). Pregnancy does not cause the formation of nodules (option 4).
Cognitive Level: Application **Client Need:** Health Promotion and Maintenance **Integrated Process:** Communication and Documentation **Content Area:** Adult Health: Reproductive **Strategy:** Recall that common breast changes during pregnancy include increased size, stretch marks, darker nipples, and development of a vascular pattern. **Reference:** D'Amico, D. & Barbarito, C. (2007). *Health & physical assessment in nursing*. Upper Saddle River, NJ: Pearson Education, Inc., p. 406.

9 **Answer: 3, 4, 5** **Rationale:** Benign breast lesions may be tender to the touch, are well-defined and have regular

borders. They are usually firm, not soft (option 1) and are not mobile (option 1). In contrast, malignant lesions are usually solid, dense, hard, and nontender with irregular and poorly defined borders. Other findings associated with malignancy may include nipple retraction, dimpling, discharge, and palpable nodes.
Cognitive Level: Analysis **Client Need:** Health Promotion and Maintenance **Integrated Process:** Teaching/Learning **Content Area:** Adult Health: Reproductive **Strategy:** Recall that cancer is usually a unilateral, nontender, solid, dense mass with an irregular border. This will help to eliminate some incorrect options. **Reference:** D'Amico, D. & Barbarito, C. (2007). *Health & physical assessment in nursing*. Upper Saddle River, NJ: Pearson Education, Inc., p. 419.

10 **Answer: 3** **Rationale:** Sitting with hands on the hips contracts the pectoralis muscle, facilitating the ability to observe for dimpling (option 3). The supine position (option 1) evenly distributes the breast tissue over the chest wall and does not accentuate dimpling. Lifting hands over the head (option 2) will permit the nurse to observe fibrosis of the breast, as one breast will lag behind the other. The lateral position (option 4) is not used during breast assessment.
Cognitive Level: Application **Client Need:** Health Promotion and Maintenance **Integrated Process:** Nursing Process: Assessment **Content Area:** Adult Health: Reproductive **Strategy:** Recall that the positions that facilitate breast assessment include supine, sitting with hands over head, and sitting with hands on hips; this will help to eliminate option 4. Next notice the critical word *best* in the question to select the option that provides optimal visualization of dimpling during skin inspection. **Reference:** D'Amico, D. & Barbarito, C. (2007). *Health & physical assessment in nursing*. Upper Saddle River, NJ: Pearson Education, Inc., pp. 410–411.

References

Bickley, L. (2010). *Bates guide to physical examination and history taking* (10th ed.). Philadelphia: Lippincott Williams & Wilkins.

D'Amico, D. & Barbarito, C. (2007). *Health & physical assessment in nursing*. Upper Saddle River, NJ: Pearson Education, Inc., pp. 397–424.

Jarvis, C. (2008). *Physical examination and health assessment* (5th ed.). St. Louis, MO: Elsevier Saunders.

Zator-Estes, M. (2009). *Health assessment and physical examination* (4th ed.). Clifton Park, NY: Delmar Cengage Learning.

Female Genitourinary Assessment

11

Chapter Outline

Health History
Present Health History
Family History

Equipment, Preparation, and
    Positioning
Examination Techniques
Expected Findings

Unexpected Findings
Lifespan Considerations
Documentation

Objectives

➤ Discuss the anatomy and physiology of the female genitourinary system.
➤ Conduct a health history and sexual history of a client.
➤ Utilize the assessment techniques necessary to complete an assessment of the genitourinary system.
➤ Differentiate normal from abnormal findings obtained during the assessment of the female genitourinary system.

NCLEX-RN® Test Prep

Visit the Companion Website for this book at www.pearsonhighered.com/hogan to access additional practice opportunities and more.

Review at a Glance

anteflexion position in which uterus is folded forward at a 90-degree angle and cervix is tilted downward

anteversion normal position of uterus in which it is tilted forward and cervix is tilted downward

Bartholin's glands vestibular glands located posteriorly at base of vestibule whose function is to produce mucus that is released into vestibule and actively promotes sperm motility and viability

cervix lowest portion of uterus that joins to vagina

cystocele a hernia that develops when bladder is pushed into vagina

hymen a thin membrane of tissue over vaginal opening in females who have not become sexually active

introitus vaginal opening

labia lip-like folds of skin on either side of vestibule and urethra; divided into labia majora and labia minora

midposition when uterus lies parallel to tailbone and cervix is pointed straight

ovaries organs located on either side of lower abdominopelvic region that produce and store ova and produce hormones progesterone and estrogen

perineum external area between vaginal opening and anus

rectocele a hernia that develops when rectum pushes into vagina

retroflexion a position in which uterus is folded backward at a 90-degree angle and cervix is tilted upward

retroversion position in which uterus is tilted backward and cervix is tilted upward

Skene's glands glands located within vestibule below urethral meatus that produce a lubricating fluid in response to sexual arousal

uterus muscular, hollow organ located in abdominal cavity between rectum and bladder and that is occupied by growing fetus during pregnancy

vagina long, muscular canal that extends from vestibule to cervix

PRETEST

1 When gathering data about a female client's reproductive health, the nurse should ask the client which questions? Select all that apply.

1. "How old were you when you first menstruated?"
2. "How long does your menstrual cycle last?"
3. "How would you describe your menstrual flow?"
4. "How do you feel during your period?"
5. "Do you have hemorrhoids?"

2 To determine problems with reproductive health the nurse should ask the client which question?

1. "Do you use tampons or pads during menstruation?"
2. "Have you ever had an illness associated with your reproductive system?"
3. "Do you achieve sexual satisfaction?"
4. "Are you sexually active?"

3 To determine information about a vaginal infection the nurse should gather data related to which item?

1. Vaginal bleeding
2. Itching of the labia
3. Vaginal surgery
4. Sexual arousal

4 To perform an examination of the female genitalia, the nurse would place the client in which acceptable position? Select all that apply.

1. Knee-chest
2. Lithotomy
3. Lateral Sims'
4. Prone
5. Standing

5 The nurse is inspecting a female client's external genitalia and notes cauliflower-like lesions. The nurse should conclude that these lesions are consistent with which health problem?

1. A cystocele
2. Pregnancy
3. Syphilitic lesions
4. Genital warts

6 During examination of a female older adult client the nurse notes a blue cyanotic cervix. The nurse concludes that this client should be evaluated for which health problem?

1. Pregnancy
2. A sexually transmitted disease
3. Congestive heart failure
4. Cancer

7 During assessment of the female genitalia the nurse would document which observation as a normal finding?

1. Sparse hair distribution
2. Yellowish fluid on Bartholin's gland
3. Cheese-like substance present in the labia folds
4. Round and closed cervical os in a nulliparous woman

8 When obtaining a Papanicolaou (Pap) smear on a female client, the nurse will obtain the sample using which method?

1. Inserting a wooden applicator to scrape cervical cells
2. Using a cotton-tipped applicator to obtain cervical cells
3. Applying material from the examiner's gloved hand to the slide
4. Obtaining a sample of secretions from the vaginal vault

9 The nurse is about to perform a bimanual examination of a female client's reproductive system. Place the following steps for performing a bimanual examination in chronological order.

1. Slip a finger into vaginal recesses to palpate fornices
2. Palpate the uterus by pushing on the abdomen between the umbilicus and symphysis pubis
3. Place a lubricated, gloved index and middle finger of the dominant hand in the vagina to palpate the cervix
4. Palpate the ovaries by placing fingers in the left vaginal fornix and pushing on the abdomen, and then repeating on the right side
5. Perform a rectovaginal examination

10 After performing a rectovaginal examination the nurse would take which action next?

1. Dispose of gloves and instruct the client to dress
2. Perform a test for occult blood on matter that is on the gloved finger
3. Discuss the findings of the examination with the client
4. Dispose of all equipment

➤ *See pages 220–222 for Answers and Rationales.*

I. HEALTH HISTORY

A. Ask the client questions about sexual and reproductive health, keeping in mind that this subjective matter is very private and personal
   1. Be sensitive to need for privacy
   2. Assure client that all information will be kept confidential

B. Begin assessment by asking general questions
   1. "Do you have concerns about your health?"
   2. "How old were you when you experienced your first period?"
      a. "What was the first day of your last period?"
      b. "How long does your menstrual cycle usually last?"
      c. "Is your menstrual cycle consistent or irregular?"
      d. "How many days does the menses last?"
      e. "How would you describe your menstrual flow?"
      f. "How do you feel when experiencing your menses?"
      g. "How do feel just before your menses?"
      h. "Do you experience cramps? If so, how do you relieve cramping?"
      i. "Do you take anything for menstrual symptoms?"
      j. "Do you use home remedies for your menses?"
   3. "Have you ever been pregnant? If so, how many times?"
      a. "Did you experience any problems during the pregnancy, delivery, or postpartum period? If yes, please describe them."
      b. "Were your deliveries vaginal or cesarean section?"
   4. "Have you ever had a miscarriage?"
      a. "Do you know what caused the miscarriage?"
      b. "Did you need to undergo surgery?"
   5. "Have you ever had an abortion?"
      a. "At how many weeks was the abortion performed?"
      b. "How has it been emotionally?"
   6. "Do you have children?"
      a. "How many children do you have? Are you the birth mother?"
      b. If none, "Have you attempted to have children? If so, for how long?"
      c. If the client has been unable to conceive after one year, "How often do you and your partner engage in intercourse?"
         1) "Have you sought assistance for fertility problems? If so what did the treatment involve?"
         2) "Has the inability to conceive placed a strain on your relationship?"
   7. "Are you sexually active?"
      a. "Are there any issues that prevent you from achieving sexual satisfaction?"
      b. "Have you ever experienced pain during intercourse?"
      c. "Have you experienced a change in your libido (sex drive)?"
         1) "Can you describe the change?"
         2) "Is the change associated with anything in particular?"
      d. "Do you use contraceptives? If yes, what type?"

C. Ask questions related to illness or infections

1. "Are you or have you ever experienced any problems associated with the female reproductive system?"
2. If so, "Have you ever been diagnosed with the following problems?" (see Box 11-1 for risk factors associated with female reproductive cancers)
   a. Dysmenorrhea
   b. Uterine fibroids
   c. Uterine cancer
   d. Cervical cancer
   e. Vulvar cancer
3. "What was the treatment for the problem?"
   a. "Was the treatment successful?"
   b. "Has the problem ever recurred?"
   c. "How do you manage the problem?"
4. "Have you ever experienced an infection such as cystitis, vaginitis, or pelvic inflammatory disease?"
   a. "If so, when?"
   b. "What treatment was prescribed for the infection?"
   c. "After treatment did you feel better?"
   d. "What other treatments, if any, have you tried for the infection?"
   e. "Has the infection ever recurred?"
   f. "Are you experiencing an infection now?"
5. "Have you ever had surgery on your reproductive system?"
   a. If so "What type? When? Where?"
   b. "What was the outcome of the surgery?"
6. "Have you ever had an abnormal Papanicolaou (Pap) smear?"
   a. If so, "How long ago was it?"
   b. "What treatment was needed?"
   c. "What was the outcome?"
7. "Have you had a sexually transmitted disease, such as herpes, gonorrhea, syphilis, human papillomavirus, or chlamydia?"
   a. "Was it treated? If so, how?"
   b. "Was your partner treated?"
8. "Have you been exposed to HIV?"
   a. If yes, "Can you describe the situation?"
   b. "Have you been tested for HIV? If so, what were the results?"

D. Ask client about symptoms associated with reproductive system

1. "Have you ever had any rashes, lesions, ulcerations, sores, or warts on your genitalia or surrounding tissue?"

Practice to Pass

What questions should the nurse ask a client to obtain information about a history of abnormal Pap smear?

!

Practice to Pass

What should the nurse ask the client to assess symptoms associated with the reproductive system?

Box 11-1	Cervical Cancer	Ovarian Cancer	Endometrial Cancer
Risk Factors Associated with Cancer	Early age sexual intercourse	Advancing age	Family history of cancer, diabetes, or hypertension
	Multiple sexual partners	Early menarche	
		Late menopause	Nulliparity
	Human papillomavirus infection	Nulliparity	Infertility
		History of infertility	Late menopause
	Cigarette smoking	History of female reproductive cancer	History of menstrual irregularities
	Onset before age 40 or 50 years	Caucasian	

Practice to Pass

A client tells the nurse that she has a discharge from the vagina. What questions should the nurse ask to assess the discharge?

2. "Have you ever had or felt any lumps or masses in any area?"
   a. If so, "Can you describe what you felt?"
   b. "Where was/is the lesion/mass?"
   c. "Was/is it soft or hard? Is it movable?"
   d. "When did you first notice the mass or lesion?"
   e. "Is it painful?"
   f. "Have you noticed any change in it since it developed?"
   g. "Have you used home remedies to treat it?"
3. "Have you seen any redness or swelling of your genitals?"
4. "Do you have any organs protruding from your vagina?"
5. "Have you ever noticed any discharge from your vagina?"
   a. If so, "What color was it?"
   b. "Is there any discharge now?"
   c. "Is there any odor to it?"
   d. "Can you describe the amount of the discharge?"
   e. "When did you first notice the discharge?"
6. "Have you ever had any itching of the **vagina** (long, muscular canal that extends from vestibule to cervix) or **labia** (lip-like folds of skin on either side of vestibule and urethra)?"
   a. If so, "When did it start?"
   b. "Has it been treated? If so, how?"
   c. "Have there been any associated urinary symptoms?"
7. "Have you ever had any vaginal bleeding outside your normal menstrual cycle?"
   a. If so, "When did it occur?"
   b. "How much bleeding occurs?"
8. "Have you ever had any problems in the rectal area, such as pain, itching, burning, or bleeding?"
   a. "When did the problem begin?"
   b. "Do you ever engage in anal intercourse?"
   c. "Do you know what is causing the problem?"
   d. "Have you been treated for the problem?"
   e. "What was the treatment? Has it helped?"
9. "Do you have any pain, tenderness, or soreness in your pelvic area?"
   a. If yes, "Can you please describe the pain?"
      1) "Is it dull, sharp, radiating, intermittent, or continuous?"
      2) "When did it start?"
      3) "Does anything make the pain better or worse?"
   b. "Are there any associated symptoms? If so, can you please describe the symptoms?"
10. "Do you routinely check your genitals? If so, how often?"
11. "How often do you get a physical examination?"
12. "Do you use tampons?"
    a. If yes, "How often do you change the tampon?"
    b. "Do you know the risks of toxic shock syndrome, a risk factor of using tampons?"
13. "What products do you use for feminine hygiene?"
14. "Are you in a monogamous relationship?"
    a. If not, "Are you aware of sexually transmitted infections?"
    b. "What precautions do you take to protect against sexually transmitted infections?"
    c. "Do you use latex condoms?"
15. "Are you able to be sexually aroused?"
16. "Are you satisfied with your sexual experiences?"
    a. If not, "Are you able to achieve an orgasm?"
    b. "Have you noticed a change in your ability to have an orgasm?"

17. "Are you able to talk to your partner about your sexual needs?"
    a. "Does your partner listen to your needs?"
    b. "Do you accept your partner's needs?"
18. "Does your family accept your relationship with your partner?"
19. "Are you and your partner using contraceptives?"
    a. If so "What type of contraceptive(s)?"
    b. "Do you use contraceptives consistently?"
20. "Have you ever been sexually abused?"
    a. "Have you ever been molested or raped?"
    b. If so, "When and by whom?"
    c. "Have you done anything about this?"
E. **Age-specific questions**
    1. Depending on client age, ask these questions of child (or caregiver as appropriate) when assessing children
       a. "Have you ever noticed any redness, swelling, or discharge that is discolored or foul smelling?"
       b. "Have you had any itching, burning, or swelling in the genital area?"
       c. "Has anyone ever touched you when you did not want them to?"
          1) "Where did they touch you?"
          2) "Has anyone ever asked you to touch them when you did not want to?"
          3) "Where did he or she ask you to touch him or her?"
          4) "Who touched you?"
          5) "How many times did this happen?"
          6) "Who else knows about this?"
    2. In addition to the preceding questions for children, ask an adolescent client, "Are you having sexual relations with anyone?"
    3. When working with an older adult, ask the following questions:
       a. "When did you begin menopause?"
       b. "What physical changes you have noticed since menopause?"
       c. "Since starting menopause, have you had any vaginal bleeding?"

II. PRESENT HEALTH HISTORY

Practice to Pass

To assess a client's current health status, what questions should the nurse ask the client?

A. **Ask client about any experience with chronic illness; have client describe illness**
B. **Ask about current prescription medication: what kind, dosage, frequency, and intended and unintended effects**
C. **Ask about any over-the-counter medications**
    1. "What medications are being taken?"
    2. "What herbal medications are being taken?"
D. **Ask about regular pelvic examinations**
    1. "When was last pelvic examination?"
    2. "When was last Papanicolaou (Pap) smear?"
    3. "What were the findings?"

III. FAMILY HISTORY

A. **The number of questions to ask the client is more limited when assessing the female reproductive system**
B. **A key area to assess is whether any female in client's family has had cancer of breast, *cervix* (lowest portion of uterus that joins to vagina), ovary, or *uterus* (muscular, hollow organ located in abdominal cavity between rectum and bladder)**

C. Another question is whether client's mother took diethylstilbestrol (DES) treatment during pregnancy
1. Daughters of mothers who took DES have had increased rates of cervical cancer, infertility, and ectopic pregnancy
2. Although drug has been off the market since 1971, effects could persist depending on age and generation of client

IV. EQUIPMENT, PREPARATION, AND POSITIONING

A. Equipment: Gather the equipment and supplies to perform an assessment of female reproductive system
1. Examination gown
2. Examination drape or flat sheet
3. Examination lamp
4. Non-sterile examination gloves
5. Lubricant
6. Endocervical (Pap smear) spatula
7. Endocervical (Pap smear) cotton-tipped applicator
8. Slide
9. Fixative
10. Speculum
11. Mirror (for client to visualize genitalia)

B. Positioning and preparation
1. Be sure to know how to operate a speculum, to lock and unlock blades
2. Warm speculum by running it under warm water
3. Select an appropriate-sized speculum; nulliparous women require a narrow Pedersen speculum
4. Provide privacy and warmth
5. Have client empty bowels and bladder
6. Permit client to change in private
7. Drape client appropriately to preserve dignity
8. Use an unhurried, deliberate approach
9. Reassure and ask client how she is doing during examination
10. Use standard precautions
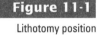 11. Position client in lithotomy position with buttocks to edge of table and feet in foot rests of stirrups (Figure 11-1)

Figure 11-1

Lithotomy position

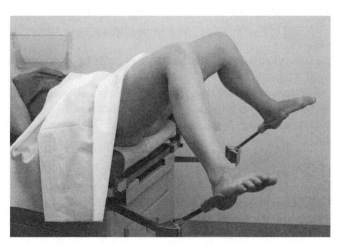

12. Explain procedure prior to beginning examination and during examination
13. Upon completion of assessment have client dress privately, and then explain findings

V. EXAMINATION TECHNIQUES

A. **Inspect pubic hair distribution; hair should be evenly distributed and may extend to umbilicus; note if client shaves pubic area and assess for infection and/or irritation**
B. **Inspect skin over mons pubis and inguinal area; inspect for lesions or infestations and for any piercings the client may have**
C. **Inspect labia majora and minora by using index finger and thumb of non-dominant hand to separate labia**
   1. Pigmentation should be darker than general skin color
   2. Inspect whether tissue is shriveled or full, gaping or closed, dry or moist; inspect for nodules, lesions, infestations, ulcerations
D. **Inspect clitoris for size**
E. **Inspect urethral meatus, vaginal *introitus* (vaginal opening), and *perineum* (external area between vaginal opening and anus)**
   1. Inspect for positioning; meatus should be midline
   2. Inspect introitus for the presence of a **hymen** (thin membrane of tissue over vaginal opening in females not yet sexually active) and discoloration; opening should be moist
   3. Inspect skin of perineum for smoothness, lesions, presence of a hymen, and discoloration
F. **Inspect anus for color, lesions, ulcerations, growths, deformities, hemorrhoids, and bleeding**
G. **Palpate labia majora by using index finger; palpate for lesions or nodules**
H. **Palpate labia minora by using index finger; palpate for lesions or nodules**
I. **Palpate *Skene's glands* (glands located within vestibule below urethral meatus that produce a lubricating fluid in response to sexual arousal) and *Bartholin's glands* (vestibular glands located posteriorly at base of vestibule that produce mucus that actively promotes sperm motility and viability) (Figures 11-2 and 11-3)**
   1. Palpate for pain, discomfort, or discharge by inserting an index finger upward into anterior vaginal wall
   2. Palpate lateral wall tissue of vagina by using index finger and thumb
J. **Palpate vaginal wall, rectum, and observe for urinary incontinence**
   1. Palpate vaginal wall and rectum for muscle tone by placing a finger in vagina and having client squeeze the vaginal orifice
   2. Remove finger and have client bear down; observe for bulging and urinary incontinence
K. **Insert a speculum (in a horizontal or oblique position) into vaginal opening**
   1. Inserting first two fingers of non-dominant hand and press down on posterior vaginal wall
   2. Wait for vaginal wall muscles to relax prior to inserting speculum lubricated with water (Figure 11-4)
   3. Do not use water-soluble lubricant, as lubricant will interfere with cytological studies
   4. Rotate speculum into a horizontal position and open blades
   5. Visualize cervical os and lock blades
L. **Inspect cervical os**
   1. Inspect for color and symmetry
   2. Inspect for smoothness and position
   3. Inspect for size and shape
   4. Inspect for discharge

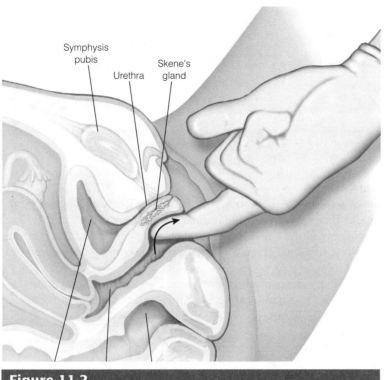

Symphysis pubis

Urethra

Skene's gland

Figure 11-2

Palpation of Skene's glands

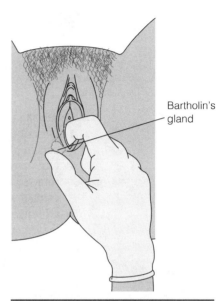

Bartholin's gland

Figure 11-3

Palpation of Bartholin's glands

Figure 11-4

Insertion of speculum into vagina

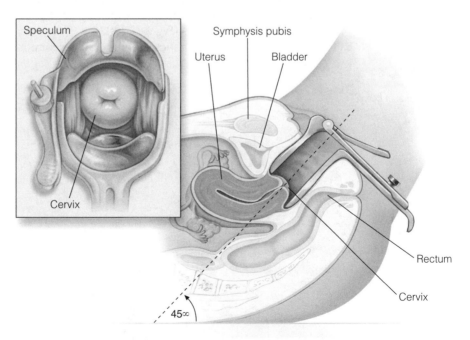

Speculum

Cervix

Symphysis pubis

Uterus

Bladder

Rectum

Cervix

45∞

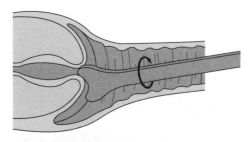

Figure 11-5

Cervical scrape

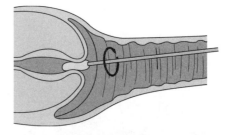

Figure 11-6

Endocervical swab

M. Obtain vaginal smears and cultures
1. Do not take smears or a culture if client took a bath, douched, or used vaginal products in past 24 hours, as these products could interfere with test results
2. Obtain cervical scraping or cultures by placing spatula against cervical os and rotating; remove and apply sample to a slide (Figure 11-5); a cervical scraping is obtained by using a wooden applicator
3. Obtain a Papanicolaou (Pap) smear or sample by placing an endocervical cotton-tipped applicator or cytology brush into cervical os and rotating applicator; then apply a thin sample on a slide (Figure 11-6)

N. Perform a bimanual examination
1. Stand at the end of examination table and lubricate index and middle finger of dominant hand
2. Insert downward pressure on posterior wall of vagina and wait for opening to relax
3. Insert a finger into introitus and palpate vaginal wall
4. Palpate cervical os with internal fingers for position, size, surface characteristics, mobility, and discomfort after placing non-dominant hand to exert downward pressure on abdomen midway between umbilicus and pubis (Figure 11-7)
5. Palpate uterus for position and size by moving fingers from cervix to anterior vagina to attempt to palpate uterus (Figure 11-8)
6. Palpate uterus for characteristics, mobility, and discomfort

Figure 11-7

Palpation of cervix

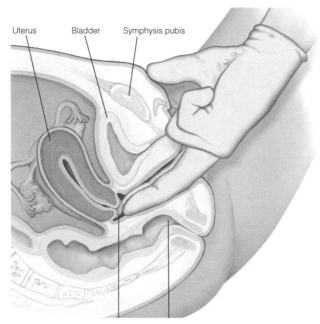

Uterus   Bladder   Symphysis pubis

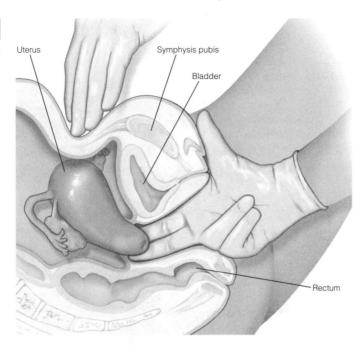

Figure 11-8

Palpation of uterus

Uterus

Symphysis pubis

Bladder

Rectum

7. Palpate adnexa and **ovaries** (organs that produce and store ova and produce hormones progesterone and estrogen) for size, shape, and discomfort by lifting upward while pressing downward on lower abdomen with the non-dominant hand (Figure 11-9)
O. **Perform a rectovaginal examination by leaving index finger in vagina and inserting middle finger in rectum by applying pressure to anus and asking client to bear down**
    1. Palpate rectal wall for surface characteristics
    2. Palpate ovaries and uterus by placing non-dominant hand on lower abdomen and applying gentle pressure while palpating rectal wall with middle finger in rectum and index finger in vagina (Figure 11-10)
    3. Palpate rectal sphincter tone prior to withdrawing finger
    4. Test any fecal matter on glove for occult blood

VI. EXPECTED FINDINGS

A. When inspecting external genitalia, pubic hair reveals an inverse triangle of hair that may extend up toward umbilicus
B. Skin over mons pubis and inguinal area should be smooth and clear without lesions
C. During inspection of labia majora and minora, darker skin pigmentation than client's skin color should be noted; labia may be full or shriveled, gaping or closed, and symmetrical; labia minora should be symmetrical and moist without lesions or sores
D. When palpating labia minora tissue should be smooth and soft
E. Clitoris should be approximately 2 cm in length
F. During inspection of urethral meatus, vaginal introitus, and perineum, nurse should find meatus to be midline and vaginal introitus should be pink and moist; perineum should be smooth and without lesions or discoloration
G. Vaginal bleeding may indicate benign masses such as fibroids (leiomyomas) or possibly reproductive cancer
H. Skin of anus should have increased pigmentation without hemorrhoids
I. During palpation of Skene's and Bartholin's glands there should be no pain or discharge
J. When evaluating vagina and rectal muscle tone a nulliparous woman should squeeze tightly around examiner's hand, whereas a multiparous woman may not be able to squeeze as tightly around examiner's finger

Figure 11-9

Variations in uterine position
    A. Anteversion,
    B. Midposition,
    C. Retroversion,
    D. Anteflexion,
    E. Retroflexion.

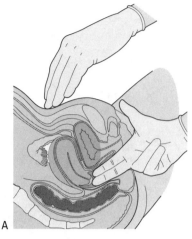

A

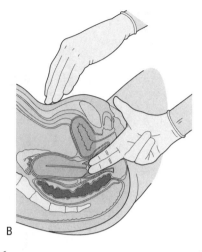

B

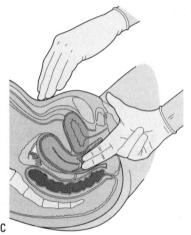

C

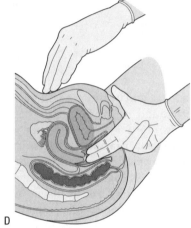

D

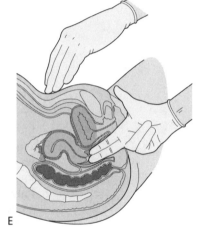

E

Figure 11-10

Retrovaginal palpation

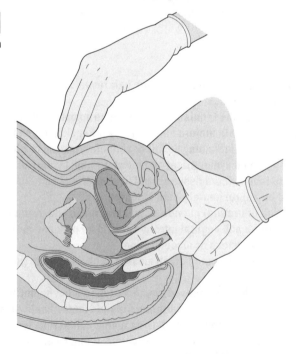

K. There should be no urinary incontinence when client bears down or coughs

L. During speculum examination the visualized cervix should be pink in color and without discharge; os resembles a closed circle in a nulliparous woman and a slit in a multiparous woman

M. When performing a bimanual examination the cervix should be firm, non-tender, and have consistency of a nose

N. Palpation of uterus should find it slightly above bladder and cervix should be slightly forward; normal uterine positions include:

Practice to Pass

When palpating the uterus, the nurse would document the position of the uterus in which manner?

1. **Anteversion**—normal variation of position in which uterus is tilted forward and cervix is tilted downward

2. **Midposition**—normal variation of position in which uterus lies parallel to tailbone and cervix points straight

3. **Retroversion**—normal variation of position in which uterus is pointed backward and cervix is pointed upward

O. During a bimanual examination, palpation of ovaries should normally not be possible; if an ovary is palpable it should be mobile, almond-shaped, smooth, and firm

P. During rectovaginal examination the rectovaginal septum should be smooth and nontender; feces should be heme negative when tested

VII. UNEXPECTED FINDINGS

A. Pubic hair should not be sparse in pattern or have signs of nits or lice infestation

B. When inspecting labia majora and minora they should be free of lesions, warts, vesicles, rashes, or ulcerations; there should be no erythema or signs of inflammation

C. A clitoris that is long may indicate that client is experiencing high levels of testosterone

D. Urine leaking from the urinary meatus when client coughs or examiner palpates the anterior vaginal wall is considered an abnormal finding

E. When inspecting vaginal introitus and perineum, uterus should not be protruding from vaginal opening; if so, client is experiencing uterine prolapse

F. It is abnormal to find bulging when palpating vaginal walls

G. When palpating Bartholin's and Skene's glands there should be no discharge

H. During visualization of cervix there should be no discharge

1. Green discharge may indicate a gonorrhea infection

2. Thick, white, cheesy discharge may indicate candida

3. Frothy, yellow-green discharge may indicate trichomoniasis

4. A chlamydial infection manifests as a yellow discharge

5. A creamy, white-gray discharge may indicate bacterial vaginosis if it has a fishy odor

I. When palpating cervix, client should not feel pain and examiner should not feel nodules

J. When palpating uterus no tenderness should be elicited in client, as that would indicate inflammation; there should be no notable masses, nodules, or bulging as this may indicate inflammation, infection, cysts, tumor, prolapse, *rectocele* (a hernia that develops when rectum pushes into vagina), or *cystocele* (a hernia that develops when bladder is pushed into vagina)

1. **Anteflexion**—abnormal variation of position in which uterus is folded forward at a 90-degree angle and cervix is tilted downward

2. **Retroflexion**—abnormal variation of position in which uterus is folded backward at a 90-degree and cervix is tilted upward

K. Ovaries usually are not palpable and should not be tender or bulging

1. Ovarian cancer may be asymptomatic in early stages, or may present with gastrointestinal disturbances (pressure, bloating, cramps, indigestion, nausea, loss of appetite, constipation, or diarrhea), calf or lower back pain or frequent urination

2. Later signs of ovarian cancer include severe abdominal pressure and bloating, ascites, constipation, urinary frequency, abnormal bleeding from vagina, and severe pain

3. Ovarian cysts (fluid-filled sacs within or on surface of ovary) may be asymptomatic or may lead to pelvic pain, abdominal distention, and lower back pain

L. It is abnormal to perform a rectovaginal examination and note tenderness, masses, nodules, or bulging

VIII. LIFESPAN CONSIDERATIONS

A. Infants and children

1. Infants have immature genitalia
   a. Cervix composes two-thirds of uterus and labia have a smooth, dry appearance; immediately after birth there may be a whitish mucoid discharge for approximately one month
   b. Internal exams are not routinely performed on infants; place infant on back and examine in frog position
2. As they age, children need to have their opinion respected as to whether or not a parent is in examination room
   a. Young children (ages 4–6) need to cooperate with help of gentle coaxing from examiner; younger children are also examined using a frog position; as child ages the lithotomy position may need to be used
   b. If internal examination needs to be performed a Pederson speculum is used; there should be no evidence of abuse

B. Adolescents

1. Should be given privacy and given an opportunity to ask questions
2. Explain all steps of examination to client and reassure confidentiality

C. Pregnant female

1. Pregnancy and accompanying changes in hormone levels cause structural changes to uterus, cervix, ovaries, and vagina
2. Uterus enlarges to a capacity of about 5 liters and weighs approximately 1 kilogram (2.2 pounds) by end of pregnancy
3. Pregnant uterus pushes up into abdominal cavity as it enlarges, displacing liver and intestines from their usual positions
4. During pregnancy Braxton Hicks contractions can occur, which are irregular in nature; they are not painful and are less intense in earlier pregnancy and can be painful and more intense during later pregnancy
5. Cervix changes appearance during pregnancy
   a. Vascularity increases in cervix, leading to softening of cervix, called Goodell's sign
   b. Vascularity also changes tissue to a bluish color, called Chadwick's sign
   c. Cervical mucus production increases to form a mucus plug at cervical os, which is a protective measure that prevents foreign matter from entering uterus
   d. Expulsion of mucus plug at beginning of labor is called "bloody show"
6. Vaginal epithelium hypertrophies during pregnancy and vagina also shows Chadwick's sign; vaginal walls soften and relax during pregnancy to allow movement of infant during birth

D. Older adults

1. Older adult clients may experience thinning and graying of pubic hair; organs of reproductive system may atrophy
2. Lithotomy position may be difficult for older client to assume, so examiner may need to modify position or use a lateral position
3. Due to dry vaginal tissue client may need additional lubricant to provide for comfort during examination; older clients may lose sphincter tone and uterus may not be palpable due to atrophy

IX. DOCUMENTATION

A. Documentation should include client's subjective complaints

B. Objective data should include the following:

1. External genitalia: presence of lesions and coloration
2. Vagina: amount and color of discharge, bleeding, presence of cytocele, rectocele or prolapse, lesions
3. Cervix: color position, parity, lesions, discharge
4. Uterus: position, mobility, texture; ovaries palpable or not, tenderness
5. Rectovaginal: tenderness, sphincter tone, masses, and hematest results

Case Study

A female older adult visits the clinic. The client states she was cleaning the kitchen, scrubbing the floor, and felt her "inside coming out." She says "it feels very uncomfortable and heavy." The nurse prepares the client for a vaginal examination and assists her into a lithotomy position. The client states that she "cannot lie like this." The nurse changes the client's position and proceeds with the assessment. The nurse observes the uterus protruding from the vagina. The cervix appears dry. The nurse also observes urinary incontinence when the client coughs.

1. What is the most appropriate position for this client?

2. What should the nurse teach the client?

3. What is the most appropriate nursing diagnosis for this client?

4. What is the most appropriate action for the nurse to take?

5. What should the nurse instruct the client to do to help with the urinary incontinence?

For suggested responses, see page 310

POSTTEST

1 The nurse observes the following during a pelvic examination. The nurse would document this finding as which of the following?

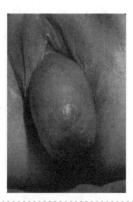

1. Skene's gland
2. Prolapsed uterus
3. Cystocele
4. Rectocele

2 A 30-year-old client who has had three normal Papanicolaou (Pap) smears asks the nurse, "How often should I get a Pap smear?" What is the nurse's best reply?

1. Every six months
2. Once a year
3. Once every two to three years
4. Every five years

3 The nurse is performing a vaginal examination and assesses wart-like lesions on the vulva. The nurse would conclude that this finding may indicate which health problem?

1. Gonorrhea
2. Chlamydia
3. Human papillomavirus
4. Fibroids

4 When palpating a client's uterus the nurse feels the tip of the cervix is tilted downward. The nurse would conclude that the uterus is in which position?

1. Midline
2. Anteversion
3. Retroversion
4. Parallel to the ovaries

5 The client tells the nurse, "I am afraid I am going to get ovarian cancer." The client then asks the nurse, "What are the early symptoms of ovarian cancer?" What is the nurse's best response?

1. "Pelvic and back pain and abdominal distention develop as early signs of ovarian cancer."
2. "Gastrointestinal discomfort and/or calf or lower back pain tend to be earlier signs of ovarian cancer."
3. "It only occurs in menopausal women; dryness, itching, and burning in the vagina occur with ovarian cancer."
4. "Redness and swelling of the vagina with a thick, cheesy discharge occur."

6 When performing a rectovaginal examination the nurse's finger is unable to penetrate the rectum. To facilitate the examination the nurse should take which action next?

1. Re-lubricate the gloved finger and try again
2. Instruct the client to bear down and as the client is bearing down insert a lubricated, gloved finger
3. Defer the examination
4. Ask the client to try and relax and attempt the procedure again in 10 minutes

7 When performing a rectovaginal examination the nurse would expect to implement which assessment procedure?

1. Palpate the ovaries
2. Palpate the fallopian tubes
3. Determine the position of the uterus
4. Compress the rectovaginal septum

8 Place in chronological order the following steps for inserting a speculum into the client's vagina. All options must be used.

1. Hold the speculum in the dominant hand
2. Select the correct speculum
3. Insert the speculum at a 45-degree angle
4. With the non-dominant hand apply pressure on the posterior aspect of the vaginal opening
5. Open the speculum and visualize the cervix

9 While inspecting the urethral orifice of a female client during an examination, the nurse observes urine leakage. What conclusion would be appropriate for the nurse to draw from this observation?

1. The client did not empty the bladder as instructed
2. There is a weakening of the pelvic muscles
3. A cystocele is present
4. A urinary tract infection is present

10 During the external examination of the labia the nurse notes some papules and a draining papule appearing like an ulcer. The nurse would expect the client to be evaluated for which condition?

1. Ovarian cancer
2. Sexually transmitted disease
3. Polyps
4. Pregnancy

➤ *See pages 222–224 for Answers and Rationales.*

ANSWERS & RATIONALES

Pretest

1 **Answer: 1, 2, 3, 4** **Rationale:** The nurse needs to gather information about the onset of menarche, the client's cycle, and if the client is experiencing discomfort through premenstrual syndrome or dysmenorrhea. The

question about hemorrhoids may provide information about symptoms but does not provide information about reproductive health (option 5).
Cognitive Level: Application **Client Need:** Health Promotion and Maintenance **Integrated Process:** Nursing Process: Assessment **Content Area:** Adult Health: Reproductive

Strategy: Eliminate any option that is not asking about reproductive health. In this question, note that option 5 refers to a gastrointestinal problem to eliminate that option. **Reference:** D'Amico, D. & Barbarito, C. (2007). *Health & physical assessment in nursing.* Upper Saddle River, NJ: Pearson Education, Inc., pp. 631–632.

2 **Answer: 2** **Rationale:** Asking if the client has ever been diagnosed with a female reproductive system problem permits the client to discuss the problem and is a comprehensive method for gathering this data (option 2). Whether a client uses tampons or pads does not provide health history data (option 1). Asking about tampon use will provide information about potential risk for toxic shock syndrome. Asking about sexual satisfaction does not provide information about sexual health (option 3). Asking about sexual satisfaction will provide information about concerns related to performance. Asking if the client is sexually active does not provide information about potential health problems; the nurse would need to ask what sex practices the client is engaging in (option 4).
Cognitive Level: Application **Client Need:** Health Promotion and Maintenance **Integrated Process:** Nursing Process: Assessment **Content Area:** Adult Health: Reproductive **Strategy:** Selecting the option that directly asks if the client has had problems associated with reproductive health gathers data related to reproductive problems. Recognize that this option is also the global option and could encompass the other options. **Reference:** D'Amico, D. & Barbarito, C. (2007). *Health & physical assessment in nursing.* Upper Saddle River, NJ: Pearson Education, Inc., p. 633.

3 **Answer: 2** **Rationale:** Itching is associated with infections such as vaginitis, dermatitis, lice, and candidiasis (option 2). Vaginal bleeding may indicate fibroids or cancer (option 1). Vaginal surgery may provide information related to reproductive problems (option 3). Sexual arousal may provide the examiner with information about the psychological health of the client (option 4).
Cognitive Level: Application **Client Need:** Health Promotion and Maintenance **Integrated Process:** Nursing Process: Assessment **Content Area:** Adult Health: Reproductive **Strategy:** Recall that signs of infection include redness, swelling, itching, discharge, and possibly pain. Recognize that option 2 is the only answer that provides information about one of these symptoms. **Reference:** D'Amico, D. & Barbarito, C. (2007). *Health & physical assessment in nursing.* Upper Saddle River, NJ: Pearson Education, Inc., p. 635.

4 **Answer: 2, 3** **Rationale:** Lithotomy is a supine position with the knees and hips flexed and the feet in stirrups, which permits visualization of the genitalia (option 2). Lateral Sims' is on the side with knee and hip flexed, which is often used for an elderly client who cannot assume the lithotomy position (option 3). The knee-chest position is not used, as it is often embarrassing

and uncomfortable for the client (option 1). Prone is a position in which the client lies on the abdomen and which will not permit palpation of the abdomen (option 4). Standing will not permit access to the genital organs (option 5).
Cognitive Level: Application **Client Need:** Health Promotion and Maintenance **Integrated Process:** Nursing Process: Implementation **Content Area:** Adult Health: Reproductive **Strategy:** Eliminate options that do not permit access to the genitalia or cause client discomfort. **Reference:** D'Amico, D. & Barbarito, C. (2007). *Health & physical assessment in nursing.* Upper Saddle River, NJ: Pearson Education, Inc., p. 641.

5 **Answer: 4** **Rationale:** Genital warts are cauliflower-like papules on the genitalia that result from infection with the human papillomavirus (option 4). Cystocele is a hernia that develops when the bladder is pushed forward into the anterior vaginal wall (option 1). A pregnant cervix will reveal a bluish tinge known as the Chadwick sign, but there are no signs of pregnancy visible on the external genitalia (option 2). Syphilis is a non-tender lesion that may have drainage (option 3).
Cognitive Level: Analysis **Client Need:** Health Promotion and Maintenance **Integrated Process:** Nursing Process: Analysis **Content Area:** Adult Health: Reproductive **Strategy:** First eliminate options 1 and 2 because these do not relate to findings on the external genitalia. Next recall that genital warts are raised, moist, cauliflower-like, painless papules that may develop on the labia, vulva, vagina, cervix, and anal areas to choose option 4 over option 3. **Reference:** D'Amico, D. & Barbarito, C. (2007). *Health & physical assessment in nursing.* Upper Saddle River, NJ: Pearson Education, Inc., p. 642.

6 **Answer: 3** **Rationale:** A client may experience a cyanotic cervix when she has congestive heart failure (option 3). A client during the second month of pregnancy may have a bluish tinge to the cervix known as Chadwick's sign (option 1). A sexually transmitted disease may produce lesions with drainage (option 2). Cancer produces ulcerations, discharge, and bleeding (option 4).
Cognitive Level: Analysis **Client Need:** Health Promotion and Maintenance **Integrated Process:** Nursing Process: Analysis **Content Area:** Adult Health: Reproductive **Strategy:** Note that the client in the question is an older adult to eliminate option 1 first. Then remember that cyanosis is usually associated with cardiovascular disease and recognize that congestive heart failure is the only cardiovascular disease in the remaining options. **Reference:** D'Amico, D. & Barbarito, C. (2007). *Health & physical assessment in nursing.* Upper Saddle River, NJ: Pearson Education, Inc., p. 656.

7 **Answer: 4** **Rationale:** The cervical os in a nulliparous woman is round and closed, whereas in a multiparous woman the os is slit-like (option 4). The adult female should have hair distribution that is full and forms an inverted triangle over the pubis (option 1). There should

be no drainage from glands (option 2). A cheese-like substance in the labia folds could indicate a candida infection (option 3).
Cognitive Level: Analysis **Client Need:** Health Promotion and Maintenance **Integrated Process:** Nursing Process: Assessment **Content Area:** Adult Health: Reproductive **Strategy:** Eliminate options that describe a problem such as lack of hair, drainage, or foreign material on the genitalia. **Reference:** D'Amico, D. & Barbarito, C. (2007). *Health & physical assessment in nursing.* Upper Saddle River, NJ: Pearson Education, Inc., p. 647.

8 **Answer: 2** **Rationale:** To obtain a Papanicolaou (Pap) smear the nurse will insert a cotton-tipped applicator or cytology brush into the cervical os and obtain a sample of cells and then place them on a slide for cytological examination (option 2). A cervical scraping is obtained by using a wooden applicator (option 1). During physical examination, the only material likely to be on an examiner's glove would be feces following a rectovaginal exam and this could be used to test for occult blood (option 3). A vaginal pool sample (from the vaginal vault) is obtained when the client has had a hysterectomy (option 4).
Cognitive Level: Application **Client Need:** Health Promotion and Maintenance **Integrated Process:** Nursing Process: Assessment **Content Area:** Adult Health: Reproductive **Strategy:** Recall that a cotton-tipped applicator is used to obtain cells for a Pap smear. Recognize that the only option that has a cotton-tipped applicator in it is option 2. **Reference:** D'Amico, D. & Barbarito, C. (2007). *Health & physical assessment in nursing.* Upper Saddle River, NJ: Pearson Education, Inc., pp. 647–649.

9 **Answer: 3, 1, 2, 4, 5** **Rationale:** The bimanual assessment is performed in the following order: palpating the cervix, the fornices, uterus, ovaries, and finally a rectovaginal examination.
Cognitive Level: Application **Client Need:** Health Promotion and Maintenance **Integrated Process:** Nursing Process: Assessment **Content Area:** Adult Health: Reproductive **Strategy:** To answer this question, remember to find an identifiable structure such as the cervix (it feels like the tip of the nose); the fornices are on either side of the cervix. The uterus is a large structure to locate next, and the ovaries are located on either side of the uterus. Finally, the rectovaginal examination is performed because the rectum is considered a contaminated orifice and the examiner would not cross-contaminate the vaginal area. **Reference:** D'Amico, D. & Barbarito, C. (2007). *Health & physical assessment in nursing.* Upper Saddle River, NJ: Pearson Education, Inc., pp. 649–653.

10 **Answer: 2** **Rationale:** After performing a rectovaginal examination, any feces on the gloved finger is evaluated for occult blood with a hematest (option 2). Not all equipment is disposable and the examination area should be cleaned up after the client goes to dress (options 1 and 4). Also, the client may need assistance in getting up after the exam. The client should be permit-

ted to dress prior to discussing the assessment findings with the examiner (option 3).
Cognitive Level: Application **Client Need:** Health Promotion and Maintenance **Integrated Process:** Nursing Process: Assessment **Content Area:** Adult Health: Reproductive **Strategy:** Eliminate option 3 first because the client should be permitted to dress prior to discussing the assessment findings with the examiner. Eliminate option 1 next because the client may need to be assisted to a sitting position before dressing and may also require assistance removing the legs from the stirrups. Finally, eliminate option 4 recalling that not all equipment is disposable and the examination area should be cleaned up after the client goes to dress. **Reference:** D'Amico, D. & Barbarito, C. (2007). *Health & physical assessment in nursing.* Upper Saddle River, NJ: Pearson Education, Inc., p. 654.

Posttest

1 **Answer: 2** **Rationale:** A prolapsed uterus occurs when the uterus protrudes downward into the vagina or perhaps even through the vaginal opening (option 2). A Skene's gland is located on the anterior wall of the vagina and should produce no discharge (option 1). A cystocele is a hernia that occurs when the bladder is pushed into the anterior wall of the vagina (option 3). A rectocele is a hernia that occurs when the rectum is pushed into the posterior wall of the vagina (option 4).
Cognitive Level: Application **Client Need:** Health Promotion and Maintenance **Integrated Process:** Communication and Documentation **Content Area:** Adult Health: Reproductive **Strategy:** Note the contour of the structure and recall the shape of the various structures indicated in the question. A clue in the picture is the central opening in the uterus that is the cervix. **Reference:** D'Amico, D. & Barbarito, C. (2007). *Health & physical assessment in nursing.* Upper Saddle River, NJ: Pearson Education, Inc., pp. 643.

2 **Answer: 3** **Rationale:** The client requires a Pap smear once every two to three years if the client has had three normal annual Pap smears in the past (option 3). Every six months is recommended for the client with dysplasia (option 1). Once a year is recommended beginning at age 21, or within three years of starting sexual intercourse (option 2). There is no recommendation for every five years (option 4).
Cognitive Level: Application **Client Need:** Health Promotion and Maintenance **Integrated Process:** Teaching/Learning **Content Area:** Adult Health: Reproductive **Strategy:** Eliminate option 1 as check ups are indicated every six months for abnormal Pap smears. Eliminate option 2 (annual Pap smears) as the client is 30 years old. Annual Pap smears should begin by age 21 and continue annually for three years if normal then the patient may have a Pap smear every three years. Eliminate option 4 (every five years) as this time frame exceeds the recommendation for this client of every three years.

Reference: D'Amico, D. & Barbarito, C. (2007). *Health & physical assessment in nursing.* Upper Saddle River, NJ: Pearson Education, Inc., p. 662.

3 **Answer: 3** **Rationale:** The Human papillomavirus produces wart-like growths that are painless and grow in clusters on the external or internal genitalia (option 3). Gonorrhea may produce bleeding or discharge although some clients are asymptomatic (option 1). The symptoms associated with chlamydia may be discharge or tenderness or the client may be asymptomatic (option 2). Fibroids are not sexually transmitted and are found on the uterus and not the vulva (option 4). **Cognitive Level:** Analysis **Client Need:** Health Promotion and Maintenance **Integrated Process:** Nursing Process: Evaluation **Content Area:** Adult Health: Reproductive **Strategy:** Eliminate fibroids as an answer because a fibroid is not a sexually transmitted disease. Next recall that chlamydia and gonorrhea do not produce wart-like lesions to eliminate these options. **Reference:** D'Amico, D. & Barbarito, C. (2007). *Health & physical assessment in nursing.* Upper Saddle River, NJ: Pearson Education, Inc., pp. 656–660.

4 **Answer: 2** **Rationale:** Anteversion is when the cervix is tilted downward and is considered an abnormal position (option 2). The uterus and cervix should be midline and parallel to the tailbone (option 1). A retroverted uterus is when the cervix is tilted upward and is considered abnormal (option 3). The uterus does not necessarily have to be parallel to the ovaries (option 4). **Cognitive Level:** Analysis **Client Need:** Health Promotion and Maintenance **Integrated Process:** Nursing Process: Assessment **Content Area:** Adult Health: Reproductive **Strategy:** Note that options 2 and 3 are opposites, so from a test-taking perspective the correct answer should be one of the two. **Reference:** D'Amico, D. & Barbarito, C. (2007). *Health & physical assessment in nursing.* Upper Saddle River, NJ: Pearson Education, Inc., p. 652.

5 **Answer: 2** **Rationale:** Ovarian cancer begins in the ovarian cells and produces signs of gastrointestinal discomfort, pain in the calves or lower back; weight loss; loss of appetite; nausea; diarrhea; constipation; and frequent urination (option 2). As the disease progresses, bleeding from the vagina begins. When the client is experiencing ovarian cysts she may have pelvic and back pain, and abdominal distention develops (option 1). In menopausal women dryness, itching, and burning in the vagina occurs with atrophic vaginitis and is not ovarian cancer (option 3). Candidiasis is associated with redness and swelling of the vagina and produces a thick, cheesy discharge (option 4). **Cognitive Level:** Application **Client Need:** Health Promotion and Maintenance **Integrated Process:** Teaching/Learning **Content Area:** Adult Health: Reproductive **Strategy:** Eliminate option 4, which is related to discharge because that implies an infective process. Option 1 is associated with cysts. Eliminate option 3 because ovarian cancer can affect all age levels. **Reference:** D'Amico,

D. & Barbarito, C. (2007). *Health & physical assessment in nursing.* Upper Saddle River, NJ: Pearson Education, Inc., pp. 658–659.

6 **Answer: 2** **Rationale:** The client should be instructed to bear down and the nurse should attempt to insert the gloved, lubricated finger (option 2). Bearing down will relax the anal sphincter. The finger is not re-lubricated to prevent contaminating the vagina or tube of lubricating jelly (option 1). The examination is not deferred as the rectovaginal assessment is an essential component of the assessment (option 3). The procedure should not be delayed as the assessment requires the client to be in lithotomy position, which may be uncomfortable and if excessive in timeframe, could pose risk for deep vein thrombosis (option 4). **Cognitive Level:** Application **Client Need:** Health Promotion and Maintenance **Integrated Process:** Nursing Process: Implementation **Content Area:** Adult Health: Reproductive **Strategy:** Eliminate deferring the examination as the client should not be inconvenienced by having to return. Eliminate options that may cause harm to the client such as excessive time in the lithotomy position and potential cross-contamination. **Reference:** D'Amico, D. & Barbarito, C. (2007). *Health & physical assessment in nursing.* Upper Saddle River, NJ: Pearson Education, Inc., p. 654.

7 **Answer: 4** **Rationale:** During the rectovaginal examination the nurse would compress the rectovaginal septum (option 4). The nurse would not expect to palpate the ovaries or fallopian tubes during a rectovaginal examination (options 1 and 2). The position of the uterus is determined by the bimanual examination (option 3). **Cognitive Level:** Application **Client Need:** Health Promotion and Maintenance **Integrated Process:** Nursing Process: Assessment **Content Area:** Adult Health: Reproductive **Strategy:** Eliminate option 3 as this is not done the during the rectovaginal part of the exam, but rather during the bimanual component of the exam. Eliminate options 1 and 2 as the ovaries and fallopian tubes are not palpable. **Reference:** D'Amico, D. & Barbarito, C. (2007). *Health & physical assessment in nursing.* Upper Saddle River, NJ: Pearson Education, Inc., pp. 653–654.

8 **Answer: 2, 1, 4, 3, 5** **Rationale:** The nurse selects the correct speculum and places it in the dominant hand. The nurse then applies pressure on the posterior aspect of the vaginal opening, inserts the speculum at a 45-degree angle and opens the speculum and visualizes the cervix. **Cognitive Level:** Application **Client Need:** Health Promotion and Maintenance **Integrated Process:** Nursing Process: Implementation **Content Area:** Adult Health: Reproductive **Strategy:** Visualize the steps of the procedure in your mind. The nurse needs to select the correct size first. An instrument is always held in the dominant hand. The non-dominant hand is used to decrease discomfort for the client and ease the speculum insertion. The cervix is visualized. **Reference:** D'Amico, D. & Barbarito, C. (2007). *Health & physical assessment in nursing.* Upper Saddle River, NJ: Pearson Education, Inc., pp. 645–647.

ANSWERS & RATIONALES

9 **Answer: 2** **Rationale:** Urinary incontinence indicates weakened pelvic musculature (option 2). The nurse should not assume the client is non-compliant and did not follow directions (option 1). A cystocele is a hernia in which the bladder is pushed into the anterior aspect of the vaginal wall (option 3). A urinary tract infection is associated with redness, inflammation, and discharge (option 4).
Cognitive Level: Application **Client Need:** Health Promotion and Maintenance **Integrated Process:** Nursing Process: Analysis **Content Area:** Adult Health: Reproductive **Strategy:** Recall that stress incontinence is due to the weakening of the pelvic muscles to easily eliminate each of the incorrect options. **Reference:** D'Amico, D. & Barbarito, C. (2007). *Health & physical assessment in nursing.* Upper Saddle River, NJ: Pearson Education, Inc., p. 652.

10 **Answer 2** **Rationale:** Syphilitic lesions are nontender papules that change into weeping ulcers (option 1). Ovarian cancer produces gastrointestinal symptoms but no lesions (option 2). A polyp is a small growth on the cervix (option 3). Pregnancy (option 4) produces a bluish tinge to the cervix.
Cognitive Level: Analysis **Client Need:** Health Promotion and Maintenance **Integrated Process:** Nursing Process: Analysis **Content Area:** Adult Health: Reproductive **Strategy:** Eliminate options that are not associated with lesions. Sexually transmitted disease produces lesions. **Reference:** D'Amico, D. & Barbarito, C. (2007). *Health & physical assessment in nursing.* Upper Saddle River, NJ: Pearson Education, Inc., p. 656

References

Bickley, L. (2010). *Bates guide to physical examination and history taking* (10th ed.). Philadelphia: Lippincott Williams & Wilkins.

D'Amico, D. & Barbarito, C. (2007). *Health and physical assessment in nursing.* Upper Saddle River, NJ: Pearson Education, Inc., pp. 624–665.

Jarvis, C. (2008). *Physical examination and health assessment* (5th ed.). St. Louis, MO: Elsevier Saunders.

Zator Estes, M. (2009). *Health assessment and physical examination* (4th ed.). Clifton Park, NY: Delmar Cengage Learning.

Male Genitourinary Assessment

12

Chapter Outline

Health History
Present Health History
Family History
Equipment, Preparation,
  and Positioning

Examination Techniques
Expected Findings
Unexpected Findings

Lifespan Considerations
Documentation

Objectives

➤ Discuss structures and functions of the male reproductive system.
➤ Describe developmental, psychosocial, cultural, and environmental
  variations in assessment techniques and findings.
➤ Review focused questions to be used to conduct a health history
  and sexual history of a client.
➤ Describe the techniques for assessing the male reproductive system.
➤ Differentiate normal from abnormal findings obtained during the
  assessment of the male reproductive system.

NCLEX-RN® Test Prep

Visit the Companion Website for this book
at www.pearsonhighered.com/hogan to
access additional practice opportunities
and more.

Review at a Glance

cremasteric reflex an involuntary response in which testis moves upward temporarily in response to a stimulus, such as cold hands, cold room, or when elicited during examination by stroking thigh

epididymis a crescent-shaped ductal system that emerges posteriorly from testis that holds sperm during maturation

epididymitis inflammation of epididymis of male reproductive system, accompanied usually by a dull, aching pain; often caused by infection

epispadias a condition present at birth in which urethral meatus is located on dorsal surface of glans penis

hernia protrusion of an organ or structure through an abnormally weakened area or opening in a muscle wall

hydrocele a nontender accumulation of fluid in scrotum, which is often benign and self-limiting, but may also indicate a more serious problem

hypospadias a condition present at birth in which urethral meatus is located on ventral surface of glans penis

orchitis inflammation of testicle

paraphimosis an uncommon condition in which foreskin, once pulled back behind glans penis, cannot be returned to

its original position; this constitutes a medical emergency to prevent tissue damage

Peyronie's disease a condition in which shaft of penis is crooked when erect

phimosis a condition in which foreskin of penis is nonretractable after age of three years

spermatocele a cyst located in epididymis

varicocele an enlargement of veins of spermatic cord that leads to a soft compressible mass in scrotum; may result in male infertility

PRETEST

1 The nurse is assessing the genitalia of an adult male client. The nurse notes that the scrotal sac is more darkly pigmented than the client's general skin color. After making this observation, what would the nurse do next as a follow-up action?

1. Palpate scrotum for masses and lesions
2. Ask client if he has experienced any pain in the scrotal area
3. Transilluminate scrotum for masses
4. Document this as a normal finding

2 The nurse is conducting a health education program for veterans. When instructing the veterans on prostate health the nurse should explain that individuals of which ethnicity have the highest incidence of prostate cancer?

1. Caucasian
2. African American
3. European American
4. Canadian

3 The client has had a prostate specific antigen (PSA) level drawn and the healthcare provider told the client that the result was 3 ng/dL. The client asks the nurse, "What does a PSA of 3 mean?" The nurse interprets this value as having which meaning?

1. Decreased value requiring retesting
2. Normal finding requiring no action
3. High value indicating probable cancer
4. Very high value requiring immediate surgery

4 The nurse is assessing an 80-year-old man being seen in the urology office reporting, "I go to the bathroom 3–4 times each night and it feels like I can't empty my bladder completely." Based on this report, the nurse expects to note which findings during evaluation of the client's prostate gland? Select all that apply.

1. Small nodule on the prostate gland
2. Firm, fixed prostate gland
3. Edematous scrotal sac
4. Soft mobile nodule in scrotal sac
5. Enlargement of the prostate gland

5 The nurse would use which procedure as the preferred method for examining the rectum of a male client?

1. Have the client stand in front of nurse, then insert a lubricated, gloved, flexed index finger into the rectum in direction of umbilicus
2. Have the client assume lateral Sim's position and insert a lubricated, gloved, flexed, index finger into the rectum toward umbilicus
3. Position the client leaning over examination table and insert a lubricated, gloved, flexed index finger into the rectum toward umbilicus
4. Position the client in a lithotomy position and insert a lubricated, gloved, flexed index finger into the rectum toward umbilicus

6 An adolescent boy is undergoing a physical examination to meet the school requirement to play sports. The nurse practitioner palpates an inguinal hernia. When the mother of the boy asks the nurse what an inguinal hernia is, what is the nurse's best response?

1. "A portion of the bladder has entered the testicular sac."
2. "A portion of the bowel is protruding through weakened abdominal muscles."
3. "The testicles have retracted into the abdominal wall."
4. "The testicles have protruded through the abdominal muscle wall."

7 The nurse is assessing the genitalia of a newborn infant. The nurse observes that the urinary meatus is on the dorsal side of the penis. The nurse would document the presence of which finding?

1. Epispadias
2. Hypospadias
3. Urethral stricture
4. Urethritis

8 The nurse would ask which priority assessment question when taking the history of a 28-year-old male client being seen in the clinic for a physical examination?

1. "Do you have nocturnal emissions when you are sleeping?"
2. "Are you getting up frequently during the night to urinate?"
3. "Are you able to achieve an erection?"
4. "Do you perform testicular self-examination (TSE)?"

9 When teaching the client to perform a testicular self-examination (TSE), the nurse would include which instruction to the client?

1. Perform the examination after intercourse monthly
2. Perform the examination in the shower monthly
3. Perform the examination while in a sitting position
4. Only report lumps that are painful to the touch to the healthcare provider

10 A 30-year-old uncircumcised male is unable to retract the foreskin so the glans of the penis can be assessed during physical examination. The clinic nurse would document the presence of which finding?

1. Hypospadias
2. Epispadias
3. Phimosis
4. Stricture

➤ *See pages 238–240 for Answers and Rationales.*

I. HEALTH HISTORY

A. It is important to take a thorough history of male reproductive and urinary systems because of dual functions of reproductive organs (see Figures 12-1 and 12-2)
B. Purpose of taking a history is to identify potential or current problems and risk factors
C. Use a concerned listening approach during health history because of sensitive nature of information needed to assess reproductive system
  1. Most clients are embarrassed to discuss personal behaviors
  2. Monitor your own verbal and nonverbal behavior to assure a nonjudgmental approach
  3. Remember that sexuality is often associated with man's sense of masculinity

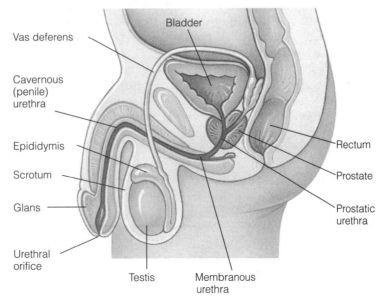

Figure 12-1

Anatomy of the male reproductive organs

Vas deferens
Bladder
Cavernous (penile) urethra
Epididymis
Scrotum
Glans
Urethral orifice
Testis
Membranous urethra
Rectum
Prostate
Prostatic urethra

Figure 12-2

Anterior view of contents of
the scrotum

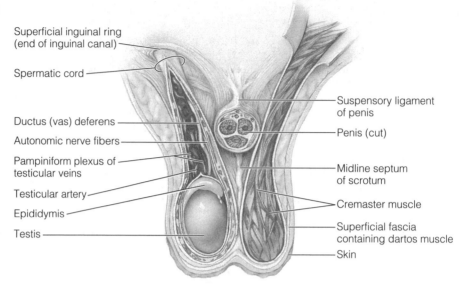

Superficial inguinal ring
(end of inguinal canal)

Spermatic cord

Ductus (vas) deferens

Autonomic nerve fibers

Pampiniform plexus of
testicular veins

Testicular artery

Epididymis

Testis

Suspensory ligament
of penis

Penis (cut)

Midline septum
of scrotum

Cremaster muscle

Superficial fascia
containing dartos muscle

Skin

D. Determine client's age because certain problems occur at different periods throughout a
client's lifespan
E. Obtain a history of all occupations throughout client's working career; chemical exposure or
physical exertion may affect client's reproductive health
F. Data about male reproductive system can be gathered by asking the following questions
(rationales included in parentheses)
1. "Have you had a childhood illness such as mumps?" (can cause sterility or infertility)
2. "Have you had undescended testes?" (may increase risk of testicular cancer)
3. "Have you ever been diagnosed with an inguinal hernia?" (may increase risk of testicular cancer; see Box 12-1 for risk factors for testicular cancer)
4. "Have you had surgeries of the reproductive system?" (surgery may alter body
image or affect sexual functioning; surgeries may include circumcision, vasectomy,
prostatectomy, orchiectomy, surgical repair on a sexual organ)
5. "Do you have regular prostate screening?" (can help detect age-related prostatic
hyperplasia or prostate cancer; see Box 12-2 for risk factors for prostate cancer)
   a. "Have you had a prostate specific antigen (PSA) level done?" (should be performed annually after age 45; normal value is 0–4 ng/mL)
   b. "Have you had regular digital rectal screenings?"
6. "Have you had any genitourinary or reproductive system trauma?" (may lead to fer-
tility problems)
7. "Have you ever had a sexually transmitted disease?" (may lead to complications or
possibly death with tertiary syphilis)

Box 12-1

**Risk Factors for
Testicular Cancer**

Cryptorchidism
Age 20–40
Family history of cancer
Mump orchitis
Inguinal hernia
Maternal history of using diethylstilbestrol (DES)

Box 12-2	Family history of prostatic cancer
Risk Factors for Prostate Cancer	Age African-American descent

Box 12-3	Alpha blockers
Medication Classes That May Affect Sexuality	Antibiotics Antidepressants Antihypertensives Antispasmodics Female hormones Narcotics Psychotropics Sedatives 5-alpha reductase inhibitors

8. "Have you had a history of urinary tract infections?" (may cause pain and spread of disease)
9. "Have you had a history of urinary or reproductive cancer?"
10. "Have you experienced any infertility issues?"
11. "Do you have any allergies to latex?" (may inhibit safe sexual practices)
12. "What medications do you take regularly or occasionally?" (may affect male sexuality; see Box 12-3 for a list of medications that can affect sexuality)
13. "Have you had any exposure to chemicals or excessive radiation in the past?" (can increase the risk of malignancy)
14. "Have you traveled recently?"

II. PRESENT HEALTH HISTORY

A. **This section outlines a detailed history; not all questions may be appropriate for every situation, depending on client and skill level of nurse (routine assessment versus advanced practice nurse examination)**
B. **Ask client about any pain; may assist in determining the nature of problem**
C. **Ask client about any genital lesions, warts, and lesions; provides information related to nature of problem**
D. **Ask client questions about the following to determine presence of a systemic disease process or systemic infection**
   1. Changes in weight
   2. Any rashes or fevers
   3. Any change in energy level (decreased energy may also reduce ability to participate in sexual activity)
   4. Need to get up at night to urinate (may provide information related to urinary problems)
   5. Any neurological problems (may be the cause of an inability to engage in intercourse)
   6. Any swollen glands or nodes (may indicate systemic infection or sexually transmitted disease)
   7. Sore throat or drainage from eyes (may indicate sexually transmitted infection)
   8. Any respiratory problems (may prevent the client from engaging in intercourse)
   9. Any cardiovascular problems (may provide information about decreased endurance or medications that can alter sexual functioning)

10. Current diagnosis of diabetes mellitus (may provide information related to neuropathy and inability to obtain erection)

11. Current diagnosis of sickle cell disease (may cause priapism, painful erection without arousal)

E. **Ask client about infertility; provide information related to diagnostic testing**

F. **Ask client about measures used to maintain a healthy reproductive system**
   1. Performance of monthly testicular self-examination (TSE)
   2. Use of safe sex practices; decreases risk of sexually transmitted infections

G. **Ask client about substance use**
   1. Drug use (may decrease libido)
   2. Alcohol use; type of alcohol and amount (alcohol may cause impotence)
   3. Tobacco use; type and amount

H. **Ask client about occupation (chemical or radiation exposure in workplace may lead to infertility and cancer)**

I. **Ask questions about sexual functioning last as this provides the nurse with period of time to develop a therapeutic relationship with client; keep in mind that not all questions may be appropriate for every client**
   1. "Are you sexually active?"
   2. "What type of sexual behavior do you engage in (oral, anal, genital)?" (provides information about risk for sexually transmitted infection; anal sex may increase risk of urinary tract infection; in cases of penile fracture, inquire also about masturbation, since simulating intercourse on a bed can be a cause)
   3. "Do you have more than one partner? If so, how many partners have you had?" (multiple partners increases risk of disease transmission)
   4. "Do you use condoms consistently?" (provides information about risk for sexually transmitted infection; follow-up with appropriate teaching as needed when assessment is completed)
   5. "Are you able to achieve an erection with stimulation?" (ability to achieve an erection is dependent on physical and psychological factors; medications and cardiovascular disease may interfere with this ability)
   6. "Are you able to maintain an erection sufficiently long enough for sexual intercourse?" (provides information about possible erectile dysfunction)
   7. "Do you experience painful bending of the penile shaft during an erection?" (may indicate **Peyronie's disease**, a condition in which shaft of penis is crooked when erect)
   8. Ask client about his ability to achieve an orgasm (may provide information as to nature of problem)
   9. "Have you ever had a sexually transmitted disease?"
   10. "Have you had any medical treatment for any urinary or sexual reproductive problem?"
   11. "Do you have a headache prior to or during an orgasm?" (an acute, first-time, severe headache can indicate cerebral hemorrhaging and should be treated as a medical emergency)

III. FAMILY HISTORY

A. **Ask client about family history of male reproductive disorders**
   1. Testicular cancer
   2. Prostate cancer
   3. Infertility

B. **Ask client about family history of systemic disorders that can directly or indirectly affect sexual function**
   1. Diabetes mellitus
   2. Cardiovascular disease, including hypertension

C. **Ask client if his mother took diethylstilbestrol (DES); if so, males have a higher incidence of infertility, hypospadias, and testicular problems**

Practice to Pass

The nurse is preparing to interview the client about maintaining healthy sexual practices. What approach should the nurse use to obtain the best data?

IV. EQUIPMENT, POSITIONING, AND PREPARATION

A. Equipment

1. Gloves
2. Lubricant
3. Penlight
4. Urethral culture swab
5. Urogenital alginate swabs
6. Culture plate for gonorrhea testing

B. Positioning and preparation

1. Room will need to be warm; have drape available for warmth and privacy
2. Provide adequate lighting to observe client
3. Have client empty bladder and bowel for comfort
4. Have client remove clothing from waist down and provide a gown for privacy
5. Explain all steps of assessment; inform client that you will be touching his genitalia; procedure should not be uncomfortable
6. Position client standing in front of examiner, who is sitting so genitals are at eye level, or position client supine with legs spread apart for examination if client is unable to stand
7. During prostate screening and rectal examination the client may stand and lean over examination table or assume a supine position if needed
8. Don gloves to implement standard precautions
9. Note: client may experience an erection, which is a normal physiological response when having genitalia examined; if this occurs, offer reassurance that this is normal and proceed with examination in a professional manner

V. EXAMINATION TECHNIQUES

A. Inspection

1. Assess genitalia then inspect rectal area
2. Assess hair distribution
3. Inspect skin of penis
4. Ask client if he is experiencing itching
5. Observe for discharge; if present then document characteristics of discharge
6. Inspect scrotum for shape, consistency, size, location, and mobility
7. Inspect urethral meatus for location of opening of meatus
8. Observe inguinal area for lumps, masses, or visible nodes
9. Inspect rectal area for bleeding, lesions, and hemorrhoids

B. Palpation

1. Stroke client's inner thigh and observe for **cremasteric reflex**, which is noted when testicle moves upward toward body on the side being tested (ipsilateral side)
2. With gloved hands, palpate penis and scrotum for tenderness
   a. Palpate penis between thumb and first two fingers along entire length of penile shaft
   b. Palpate for pulsations
   c. If client is uncircumcised then retract foreskin or ask client to retract foreskin (being sure to replace it when finished with exam)
   d. Squeeze glans of penis, if discharge is present then obtain culture
      1) Position client sitting or standing
      2) Hold penis with non-dominant hand
      3) With dominant hand wipe penis with sterile gauze
      4) Insert urogenital alginate swab 1–2 cm into meatus and rotate swab side to side
      5) Leave swab in place for several seconds
      6) Place some of discharge on Thayer-Martin plate
      7) Gram stain may be performed, followed by a culture

Practice to Pass

What precautions does the nurse need to take prior to performing a reproductive assessment?

Box 12-4	Hard, fixed mass not visible with penlight
Clinical Manifestation of Testicular Cancer	Nontender
	Swelling

    8) Note that some laboratories will use one specimen swab; others will require two swabs

    9) Change gloves to proceed with remainder of examination

3. Palpate inguinal and femoral areas for masses or enlarged nodes by having client stand in front of examiner; when palpating right area have client shift weight to left leg and when assessing left area have client shift weight to right leg; feel triangular slit when in inguinal area

4. Palpate bulbourethral gland for tenderness, masses, or swelling

5. Palpate scrotum between thumb and first two fingers

    a. Palpate for size, consistency, and masses

    b. Palpate **epididymis** (a crescent-shaped ductal system that emerges posteriorly from testis and holds sperm during maturation) by feeling for crescent shape structure on posterior side of each testis

    c. Palpate spermatic cord from epididymis to external ring for tenderness or masses; vertical cord-like structure

    d. If a mass is felt then use a penlight to illuminate mass after darkening room; begin with unaffected testis then proceed to testis with mass (see Box 12-4 for signs of testicular cancer)

6. Palpate inguinal and femoral area for nodes; observe nodes for size, consistency, and tenderness

7. Palpate inguinal and femoral area for presence of **hernia** (protrusion of an organ or structure through an abnormally weakened area or opening in a muscle wall) by asking client to bear down and place index finger of dominant hand in scrotal sac above testis and press in until reaching external ring; ask client to bear down to continue to palpate for masses

8. Palpate for a femoral hernia by having client cough; this increases intra-abdominal pressure to make hernia more palpable

9. Perform rectal examination by inserting lubricated gloved finger into rectum with client standing and leaning forward, placing hands on examination table for support

    a. Have client bear down to facilitate insertion of finger using gentle pressure during insertion

    b. Palpate anterior and posterior rectal walls

    c. Palpate prostate gland and assess size, shape, consistency, mobility, and tenderness (see Box 12-5 for signs of prostate cancer and Table 12-1 for grading of prostate cancer)

    d. If fecal matter is on glove then perform a test for occult blood

    e. With finger in rectum perform bimanual examination by pressing thumb into perianal area while palpating bulbourethral gland for tenderness or masses

Box 12-5	Dysuria
Clinical Manifestations of Prostate Cancer	Frequency
	Nocturia
	Urinary hesitancy
	Hematuria
	Urinary retention
	Dribbling of urine

Table 12-1	Grade 1	Less than 1 cm protrusion into rectum
	Grade 2	1–2 cm protrusion into rectum
Grading System for	Grade 3	2–3 cm protrusion into rectum
Prostate Cancer	Grade 4	Greater than 4 cm into rectum

    f. Remove gloves and assist client to full upright position

    g. Give client tissues to wipe perianal area or assist client as needed

    h. Wash hands

10. Auscultate any scrotal mass both in supine and standing position; if bowel sounds are heard this indicates presence of a hernia

VI. EXPECTED FINDINGS

A. Inspection

Practice to Pass

The nurse observes a client scratching the tissue surrounding the penis. The nurse should assess the client for which manifestations?

1. Pubic hair should be formed in triangular shape with coarse texture; hair may be present on thighs and scrotum; no hair should be present on shaft of penis

2. Skin should be without lesions, swelling, and inflammation

3. There should be no itching

4. Penis should have no drainage or discharge, even with squeezing of glans of penis

5. Skin on penis shaft should be loose and free of lesions

6. Penis should be nontender without masses

7. Client may be circumcised or not; uncircumcised client's foreskin should be able to be retracted

8. Scrotum should have deeper skin pigmentation than skin on body; skin should be free of lesions, nodules, swelling, and inflammation

9. Left scrotal sac is usually situated lower than right

10. Urinary meatus should be centrally located without discharge and pink in color; presence of a white cheesy material, known as smegma, is a normal finding

11. Inguinal area should have no edema and there should be no palpable lymph nodes

12. Rectal area should not have any lesions, bleeding, hemorrhoids, or fissures

13. Cremasteric reflex will be present; testicles will draw close to body due to contraction of cremaster muscle

B. Palpation

1. There should be no drainage from meatus when penis is squeezed

2. Pulsation may be present on underside of penis

3. Scrotum should have a testis and epididymis on each side of sac

4. Fluid in scrotal sac is able to be illuminated

!

5. Testicle should be firm, oval, smooth, and roughly the same size bilaterally without tenderness

6. Epididymis should be nontender

7. Spermatic cord should be round and feel smooth

8. If lymph nodes are palpable, they should be nontender, less than 1 cm, and mobile

9. Inguinal and femoral canal should have no masses

10. Cremasteric reflex should be present

11. Rectum should be smooth and nontender

12. Anal sphincter tone should be present

13. Prostate should be nontender, smooth, small, and mobile

14. Medial sulcus of prostate should be palpable

15. Stool that is tested for occult blood should be hematest negative (no blood present)

C. Auscultation

1. If a scrotal mass is found, nurse should auscultate for bowel sounds

2. Should be no bowel sounds present

VII. UNEXPECTED FINDINGS

A. Inspection

1. Hair should be present; alopecia could be due to genetic predisposition; chemical exposure; aging; or disease process such as cancer, endocrine, or metabolic disorders
2. Cremasteric reflex that is not present may indicate neurological issue
3. Itching may indicate lice or scabies
4. Penile discharge could be the result of a sexually transmitted infection such gonorrhea (associated with purulent white to green discharge)

5. Lesions on penis could be caused by syphilis, *condyloma acuminatum* (genital warts), *haemophilus* infection, candida, herpes simplex I and II, and *tinea cruris*
   a. Syphilis produces an ulcerated round or oval nontender lesion that has a red halo and is edematous
   b. Chancroid is a cauliflower-like reddish pink lesion
   c. Condyloma acuminatum (genital warts) is associated with tannish, brown to purplish white lesions that are macular or papular
   d. Gonorrhea produces purulent, copious drainage
   e. Haemophilus infections produce painful, pinkish red lesions
   f. Candida occurs in warm moist areas and is associated with red papular lesions that occasionally become pus filled

   g. Genital herpes (Herpes simplex I and II) manifests as painful pustules and vesicles and is associated with fever, dysuria, and other viral symptoms
   h. Fungal skin infection, such as tinea cruris (jock itch) produces an itchy, red rash in warm moist areas; prostatitis is associated with thin watery, blood-tinged drainage

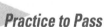

6. Scrotal edema or swelling can occur because of conditions such as malignancies, hernia, **hydrocele** (nontender accumulation of fluid in scrotum), **varicocele** (enlargement of spermatic cord veins that leads to a soft compressible mass in scrotum; may result in male infertility), or **spermatocele** (a cyst located in the epididymis)
   a. A spermatocele is a nontender cyst-like mass on testis or epididymis; it can be illuminated with a penlight
   b. Hydrocele is a nontender accumulation of fluid in the scrotum, which is often benign and self-limiting, but may also be caused by malignancy, trauma, surgical procedures, or **epididymitis** (inflammation of the epididymis, often caused by infection); able to be illuminated with penlight
   c. Varicocele is varicosities of the spermatic cord that, when palpated, feel cord-like and disappear when scrotal sac is elevated; clients often report dull aching pain; varicocele of right scrotal sac may indicate obstruction of vena cava
   d. Sebaceous cysts manifest as smooth, round, firm, nontender mass; cyst in skin of scrotum indicative of decreased circulation or obstruction of sebaceous glands
7. Examination of urinary meatus may reveal that opening is not centrally located
   a. **Epispadias** is when urethral opening is on dorsal aspect of penis
   b. **Hypospadias** is when urethral opening is on ventral aspect or underside of penis
8. Bulging observed in inguinal or femoral area indicates hernia or lymph node enlargement

B. Palpation

1. An abnormal finding during palpation of penis is a decreased pulse, which may be due to decreased circulation from disease or trauma
2. **Phimosis** is an inability to retract foreskin
3. **Paraphimosis** is an inability to return retracted foreskin to its original position; this constitutes a medical emergency to prevent tissue damage
4. Purulent drainage is indicative of infection
5. A palpable mass in one testis or testicle is usually indicative of malignancy

Practice to Pass

The client is experiencing tinea cruris. What would the nurse instruct the client to do as basic hygiene measures?

Practice to Pass

The nurse palpates fluid in the scrotal area. What assessment should the nurse perform?

6. A tender testis or testicle that is retracted is a significant finding; evaluate client for testicular torsion

7. An epididymis that is hard and inflamed (warmth, edema) or is accompanied by scrotal pain or tenderness would indicate epididymitis

8. Undescended testicles are always considered abnormal; if testis and epididymis is undescended this is known as cryptorchidism

9. If nurse palpates scrotal or inguinal mass and client reports pain or tenderness then this may indicate **orchitis** (a painful testis or testicle that has edema and is warm)

10. Enlarged lymph nodes, especially unilaterally, are associated with infection or cancer

11. Presence of a hernia
    a. If client has an indirect inguinal hernia then hernia will be palpable in inguinal ring or scrotum
    b. If client has direct hernia, when client coughs the hernia will enlarge in scrotum
    c. If client has a femoral hernia, examiner will palpate hernia in area between femoral blood vessels and inguinal ligament

12. Fluid may be illuminated with penlight; masses are not able to be illuminated

13. Palpation of prostate may reveal benign prostatic hyperplasia (BPH) or cancer
    a. Enlarged soft, nontender prostate may indicate prostatic hyperplasia
       1) Risk increases with age
       2) Firm enlarged prostate
       3) Changes in urinary pattern such as hesitancy, dribbling, nocturia, decreased force of stream, incontinence, and retention
    b. Prostate gland mass that is firm and tender may indicate prostatitis or infection
    c. Prostatitis may also be manifested as tender, warm, painful mass; client may have a fever
    d. Prostate cancer manifests as firm, hard mass

14. Occult blood or visible blood in stool would indicate bleeding in gastrointestinal tract; may be caused by hemorrhoids or other pathology

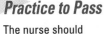

Practice to Pass

The nurse should expect to document which findings in a client with prostatitis?

VIII. LIFESPAN CONSIDERATIONS

A. Circumcision in males is a cultural preference; this practice is prevalent in groups who practice Judaism or are of Muslim faith

B. Infants
1. Any child in breech position may experience scrotal edema and bruising
2. A premature infant may have undescended testes and there may be few rugae on scrotum; term infants should have testes descended into scrotal sac
3. Urinary meatus should be centrally located; many children need surgical correction for epispadias or hypospadias

C. Children
1. Hydrocele is common in children under two years of age
2. Evaluate child's genitalia for masses, pain, and infection
3. Assess for ability to urinate

D. Adolescents
1. Assessment is same as adult
2. Assess for understanding of sexuality; sexual information should be provided if needed
3. Examination findings will vary according to the Tanner stage (see Table 12-2)

E. Older adults
1. Hair distribution is sparser and color is gray
2. Testicles are smaller and softer
3. Prostate almost always enlarges
4. Force of ejaculation decreases with age

Table 12-2 **Tanner Stages of Male Maturation**	**Stage 1.** Preadolescent; hair present is no different than that on abdomen. Testes, scrotum, and penis are the same size and shape as young child.	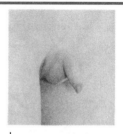 I
	Stage 2. Pubic hair slightly pigmented, longer, straighter hair, often still downy usually at base of penis, sometimes on scrotum; enlargement of scrotum and testes.	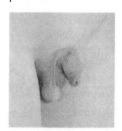 II
	Stage 3. Pubic hair dark, definitely pigmented, curly around base of penis; enlargement of penis, especially in length, further enlargement of testes, descent of scrotum.	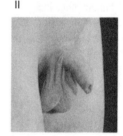 III
	Stage 4. Pubic hair definitely adult in type but not in extent, spread no further than inguinal fold. Continued enlargement of penis and sculpturing of glans, increased pigmentation of scrotum.	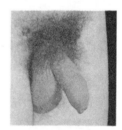 IV
	Stage 5. Hair spread to medial surface of thighs in adult distribution. Adult stage, scrotum ample, penis reaching nearly to bottom of scrotum.	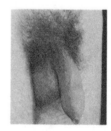 V

Source: D'Amico, D. & Barbarito, C. (2007). *Health & physical assessment in nursing.* Upper Saddle River, NJ: Pearson Education, Inc., p. 588, Table 21.2.

5. Time to achieve erection increases
6. Frequency of erectile dysfunction increases with age, but is not a normal change associated with aging

IX. DOCUMENTATION

   A. **Subjective complaint/report of client**
   B. **Activity and medication history**
   C. **History of symptoms**
   D. **Use of condoms**
   E. **Physical assessment findings**

Case Study

A 20-year-old male college student goes to the college health center with a burning pain upon urination. He tells the nurse that this began three days ago and is getting worse. He reports to the nurse that he had gonorrhea two weeks ago. He was given an antibiotic but did not finish the prescription as his symptoms went away. He states, "I did not tell my girlfriend about the infection." The client denies doing any lifting.

1. What additional data should the nurse obtain when assessing this client?

2. What education should the nurse provide to this client?

3. What other nursing interventions should the nurse plan to implement?

4. When will the nurse ask the client to return to the health center?

5. What is the most appropriate nursing diagnosis for this client?

For suggested responses, see page 311

POSTTEST

1 The nurse is performing a school physical on a 16-year-old male. Which questions are essential for the nurse to ask during the reproductive evaluation of this client? Select all that apply.

1. "Do you have nocturnal emissions?"
2. "Do you have urinary frequency?"
3. "Are you sexually active?"
4. "Do you use condoms?"
5. "Are you performing testicular self examination (TSE)?"

2 A man presents to the ambulatory clinic reporting presence of a hernia. What instruction does the nurse give the client in order to assess the area?

1. Assume lateral position to push bowel contents closer to abdominal wall
2. Bear down while nurse is palpating inguinal area
3. Assume lateral side lying position so the nurse may perform rectal examination
4. Assume position leaning over examination table while the nurse performs rectal examination

3 A 50-year-old male having an annual physical examination tells the nurse that he is unable to achieve an erection since his last exam one year ago. The nurse notes that at that visit he was placed on several medications. The nurse would conclude that which type of medication prescribed at that time is the most likely cause of his erectile dysfunction?

1. Aspirin
2. Antihypertensive
3. Cardiac glycoside
4. Diuretic

POSTTEST

4 The nurse assigned to the newborn nursery has made an admission assessment of a term newborn. The nurse would refer the newborn, who was born breech, for further evaluation and follow-up after assessing which clinical manifestation?

1. Scrotal edema
2. Absent testes
3. Positive urinary stream
4. Presence of smegma

5 The nurse is able to transilluminate the scrotum of a man during a physical examination. What term would the nurse use to document the finding that is associated with this result?

1. Mass
2. Varicocele
3. Hydrocele
4. Orchitis

6 When examining the genitalia of a 30-year-old male, the nurse would document which finding as normal?

1. Scrotal sac that has an inelastic texture
2. Firm smooth scrotal sac
3. Firm smooth testes
4. Light colored scrotal sac

7 During an annual physical examination, a 64-year-old male client asks the nurse, "What are the signs of benign prostatic hyperplasia?" What would the nurse include in a response to the client?

1. Hesitancy, weak stream, dribbling, and frequency
2. Mass in the scrotal sac
3. Fluid in the scrotal sac
4. Hard nodules in the inguinal area

8 The nurse is finishing a rectal examination of a male client. After withdrawing the gloved finger from the rectum, what would the nurse do next?

1. Dispose of gloves in red infectious waste bag
2. Wash gloves prior to disposal to prevent contamination of housekeeping staff
3. Test material on glove for occult blood
4. Show client the bathroom where he can empty his bowel

9 The nurse is examining the genitalia of a male client and observes urethral discharge. What is the most appropriate action for the nurse to take?

1. Put on gloves to avoid contamination of nurse's hands
2. Have client squeeze some discharge onto a slide to observe its characteristics
3. Insert a sterile applicator into the urinary meatus to collect discharge for culture and sensitivity testing
4. Ask the healthcare provider to write an order for broad spectrum antibiotic therapy

10 During an examination of the genitalia, a male client develops an erection. What is the most appropriate action for the nurse to take?

1. Leave the room for a few minutes until client is not aroused
2. Send in another nurse or healthcare provider to continue assessment
3. Apologize to client and continue with examination
4. Reassure client about this normal response and continue with examination

➤ *See pages 240–242 for Answers and Rationales.*

ANSWERS & RATIONALES

Pretest

1 **Answer: 4** **Rationale:** The scrotum of an adult male should be more deeply pigmented than the general color of the client's skin (option 4). The skin of the scrotum should also be wrinkled. The scrotum should be palpated for masses and lesions during the exam but this not related to the color of the scrotum (option 1). The nurse should ask the client if he is experiencing any pain in the genitalia as this is an essential aspect of the assessment, but again this is not related to the color of the scrotal skin (option 2). Transillumination (option 3) is not related to the color of the scrotum.

Cognitive Level: Application Client Need: Health Promotion and Maintenance Integrated Process: Nursing Process: Implementation Content Area: Adult Health: Reproductive Strategy: Recall that normal skin color varies on different areas of the body. Then recall that the scrotum is slightly more pigmented than the surrounding skin. Knowing that expected findings need merely to be documented, you can eliminate all options except option 4. Reference: D'Amico, D. & Barbarito, C. (2007). *Health & physical assessment in nursing.* Upper Saddle River, NJ: Pearson Education, Inc., p. 600.

2 Answer: 2 Rationale: The African-American population has the highest incidence of prostate cancer. The Caucasian, Canadian, and European-American populations have a lower risk of cancer than the African-American population.
Cognitive Level: Comprehension Client Need: Health Promotion and Maintenance Integrated Process: Nursing Process: Implementation Content Area: Adult Health: Reproductive Strategy: Note that the question calls for factual information. To choose correctly, it is necessary to know that the African-American population has the highest incidence of prostate cancer. Reference: D'Amico, D. & Barbarito, C. (2007). *Health & physical assessment in nursing.* Upper Saddle River, NJ: Pearson Education, Inc., p. 589.

3 Answer: 2 Rationale: A normal level for prostate specific antigen is less than 4 ng/dL. Thus, a level of 3 ng is within accepted limits and requires no action (option 2). A low value (option 1) would not require any further investigation other than repeating the routine diagnostic study in one year. A high value (above 4 ng/dL) requires further investigation (options 3 and 4).
Cognitive Level: Analysis Client Need: Health Promotion and Maintenance Integrated Process: Nursing Process: Implementation Content Area: Adult Health: Reproductive Strategy: Note the similarity in options 3 and 4. With this in mind, eliminate these first. Next recall that the normal PSA is 1–4ng/dL to choose correctly. Reference: D'Amico, D. & Barbarito, C. (2007). *Health & physical assessment in nursing.* Upper Saddle River, NJ: Pearson Education, Inc., p. 620.

4 Answer: 2, 5 Rationale: As the prostate gland enlarges with age, it becomes firm, fixed, and hard (option 2). Although the gland is enlarged (option 5), small nodules are not present (option 1) and there would be no edema or nodules in the scrotal sac (options 3 and 4).
Cognitive Level: Analysis Client Need: Health Promotion and Maintenance Integrated Process: Nursing Process: Assessment Content Area: Adult Health: Reproductive Strategy: Consider that the client's symptoms could be caused by an enlarged prostate gland either as part of the aging process or because of prostate cancer. Eliminate options 3 and 4 because they refer to the scrotal sac and the prostate gland surrounds the urethra. Next recall that with prostate cancer the client will report

frequency, hesitancy, nocturia, dribbling incontinence, and urinary retention. Upon palpation the prostate will feel hard, fixed, and enlarged. Reference: D'Amico, D. & Barbarito, C. (2007). *Health & physical assessment in nursing.* Upper Saddle River, NJ: Pearson Education, Inc., p. 597.

5 Answer: 3 Rationale: The correct procedure to assess the rectum of the male client is to first position the client standing and leaning against the examination table. The nurse then places a lubricated, gloved, flexed finger against the anal sphincter and presses inward. The anal sphincter will tighten and then relax; as the sphincter relaxes the nurse inserts the finger into the anus toward the direction of the umbilicus (option 3). The client should not stand without support (option 1) when examining the rectum as the client may experience a vagal response during the examination, and leaning on the table will protect the client from injury. Sim's position may be used but it is not the preferred position for the examination of the male (option 2). Lithotomy position (option 4) is used for the examination of the female client.
Cognitive Level: Application Client Need: Health Promotion and Maintenance Integrated Process: Nursing Process: Assessment Content Area: Adult Health: Reproductive Strategy: The critical words in the question are *preferred procedures.* Eliminate options 2 and 4 first recalling that the client is usually in a standing position for a rectal examination. Next recall either that the client would benefit from physical support during the exam to choose option 3, or visualize that the exam would be difficult to perform with the client standing erect to eliminate option 1. Reference: D'Amico, D. & Barbarito, C. (2007). *Health & physical assessment in nursing.* Upper Saddle River, NJ: Pearson Education, Inc., pp. 606–608.

6 Answer: 2 Rationale: An inguinal hernia is caused when there is weakening of the abdominal muscles, which allows the intestine to protrude through the abdominal muscle into the inguinal canal. The bladder does not enter the testicular sac (option 1). When the testes retract into the abdominal wall (option 3) it is known as undescended testes. Testes do not usually protrude through the abdominal wall (option 4).
Cognitive Level: Comprehension Client Need: Health Promotion and Maintenance Integrated Process: Communication and Documentation Content Area: Child Health Strategy: Recall that inguinal hernias occur when the bowel protrudes through the abdominal wall muscle. This will help you to eliminate each of the incorrect options systematically. Reference: D'Amico, D. & Barbarito, C. (2007). *Health & physical assessment in nursing.* Upper Saddle River, NJ: Pearson Education, Inc., p. 587.

7 Answer: 1 Rationale: Epispadias is the term used to describe when the urinary meatus opens on the dorsal aspect of the penis as opposed to being centrally located (option 1). Hypospadias (option 2) is a term to describe a urinary meatus that is located on the ventral aspect of

the penis. A urethral stricture (option 3) is an abnormally small urinary meatus. Urethritis (option 4) is an infection of the urethra.
Cognitive Level: Application **Client Need:** Health Promotion and Maintenance **Integrated Process:** Communication and Documentation **Content Area:** Maternal-Newborn **Strategy:** First eliminate option 4 because the suffix *-itis* indicates inflammation. Next recall that a stricture is a narrowing to eliminate option 3. To choose correctly between the remaining two options, associate the prefix *hypo-* in hypospadias with the ventral aspect of the penis to eliminate option 2. **Reference:** D'Amico, D. & Barbarito, C. (2007). *Health & physical assessment in nursing.* Upper Saddle River, NJ: Pearson Education, Inc., p. 586.

8 **Answer: 4** **Rationale:** Young males are most at risk for testicular cancer and should be performing TSE (option 4). Nocturnal emissions are common in males, and most 20- to 30-year-old men are able to achieve an erection, so options 1 and 3 are not the priority. Frequent urination (option 2) is common in older adult males who are experiencing prostate enlargement, and is not seen in young adult males.
Cognitive Level: Application **Client Need:** Health Promotion and Maintenance **Integrated Process:** Nursing Process: Assessment **Content Area:** Adult Health: Reproductive **Strategy:** The critical word in the question is *priority*. This tells you that more than one option may be plausible but that one is more important than the others. To choose correctly, recall that men should begin performing monthly TSE in their teen years for early cancer detection. **Reference:** D'Amico, D. & Barbarito, C. (2007). *Health & physical assessment in nursing.* Upper Saddle River, NJ: Pearson Education, Inc., p. 589.

9 **Answer: 2** **Rationale:** TSE should be performed monthly. It is commonly recommended to perform the exam while taking a shower so the testicles are relaxed (option 2). The examination should not be performed after intercourse or in a sitting position (options 1 and 3). Any lump or hard lesion should be reported to the health-care provider (option 4).
Cognitive Level: Application **Client Need:** Health Promotion and Maintenance **Integrated Process:** Nursing Process: Implementation **Content Area:** Adult Health: Reproductive **Strategy:** Recall that TSE should be performed monthly in the shower and any enlargements or changes reported immediately to the health-care provider. This will help you to eliminate each of the incorrect options systematically. **Reference:** D'Amico, D. & Barbarito, C. (2007). *Health & physical assessment in nursing.* Upper Saddle River, NJ: Pearson Education, Inc., p. 589.

10 **Answer: 3** **Rationale:** Phimosis is the term used to describe the inability to retract the foreskin of the penis (option 3). Hypospadias is a condition in which the urinary meatus is on the ventral aspect of the penis (option 1). Epispadias is a condition in which the urinary meatus is located on the

dorsal aspect of the penis (option 2). A stricture is a narrowing of the meatus, a vessel, or other opening (option 4).
Cognitive Level: Comprehension **Client Need:** Physiological Integrity: Physiological Adaptation **Integrated Process:** Communication and Documentation **Content Area:** Adult Health: Reproductive **Strategy:** To answer this question correctly, it is necessary to know medical terminology. Recall that the condition is known as phimosis if the foreskin of the penis is unable to be retracted. **Reference:** D'Amico, D. & Barbarito, C. (2007). *Health & physical assessment in nursing.* Upper Saddle River, NJ: Pearson Education, Inc., p. 586.

Posttest

1 **Answer: 3, 4, 5** **Rationale:** A 16-year-old male may be sexually active. If so, then it is essential that the nurse assess if he is using condoms. Adolescent boys should start to perform TSE around 15 years of age. It is normal for an adolescent boy to have nocturnal emissions (option 1), so this question is not necessary. Urinary frequency (option 2) is often associated with an enlarged prostate gland, which is not common in the adolescent.
Cognitive Level: Analysis **Client Need:** Health Promotion and Maintenance **Integrated Process:** Nursing Process: Assessment **Content Area:** Child Health **Strategy:** Remember that the critical word *essential* indicates you should look for options that maintain client safety and/or promote health. An adolescent boy may be sexually active; if so then instruction on condoms and sexually transmitted disease may be necessary. Adolescent boys should be taught testicular self examination. **Reference:** D'Amico, D. & Barbarito, C. (2007). *Health & physical assessment in nursing.* Upper Saddle River, NJ: Pearson Education, Inc., p. 595.

2 **Answer: 2** **Rationale:** Bearing down will push the hernia into the inguinal area making it easier to palpate the hernia (option 2). A lateral position (option 1) will not push the bowel contents against the abdominal wall. While a rectal examination will be performed during the assessment of the male genitalia (options 3 and 4), it will not detect a hernia. A rectal examination allows for palpation of the prostate gland and the rectal area for masses.
Cognitive Level: Application **Client Need:** Health Promotion and Maintenance **Integrated Process:** Nursing Process: Assessment **Content Area:** Adult Health: Reproductive **Strategy:** First eliminate options 3 and 4 because they are both appropriate methods to assess the rectum and both options cannot be correct. Next eliminate option 1 because a lateral position is not used in the examination of the male genitalia. Alternatively, recall that bearing down will push the hernia into the inguinal canal to choose option 2. **Reference:** D'Amico, D. & Barbarito, C. (2007). *Health & physical assessment in nursing.* Upper Saddle River, NJ: Pearson Education, Inc., p. 606.

3 **Answer: 2** **Rationale:** Antihypertensive medications may inhibit sexual functioning. Aspirin, cardiac glycosides, and diuretics do not interfere with sexual functioning. **Cognitive Level:** Analysis **Client Need:** Physiological Integrity: Pharmacological and Parenteral Therapies **Integrated Process:** Nursing Process: Assessment **Content Area:** Adult Health: Reproductive **Strategy:** Specific knowledge of the side effects of several drug classes is needed to answer this question. Recall that antihypertensives may inhibit the sexual performance in males to help direct you to the correct option. **Reference:** D'Amico, D. & Barbarito, C. (2007). *Health & physical assessment in nursing*. Upper Saddle River, NJ: Pearson Education, Inc., p. 588.

4 **Answer: 2** **Rationale:** The critical words in the question are *term newborn*. In infants born at term, the testes should be in the scrotal sac (option 2). Scrotal edema is common in the male infant born breech (option 1). A urinary stream indicates an intact urinary system (option 3). Smegma is a benign cheese-like substance (option 4). **Cognitive Level:** Application **Client Need:** Health Promotion and Maintenance **Integrated Process:** Nursing Process: Assessment **Content Area:** Maternal-Newborn **Strategy:** Note that all of the incorrect options constitute normal findings for a breech infant except for an empty scrotal sac. Recall that undescended testes require further evaluation to help you to choose correctly. **Reference:** D'Amico, D. & Barbarito, C. (2007). *Health & physical assessment in nursing*. Upper Saddle River, NJ: Pearson Education, Inc., p. 600.

5 **Answer: 3** **Rationale:** Scrotal fluid is able to be illuminated. Light does not penetrate masses (option 1). A varicocele (option 2) is a distended cord and does not permit light to penetrate. Orchitis (option 4) is an infection and light will not penetrate an infected testis. **Cognitive Level:** Application **Client Need:** Health Promotion and Maintenance **Integrated Process:** Communication and Documentation **Content Area:** Adult Health: Reproductive **Strategy:** Remember that light can penetrate fluid. Then associate the word *fluid* with the prefix *hydro-* in the correct option. Alternatively, recall that any solid tissue (options 1, 2, and 4) is dense and light cannot penetrate it to choose correctly. **Reference:** D'Amico, D. & Barbarito, C. (2007). *Health & physical assessment in nursing*. Upper Saddle River, NJ: Pearson Education, Inc., p. 602.

6 **Answer: 3** **Rationale:** Testes usually have a firm, smooth, and possibly rubbery feeling. The scrotal sac should have rugae (rather than smooth as in option 2) and should feel like skin, rather than having an inelastic texture (option 1). The scrotal sac should have a darker pigmentation than other areas of skin (option 4). **Cognitive Level:** Application **Client Need:** Health Promotion and Maintenance **Integrated Process:** Communication and Documentation **Content Area:** Adult Health: Reproductive **Strategy:** Note that three of the options refer to the scrotum; one option deals with the testes. A test-taking strategy would be to select the option that is different.

Recall that testes should feel firm to confirm option 3 as the correct choice. **Reference:** D'Amico, D. & Barbarito, C. (2007). *Health & physical assessment in nursing*. Upper Saddle River, NJ: Pearson Education, Inc., p. 604.

7 **Answer: 1** **Rationale:** Benign prostatic hyperplasia (BPH) is an enlarged prostate gland that may cause the client to experience frequency, hesitancy, dribbling, difficulty initiating a urinary stream, a weak stream, and urinary retention or incontinence (option 1). With BPH, there would be no fluid or masses in the scrotal sac (options 2 and 3) and no nodules in the inguinal area (option 4). **Cognitive Level:** Application **Client Need:** Health Promotion and Maintenance **Integrated Process:** Nursing Process: Implementation **Content Area:** Adult Health: Reproductive **Strategy:** First recall that the prostate gland surrounds the upper urethra, making symptoms of hypertrophy urinary in nature. This will help you to eliminate options 2 and 3, which focus on the scrotal sac, and option 4, which focuses on the inguinal area. **Reference:** D'Amico, D. & Barbarito, C. (2007). *Health & physical assessment in nursing*. Upper Saddle River, NJ: Pearson Education, Inc., p. 589.

8 **Answer: 3** **Rationale:** At the end of a rectal exam, the nurse should perform a test for occult blood (option 3). The nurse should turn the glove inside out and dispose of it only after the stool on the glove is tested for occult blood (option 1). Gloves should not be washed prior to being discarded (option 2). During the rectal examination, the client may have a temporary sensation of fullness but should not need to empty the bowel (option 4). **Cognitive Level:** Application **Client Need:** Health Promotion and Maintenance **Integrated Process:** Nursing Process: Implementation **Content Area:** Adult Health: Gastrointestinal **Strategy:** The critical word in the question is *next*. Visualize the sequence of events during a rectal examination and recall that, immediately upon completion of the rectal examination, the nurse should test the feces on the glove for occult blood. **Reference:** D'Amico, D. & Barbarito, C. (2007). *Health & physical assessment in nursing*. Upper Saddle River, NJ: Pearson Education, Inc., p. 609.

9 **Answer: 3** **Rationale:** The discharge should be cultured to identify microorganisms that are responsible for the discharge (option 3). Gloves should be applied prior to initiating the examination (option 1). A slide is made of glass and is sharp therefore the penis should not be placed near the slide; option 2 represents incorrect technique and risks contamination of the client's hands. Antibiotics (option 4) are not initiated until a culture is obtained to avoid interfering with the test results. **Cognitive Level:** Application **Client Need:** Health Promotion and Maintenance **Integrated Process:** Nursing Process: Implementation **Content Area:** Adult Health: Reproductive **Strategy:** Eliminate option 1 first because the gloves should be applied prior to beginning the examination. Next eliminate option 4, because starting antibiotics prior to obtaining the culture is a clear violation of principles of antibiotic therapy. Consider basic principles of obtaining a culture to eliminate option 2. **Reference:** D'Amico, D. & Barbarito, C. (2007). *Health & physical assessment in nursing*. Upper Saddle River, NJ: Pearson Education, Inc., p. 603.

10 **Answer: 4** **Rationale:** It is normal for a client to obtain an erection during the assessment of the genitalia (option 4). This response is physiologic in nature and is not under the client's control. The nurse should provide reassurance and proceed with the examination in a professional manner. The nurse should not leave the room (option 1) or send in another examiner (option 2) as these behaviors could cause the client further embarrassment. The nurse should not apologize (option 3) as this is a physiological response.

Cognitive Level: Application **Client Need:** Health Promotion and Maintenance **Integrated Process:** Nursing Process: Assessment **Content Area:** Adult Health: Reproductive **Strategy:** Begin to answer the question by recalling that an erection is a physiological response during an exam and choose the option that addresses this principle. Options 1 and 2 do not take this principle into consideration and are likely to cause the client psychological discomfort; because of this, eliminate them both. Next note that options 3 and 4 have two parts to them and recall that both parts must be correct for the option to be correct. Choose the most therapeutic professional response, which is to reassure the client and proceed with the exam. **Reference:** D'Amico, D. & Barbarito, C. (2007). *Health & physical assessment in nursing*. Upper Saddle River, NJ: Pearson Education, Inc., p. 599.

References

Bickley, L. (2010). *Bates guide to physical examination and history taking* (10th ed.). Philadelphia: Lippincott Williams & Wilkins.

D'Amico, D. & Barbarito, C. (2007). *Health and physical assessment in nursing*. Upper Saddle River, NJ: Pearson Education, Inc., pp. 348–396.

Jarvis, C. (2008). *Physical examination and health assessment* (5th ed.). St. Louis, MO: Elsevier Saunders.

Zator-Estes, M. (2009). *Health assessment and physical examination* (4th ed.). Clifton Park, NY: Delmar Cengage Learning.

Skin, Hair, and Nails Assessment

13

Chapter Outline

Health History
Present Health History
Family History

Equipment, Preparation, and
  Positioning
Examination Techniques
Expected Findings

Unexpected Findings
Lifespan Considerations
Documentation

Objectives

➤ Identify basic structures and functions of the skin, hair, and nails.
➤ Describe developmental, psychosocial, cultural, and environmental
  variations in assessment techniques and findings.
➤ Review focused questions to be used during data collection.
➤ Describe the techniques for assessing the skin, hair, and nails.
➤ Differentiate between normal and abnormal findings of skin, hair,
  and nails.
➤ Discuss nursing measures to promote health as presented in
  Healthy People 2010.

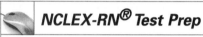

NCLEX-RN® Test Prep

Visit the Companion Website for this book
at www.pearsonhighered.com/hogan to
access additional practice opportunities
and more.

Review at a Glance

basal cell carcinoma abnormal
skin cell growth that develops as a
translucent papule with rounded, pearly
borders and central red ulcer; most common but least malignant form of skin cancer; superficial basal cell cancer can
appear as a red patch; infiltrative morpheaform can appear as a skin thickening

cyst elevated, encapsulated, and fluid-filled, semisolid, or air-filled mass usually
1 cm or larger

ecchymosis flat, irregularly shaped
lesion, changing in color from bluish-purple to greenish-yellow caused by
blood loss from a ruptured blood vessel

hemangioma raised, bright red
lesion ranging from 2 to 10 cm in diameter due to immature capillaries; can also
be a benign self-involuting tumor of
endothelial cells that line blood vessels;
cause is unknown

hematoma raised, irregularly shaped
lesion caused by a ruptured blood vessel
that leaks into surrounding tissue

Kaposi's sarcoma malignant, painless, soft lesions, ranging from pink/
purple to red/brown in color; commonly
seen in clients with human immunodeficiency virus (HIV) and caused by human
herpesvirus (HHV8); also seen in elderly
men of Mediterranean or Eastern
European descent

macule flat, non-palpable primary skin
lesion with a skin color change measuring less than 1 cm

malignant melanoma irregularly
shaped skin tumor with notched borders;
variations in color range from
black/brown to red/purple; spreads
rapidly to lymph and blood vessels

nodule elevated, solid mass with circumscribed border that ranges from
0.5 to 2 cm in diameter

papule elevated, solid, palpable mass
with circumscribed border less than 0.5 cm
in diameter

petechiae flat, round, red or purple
hemorrhages, from 1 to 3 mm in diameter,

caused by bleeding from superficial
capillaries

plaque groups of papules that form
lesions larger than 0.5 cm in diameter

port-wine stain flat, irregularly
shaped lesion ranging in color from pale
red to deep purple/red

purpura flat, extensive patches of
petechiae and ecchymoses

pustule elevated, pus-filled vesicle or
bulla with circumscribed border

scales shedding flakes of greasy, keratinized skin tissue

spider angioma flat, bright red, star-shaped marking with solid, circular center

squamous cell carcinoma
cancerous lesion that may appear as erythematous scaly patches that form shallow ulcer with sharp margins; may be 1 cm
or more in size, may also appear as an
ulcer or reddish skin patch with intermittent bleeding

venous lake flat, blue lesion with
radiating, cascading, or linear veins

extending from the center; size ranges from 3 to 25 cm; caused by a type of telangiectasis (vascular dilatation) caused by increased intravenous pressure in superficial veins

vesicle (bulla) elevated, fluid-filled, round or oval-shaped, palpable mass with thin, translucent walls and circumscribed borders, less than 0.5 cm in size; bulla is larger than 0.5 cm in size

wheal elevated, erythematous area of skin with an irregular border due to edema in tissues, may be accompanied by itching

PRETEST

1 A client comes to the healthcare provider's office for an annual checkup. Which question is best for the nurse to ask to obtain information about illness or infection of the client's skin?

1. "Have you recently had a skin infection?"
2. "Have you noticed any rashes on your body?"
3. "Can you tell me about any skin problems you have had?"
4. "Have you ever sunbathed?"

2 To best detect skin color changes when assessing a dark-skinned client, the nurse should inspect which area of the client's body?

1. Face
2. Lips
3. Neck
4. Trunk

3 What approaches would the nurse use to prepare a Caucasian client for a skin, hair, and nail assessment? Select all that apply.

1. Provide a warm, private environment
2. Be sensitive to cultural issues
3. Use tangential lighting only
4. Use standard precautions throughout the assessment
5. Bathe the client

4 To prevent complications during pregnancy, what question during a health assessment of a pregnant client in her first trimester would be most important for the nurse to ask?

1. "How have you been feeling lately?"
2. "Have you ever been pregnant before?"
3. "Do you have other children at home?"
4. "Do you use any topical medications?"

5 What would be the most appropriate question for the nurse to ask a female client who is seeking treatment for a skin rash on her hands that developed recently after starting a new job?

1. "Do you wear gloves at work?"
2. "How would you describe your level of stress?"
3. "Have you recently been exposed to extremes in temperature?"
4. "Do your hands usually perspire?"

6 Which nursing diagnosis has the highest priority for a client who has a skin tone change from normal to cyanosis?

1. Impaired skin integrity
2. Ineffective tissue perfusion
3. Risk for infection
4. Impaired spontaneous ventilation

7 During a physical examination, the nurse observes a dark, pigmented band on the nail bed of the client's left forefinger. What action by the nurse is most important?

1. Document finding as a splinter hemorrhage
2. Evaluate nail beds for clubbing
3. Refer the client for further evaluation by a healthcare provider
4. Ask the client further questions related to nail trauma

8 In assessing a young client's hair, the nurse notes the texture is very coarse, dry, and brittle. What condition should the nurse consider as a potential cause for this type of abnormality?

1. Alopecia areata
2. Hypothyroidism
3. Pediculosis capitis
4. Seborrheic dermatitis

9 The nurse finds enlarged nail beds and a spongy quality at the nail base during an assessment of a client with a diagnosis of chronic obstructive pulmonary disease (COPD). How would the nurse document this finding?

1. Clubbing
2. Onycholysis
3. Paronychia
4. Spoon nails

10 A foreign exchange student is admitted to the hospital with the onset of an acute skin condition. What action should the nurse implement to avoid miscommunication or misinterpretation of health-related information?

1. Call the client's family
2. Enlist the aid of a medical interpreter
3. Use sign language
4. Use a picture chart

➤ *See pages 260–262 for Answers and Rationales.*

I. HEALTH HISTORY

A. Anatomy and physiology review

1. Skin structures
   a. Epidermis: layer of epithelial tissue that comprises outermost portion of skin
      1) Keratin: fibrous protein that gives epidermis its tough, protective qualities
      2) Melanin: skin pigment produced by melanocytes
   b. Dermis: layer of connective tissue that lies just below the epidermis; composed of lymph vessels, blood vessels, and nerve fibers
   c. Subcutaneous tissue (hypodermis)
      1) Loose connective tissue that stores fat cells for energy, protects body against trauma, and insulates the body from heat loss
      2) Contains cutaneous or sweat glands, which include eccrine glands (located on forehead, hands, and soles of feet and produce clear perspiration of water and salts), apocrine glands (located in axillary and anogenital regions, which during puberty begin to produce secretion composed of water, salts, fatty acid, and proteins), and sebaceous or oil glands (located throughout body and which secrete sebum, an oily secretion composed of fat and keratin into hair follicles)

2. Major functions of skin (see Box 13-1)
3. Hair structures: hair is a thin, flexible, elongated fiber composed of dead, keratinized cells
   a. Vellus hair: pale, fine, short strands that covers most of body
   b. Terminal hair: darker, coarser, and longer that covers eyebrows and scalp
4. Major functions of hair (see Box 13-2)
5. Nail structures
   a. Composed of a thin plate of keratinized epidermal cells that protect distal ends of fingers and toes
   b. Lunula: moon-shaped crescent over thickened nail matrix
   c. Cuticle: fold of epidermal skin that protects root and side of each nail

▶ *Practice to Pass*

The client reports having a history of dermatological candida infections. The nurse should include this information in which section of the interview?

Box 13-1		
Major Functions of the Skin	Feels touch, pressure, temperature, and pain	Repairs surface wounds
		Synthesizes vitamin D
	Protects body and internal structures from damage and loss of fluids and electrolytes	Allows for identification through facial contours, skin and hair color, and fingerprints
	Regulates body temperature	

Box 13-2		
Major Functions of the Hair	Insulates against heat and cold	Protects eyes from sweat
	Protects against ultraviolet and infrared rays	Protects nasal passages and ear canals from foreign particles
	Perceives movement or touch	

B. Past medical history pertaining to skin, hair, and nails; ask client about previous history of the following disorders, including treatment, its effectiveness, whether problem has recurred, and how the client currently treats it if it is a chronic problem

1. Skin cancer, skin lesions, burns, or rashes
2. Chronic skin conditions such as lupus erythematosus, eczema or psoriasis
3. Infections of the skin or nails, such as warts, candida, acne, herpes simplex, or herpes zoster
4. Infestations of skin or hair

II. PRESENT HEALTH HISTORY

A. Skin

1. General questions about skin
   a. "How would you describe the condition of your skin now? How does it compare to what it was like 2 months ago? Two years ago?"
   b. "How easily and how much do you sweat? Do you have increased sweating at certain times, such as at night?" (Too much sweat loss can contribute to heat stroke or may be a side effect of medications; sweating at specific times, such as at night, can indicate infection)
   c. "Do you have difficulty at times controlling body odor?" (May be related to activity or diet, or may be associated with a systemic disorder)
   d. "Have you noticed any color changes in your skin? If so, is it over your entire body or in one area?"
   e. "Have you noticed if your skin is either oilier or drier than it used to be? Are there any other changes in how your skin feels?"
2. Questions about skin symptoms
   a. "Do you have any itching of your skin? If so, when does it occur and how severe is it?"
   b. "Do you have skin rashes anywhere on your body?"
      1) "When did you first notice it?"
      2) "Has it spread from its original location?"
      3) "Did any other symptoms, such as chills or fever, occur at about the same time?"
      4) "Did the rash start after using any new medications or skin products?"
      5) "Does it occur in relation to specific activities, such as wearing certain clothes, jewelry, or cosmetics?"
   c. "Do you have any broken areas on your skin, such as sores, ulcers, boils, or skin infections? If so, where? Are they are healing more slowly than they should?"
   d. "Do you have any areas of the skin that have drainage? If so, describe where, how much, any odor, and if other symptoms also occur."
   e. "Do you have any birthmarks or moles that have changed in size, color, shape, or overall appearance? If so, what was the change and when did it occur? Does the area have pain, itching, or bleeding?"
   f. "Do you have any other bruises, lumps or bumps, or areas of pain on your skin? If so, where are they, when did they occur, and have they spread?"
   g. "What have you done to treat your current skin condition (if applicable)? When did you begin treatment and how has it worked?"
3. Questions about pain in a specific area of the skin or in skin folds: perform a typical pain assessment including location, duration, intensity (1–10 rating scale), frequency of pain episodes, whether the pain is constant or intermittent, aggravating factors or triggers, and alleviating or relieving factors
4. Questions about behaviors that affect risk for skin problems: sun exposure, cleansers, tattoos, or piercings
   a. "Do you currently sunbathe or have you in the past? If so, how often?"

Practice to Pass

The client informs the nurse about a red rash that has appeared on the skin. What additional information should the nurse gather?

    b. "Do you go to the tanning salon? If so, how often?"

    c. "Do you recall ever having a sunburn that left blisters?"

    d. "Do you spend time in the sun working, playing sports, or exercising?"

    e. "Do you use sunscreen when you are outside? If so, what sun protection factor (SPF) does it have? Do you reapply it after a certain amount of time or after swimming?"

    f. "How frequently do you bathe or shower? What kind(s) of soap, cleanser, toner, or other skin product do you use?"

    g. "What type of detergent do you use to clean your clothes?"

    h. "Do you have any tattoos? If so, where and how long have you had it (them)? Have you had any problems with that area of skin? If so, how was it treated and what was the outcome?"

    i. "Do you have any piercings? If so, where and how long have you had it (them)? Have you had any problems with the skin piercing site? If so, how was it treated and what was the outcome? Have any piercing areas closed?"

5. Questions about the internal body environment (stress) that can aggravate skin disorders

    a. "How would you describe your usual level of stress? Has it changed in the past few weeks or months? If so, how?"

    b. "Either now or in the past, have you had intermittent or constant and prolonged emotional upsets or anxiety? If so, can you describe the situation(s)? What precipitates the skin problem? Do you seek care for this or do something specific when it occurs?"

    c. "Have you changed your diet recently or had any unfamiliar foods or beverages? If so, describe."

    d. "Do you take any medications, either prescribed or over-the-counter?"

    e. "Has the condition of your skin affected how you interact with other people in any way or limited you in any way? If so, how?"

6. Questions about external (physical) environment that can irritate skin

    a. "What is the usual temperature of your home environment? Of your work environment?"

    b. "Have you been exposed to extremes in temperature recently? If so, what were the circumstances, and when did it occur and for how long?"

    c. "Are x-rays or radioisotopes used in your work area? If so, how vigilant are you in using protective equipment and following workplace precautions?"

    d. "Do you wear gloves at work? If so, what kind and how often do you need to wear them?"

    e. "Do you work with any chemicals routinely during your job or any hobby? Does the job or hobby require you to wear a specific type of helmet, hat, gloves, goggles, or shoes? If so, do they fit well and cause no skin irritation?"

    f. "Have you traveled recently? If so, where? Have you come into contact with someone who has a similar skin problem (rash)?"

    g. "Do you participate in sports and use protective equipment such as pads, protectors, ear covers, and helmets?" (chafing, rashes, fungal infections, and irritation may occur)

B. Hair

  1. "How would you describe the condition of your hair now? How does it compare to what it was like 2 months ago? Two years ago?"

  2. "How often do you wash your hair? What types of shampoo do you use? Do you experience dandruff? If so, how do you treat it and is it effective?"

  3. "Have you noticed increased hair loss recently? If so, how has the hair fallen out? Have you had an illness within the last few months?"

  4. "What products or tools do you use to style your hair?"

5. "Do you use any chemicals on your hair, such as bleach, color, perm, or chemical straighteners? If so, how often do you use them and when was the last use?"
6. "Do you pluck your eyebrows or facial hair? Do you shave or use chemical hair removers to remove hair on any part of your body?"
7. "Do you swim regularly? If so, in what type of water (fresh water, salt water, chlorinated pools)?"

C. Nails
1. "How would you describe the condition of your nails now? How does this compare to 2 months ago? Two years ago?"
2. "Have you had any pain, swelling, or drainage around the cuticles? If so, when did you notice this? What do you think is the cause?"
3. "Have you been ill recently?" (illness can lead to nail changes such as discoloration, grooves, or ridges)
4. "Do you wear nail polish/enamel, artificial fingernails, tips, or wraps?" (enamel can lead to drying or discoloration of the nails; artificial nails may increase the risk of fungal infections)
5. "When you are at home or at work, are your hands submerged in water often or for long periods?" (this can increase the risk of bacterial or fungal infections of cuticles)

III. FAMILY HISTORY

A. **Determine family history of chronic skin problems, which may recur in other family members; examples include allergies, rashes, psoriasis, eczema, or skin cancer**
B. **Assess for the preceding problems by asking the following:**
1. "What is the skin disorder or problem?"
2. "Who in the family has this problem?"
3. "When was this problem diagnosed?"
4. "What treatments have been used?"
5. "How effective have the treatments been?"

IV. EQUIPMENT, PREPARATION, AND POSITIONING

A. **Equipment**
1. Examination gown and drape
2. Examination gloves (clean, nonsterile)
3. Examination light and penlight
4. Centimeter ruler
5. Magnifying glass
6. Wood's lamp (provides filtered ultraviolet light for special procedures)
B. **Client preparation and positioning**
1. Provide a comfortably warm and private environment
2. Use draping techniques to increase client comfort and maintain client dignity; only expose the areas of skin needed for the current area being assessed
3. Explain procedure and the need to remove clothing, jewelry, hairpieces, and possibly nail enamel
4. Be aware of and sensitive to possible cultural issues, such as not exposing skin; touching of skin by members of opposite gender; or removal of coverings of face, hair, or head; make provisions if another female needs to be present during the examination
5. Place client in a sitting position for examination of skin
6. Since skin conditions may negatively affect self-image, monitor own verbal and non-verbal reactions to skin findings during examination

V. EXAMINATION TECHNIQUES

A. Skin inspection

1. Place client in a sitting position after client puts on an examination gown
2. Explain procedure to client
3. Observe for cleanliness and use sense of smell to determine body odor; urea and ammonia salts found on skin can be related to kidney disorders
4. Observe client's skin tone and evaluate any changes in color such as cyanosis, pallor, erythema, or jaundice; cyanosis or pallor indicates abnormally low plasma oxygen; pallor is also seen in anemia; see Table 13-1 for evaluation of color variations in light- and dark-skinned clients
5. Inspect skin for even pigmentation; uneven pigmentation is caused by differences in the distribution of melanin; vitiligo is patchy, depigmented areas over face, neck, hands, feet, and body folds
6. Inspect skin for superficial arteries and veins; where skin is thin, a fine network of veins or a few dilated blood vessels may be visible

B. Skin palpation

1. Explain to client that examination will involve touching in various areas
2. Determine client's skin temperature
    a. Use dorsal surface of hand, which is more sensitive to temperature
    b. Palpate forehead or face first
    c. Continue to palpate inferiorly, including hands and feet
    d. Compare right and left sides
        1) Temperature will be higher than normal when a systemic infection or metabolic disorder is present (hyperthyroidism), after strenuous exercise, and when the environmental temperature is warm
        2) In metabolic disorders, temperature of skin is lower than normal (hypothyroidism); localized coolness occurs as result of decreased circulation due to vasoconstriction or occlusion from peripheral arterial insufficiency
        3) Unilateral difference in temperature may indicate a lack of circulation on the cooler side due to compression, immobilization, or elevation
3. Assess amount of moisture on skin surface
4. Palpate skin for texture
5. Palpate skin to determine its thickness
6. Palpate skin for elasticity
7. Inspect and palpate skin for lesions
8. Palate skin for sensitivity

C. Inspection and palpation of hair and scalp

1. Explain procedure to client
2. Observe for cleanliness
3. Observe client's hair color
4. Assess hair texture
5. Observe amount and distribution of hair throughout the scalp
6. Inspect scalp for condition and presence of lesions

D. Inspection and palpation of nails

1. Explain procedure to the client
2. Assess for hygiene
3. Inspect nails for even, pink undertone
4. Assess capillary refill
5. Inspect and palpate nails for shape and contour
6. Palpate nails to determine thickness, regularity, and attachment to nail bed
7. Inspect and palpate cuticles

Table 13-1 **Color Variations in Light- and Dark-Skinned Clients**

Color Variation	Possible Causes	Appearance in Light Skin	Appearance in Dark Skin
Pallor, loss of color in skin	Peripheral vasoconstriction, decrease in tissue perfusion	Loss of rosy tone, naturally yellow-toned skin may appear slightly jaundiced	Loss of red undertone, ash-gray appearance, brown skin appears yellow-tinged and dull
Absence of color, loss of pigment	Albinism, vitiligo, tinea versicolor	White skin with white or pale blonde hair and pink irises; vitiligo appears as patchy milk-white areas; tinea versicolor appears as patchy areas paler than surrounding skin	Same appearance as in light skin
Cyanosis, mottled blue color due to inadequate tissue perfusion	**Systemic or central**: cardiac and pulmonary disease, heart malformations, low levels of hemoglobin **Localized or peripheral:** vasoconstriction, exposure to cold, emotional stress	Blue-tinged appearance on skin, lips, and mucous membranes; blue-tinged appearance on conjunctiva and nail beds	Skin may appear a shade darker, color changes best detected on lips, tongue, and oral mucosa, which may appear pale or blue-tinged
Reddish-blue tone, ruddy tone due to increased hemoglobin and blood stasis in capillaries	Polycythemia vera	Reddish-purple hue	Inspect lips for redness, normal skin color may appear darker
Erythema, redness of skin due to increased visibility of normal oxyhemoglobin	Hyperemia, fever, warm environment, local inflammation, allergy, emotions, extreme cold exposure, alcohol consumption, dependent position of body extremity	Identifiable over entire body, local inflammation and redness, temperature may be higher at site	Generalized redness more difficult to detect, local areas may appear purple or darker than surrounding skin, may have higher temperature, hardness, swelling
Jaundice, yellow tone due to increased bilirubin	Liver disease, biliary obstruction, hemolytic disease following infections, severe burns, or from sickle cell anemia or pernicious anemia	Generalized undertone, also visible in sclera, oral mucosa, hard palate, fingernails, palms of hand, and soles of feet	More visible in sclera, oral mucosa, hard and soft palate junction, and palms of hands and soles of feet
Carotenemia, yellow-orange tinge due to increased levels of carotene in blood and skin	Ingestion of foods high in carotene, seen in endocrine disorders (diabetes mellitus, myxedema, and hypopituitarism)	Yellow-orange visible in forehead, palms, and soles of feet; no yellow undertone of sclera or mucous membranes	More visible in sclera, oral mucosa, hard and soft palate junction, palms of hands and soles of feet
Uremia, pale yellow tone due to retention of urinary chromogens in blood	Chronic renal disease	Generalized pallor and yellow tinge, skin may show bruising	Not distinctively discernable since yellow tinge is very pale and does not affect conjunctivae
Brown, increase in production and deposition of melanin	Addison's disease, pituitary tumor, local change may be caused by hormonal changes of pregnancy, use of birth control pills, exposure to ultraviolet radiation	General bronzed skin with endocrine disorders; hyper-pigmentation in nipples, palmar, creases, genitals, and pressure points; red tinge in pale skin and minimal to no reddening in olive-tone skin from sun exposure	Deepening skin tone with endocrine disorders; hyper-pigmentation in nipples, genitals, and pressure points; brown to black skin tone from sun exposure

VI. EXPECTED FINDINGS

  A. Skin inspection

    1. Skin is clean and generally free of odor

    2. Skin has normal variations according to whether skin is light or dark; skin is free of pallor, cyanosis, erythema, or jaundice

3. Skin has even pigmentation except for normal deeper pigmentation in areas of body that have more melanin, such as margins of lips, areolae, nipples, and external genitalia

4. Presence of skin freckles or nevi (congenital marks) are normal variations

5. Visible veins (few in number or a fine network) may be a normal finding when skin is thin, such as on abdomen or eyelids

B. **Skin palpation**

1. Skin is evenly warm on both sides of body

2. Hands or feet may be cooler than other areas of the body according to ambient temperature, but are similar bilaterally

3. Fine perspiration may be noted in expected areas such as face, skin folds, axillae, palms, and soles of feet

4. Skin may have a fine sheen of oil in some clients

5. Dry skin may be an expected finding if the climate is especially cold or dry

6. Skin texture should be smooth, firm, and even

7. Skin thickness is generally thin but firm; thicker skin is a normal finding on palms, soles of feet, elbows, and knees, while thinner skin is expected on lips and over eyelids

8. Skin has expected elasticity (includes both mobility [skin can be lifted] and resiliency [skin can return to normal position]); the skin under the clavicle or medial wrist returns to normal shape and position quickly after being grasped between the forefinger and thumb

9. Skin is free of edema, especially noted in feet, ankles, and sacrum

10. Skin is smooth and free of lesions (except for expected variations such as freckles, healed scars, certain birthmarks, and insect bites)

11. Skin is free of discomfort or sensitivity during palpation of skin in various areas of the body

C. **Inspection and palpation of hair and scalp**

1. Hair color is expected to vary according to level of melanin production, and graying occurs according to genetic influence

2. Hair texture may be thick or fine (thin) and may be straight, wavy, or curly

3. Hair is evenly distributed across the scalp, except for an expected variation of male pattern baldness, which is a progressive loss of hair beginning at anterior hairline

4. Hair is free of lesions during examination of scalp by parting the hair and is free of areas of fluorescent glow when shining a Wood's lamp on various areas of scalp

D. **Inspection and palpation of nails**

1. Nails are clean and well groomed (variations may be due to self-care deficit or to occupation)

2. Nails have an even, pink undertone except for expected variation of small white markings caused by minor trauma

3. During palpation for capillary refill, nail edges should blanche briefly with pressure, with color returning rapidly (within three seconds) upon release of pressure to nail bed

4. Nails are free of clubbing (diamond-shaped opening is seen between nails during assessment using Shamroth technique)

5. Nails are smooth, strong, and regular in appearance; they are firmly attached to nail bed with only slight mobility

6. Cuticles of nails are smooth and flat

VII. UNEXPECTED FINDINGS

A. **Vascular lesions of the skin**

1. **Hemangioma**—bright red, raised lesion, 2–10 cm in diameter; caused by a cluster of immature capillaries

2. **Port-wine stain**—flat, irregularly shaped lesion ranging in color from pale red to deep red; caused by a large, flat mass of blood vessels on the skin surface

3. **Spider angioma**—flat, bright red dot with tiny radiating blood vessels ranging in size from a pinpoint to 2 cm; caused by a type of telangiectasis (vascular dilatation) caused by elevated estrogen levels, pregnancy, estrogen therapy, vitamin B deficiency, or liver disease, or may not be pathologic

4. **Venous lake**—flat, blue lesion with radiating, cascading, or linear veins extending from the center; size ranges from 3 to 25 cm; caused by a type of telangiectasis (vascular dilatation) caused by increased intravenous pressure in superficial veins

5. **Petechiae**—flat, red or purple rounded "freckles" approximately 1–3 mm in diameter; caused by minute hemorrhages resulting from fragile capillaries caused by septicemias, liver disease, or vitamin C or K deficiency; also caused by anticoagulant therapy

6. **Purpura**—flat, reddish-blue, irregularly shaped extensive patches of varying size; caused by bleeding disorders, scurvy, and capillary fragility in older adult (senile purpura)

7. **Ecchymosis**—flat, irregularly shaped lesion of varying size with no pulsation
   a. In light skin it begins as a bluish-purple mark that changes to greenish-yellow; in darker skin it varies from blue to deep purple, and in darkest skin it appears as a darkened area
   b. Caused by a release of blood from superficial vessels into surrounding tissue due to trauma, hemophilia, liver disease, or deficiency of vitamins C or K

8. **Hematoma**—raised, irregularly shaped lesion similar to ecchymosis except that it elevates the skin and looks like swelling; caused by leakage of blood into the skin and subcutaneous tissue as result of trauma or surgical incision

B. **Primary lesions of skin**

1. **Macule** and patch—flat, non-palpable changes in skin color; macules are less than 1 cm with a circumscribed border (examples include freckles, measles, and petechiae); patches are larger than 1 cm and may have an irregular border (examples include Mongolian spots, port-wine stains, vitiligo, and chloasma) (see Figure 13-1A)

2. **Papule** and **plaque**—elevated, solid, palpable mass with circumscribed border; papules are smaller than 0.5 cm (examples include elevated moles, warts, and lichen planus); plaques are groups of papules that form lesions larger than 0.5 cm (examples include psoriasis, actinic keratosis, and also lichen planus) (see Figure 13-1B)

3. **Nodule** and tumor—elevated, solid, hard or soft palpable mass extending deeper into dermis than a papule; nodules are 0.5–2 cm with circumscribed borders (examples include small lipoma, squamous cell carcinoma, fibroma, and intradermal nevi); tumors are larger than 2 cm and may have irregular borders (examples include large lipoma, carcinoma, and hemangioma) (see Figure 13-1C)

4. **Vesicle** and **bulla**—elevated, fluid-filled, round or oval-shaped, palpable mass with thin, translucent walls and circumscribed borders; vesicles are smaller than 0.5 cm (examples include herpes simplex/zoster, early chickenpox, poison ivy, and small burn blisters); bullae are larger than 0.5 cm (examples include contact dermatitis, friction blisters, and large burn blisters) (see Figure 13-1D)

5. **Wheal**—elevated, often reddish area with an irregular border caused by diffuse fluid in tissues rather than free fluid in a cavity, as in vesicles; size varies; examples include insect bites and hives (see Figure 13-1E)

6. **Pustule**—elevated, pus-filled vesicle or bulla with circumscribed border; size varies; examples include acne, impetigo, and carbuncles (see Figure 13-1F)

7. **Cyst**—elevated, encapsulated, fluid-filled or semisolid mass originating in subcutaneous tissue of dermis, usually 1 cm or larger; examples include sebaceous cysts and epidermoid cysts (see Figure 13-1G)

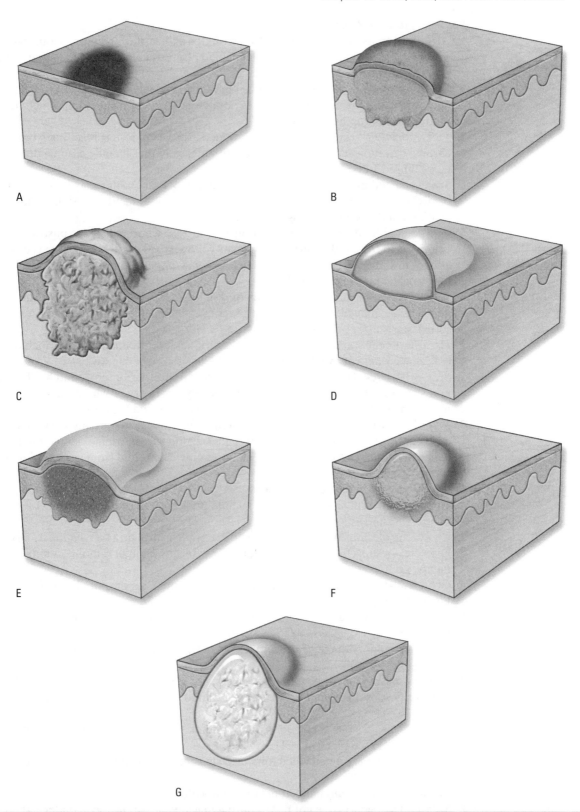

Figure 13-1

Primary skin lesions. A. Macule. B. Papule, plaque. C. Nodule, tumor. D. Vesicle, bulla. E. Wheal. F. Pustule. G. Cyst.

C. **Secondary lesions of skin**

1. **Atrophy**—translucent, dry, paper-like, wrinkled skin surface resulting from thinning or wasting of skin due to loss of collagen and elastin; examples include striae, aged skin (see Figure 13-2A)

2. *Erosion*—wearing away of superficial epidermis, causing moist, shallow depression; heals without scarring because it does not extend into dermis; examples include scratch marks, ruptured vesicles

3. *Lichenification*—rough, thickened, hardened area of epidermis resulting from chronic irritation such as scratching or rubbing; examples include chronic dermatitis (see Figure 13-2B)

4. **Scales**—shedding flakes of greasy, keratinized skin tissue; color may be white, gray, or silver; texture may vary from fine to thick; examples include dry skin, dandruff, psoriasis, and eczema (see Figure 13-2C)

5. *Crust*—dry blood, serum, or pus left on skin surface when vesicles or pustules burst; colors range from red-brown to orange or yellow; scabs occur when large crusts adhere to skin surface; examples include eczema, impetigo, herpes, or scabs following abrasion (see Figure 13-2D)

6. *Ulcer*—deep, irregularly shaped area of skin loss extending into dermis or subcutaneous tissue; may bleed or leave scar; examples include decubitus ulcers (pressure sores), stasis ulcers, chancres (see Figure 13-2E)

7. *Fissure*—linear crack with sharp edges, extending into dermis; examples include cracks at corners of mouth or in hands, athlete's foot (see Figure 13-2F)

8. *Scar*—flat, irregular area of connective tissue left after lesion or wound has healed; new scars may be red or purple; older scars may be silvery or white; examples include healed surgical wound or injury, healed acne (see Figure 13-2G)

9. *Keloid*—elevated, irregular, darkened area of excess scar tissue caused by excessive collagen formation during healing; extends beyond site of original injury; higher incidence in people of African descent; examples include keloid from ear-piercing or surgery (see Figure 13-2H)

D. **Configurations and shapes of skin lesions**

1. Annular—circular shape; examples include tinea corporis, pityriasis rosea (see Figure 13-3A)

2. Confluent—lesions that run together; an example is urticaria (see Figure 13-3B)

3. Discrete—lesions that are separate and discrete; an example is molluscum (see Figure 13-3C)

4. Grouped—lesions that appear in clusters; an example is a purpura lesion (see Figure 13-3D)

5. Gyrate—lesions that are coiled or twisted; an example is a gyrate lesion (see Figure 13-3E)

6. Target—lesions with concentric circles of color; an example is erythema multiforme (see Figure 13-3F)

7. Linear—lesions that appear as a line; an example is scratches (see Figure 13-3G)

8. Polycyclic—lesions that are circular but united; an example is psoriasis (see Figure 13-3H)

9. Zosteriform—lesions arranged in linear manner along a nerve route; an example is herpes zoster (see Figure 13-3I)

E. **Common skin lesions (see attached Nursing Notes card for illustrations of common skin lesions)**

1. Tinea—fungal infection affecting body and scalp or feet

2. Measles (Rubeola)—rash of red to purple macules or papules seen on face, then progress to neck, trunk, arms, and legs; occurs most frequently in children

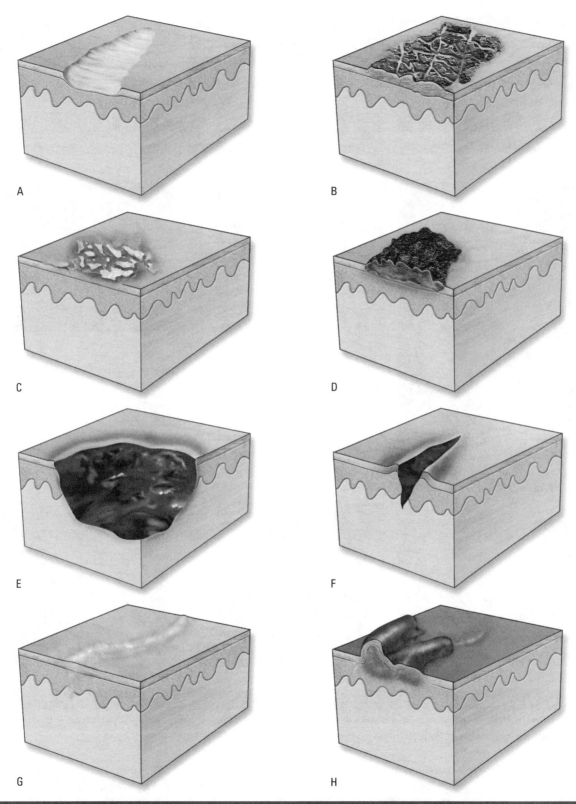

Secondary skin lesions. A. Atrophy. B. Lichenification. C. Scales. D. Crust. E. Ulcer. F. Fissure. G. Scar. H. Keloid.

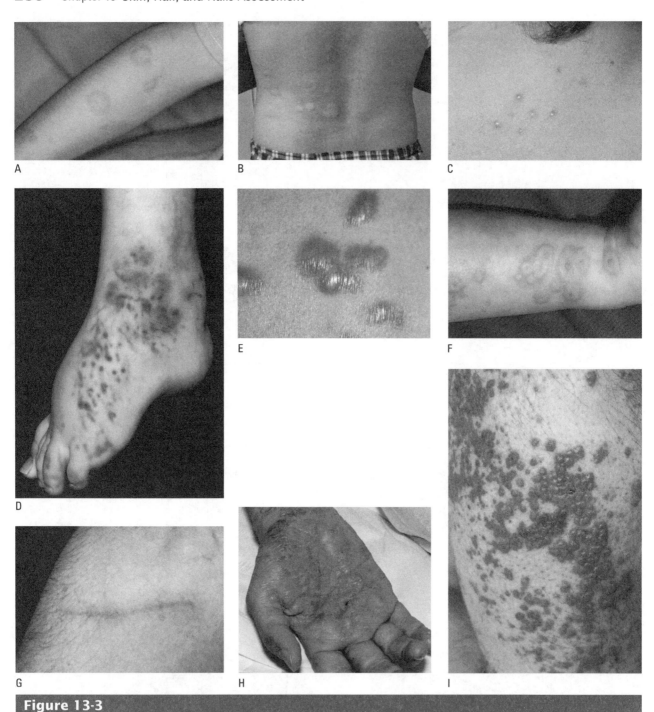

Figure 13-3

Lesions classified by shape or configuration. A. Annular lesion. B. Confluent lesions. C. Discrete lesions. D. Grouped lesions. E. Gyrate lesions. F. Target lesions. G. Linear lesions. H. Polycyclic lesions. I. Zosteriform lesions.

3. German measles (Rubella)—pink, popular rash similar to measles but paler; begins on face, then spreads over body; may be accompanied by swollen glands; occurs most frequently in children

4. Chickenpox (Varicella)—small, red, fluid-filled vesicles, usually on trunk, then progresses to face, arms, and legs; vesicles erupt over several days, forming pustules,

then crusts; may cause intense itching; occurs most frequently in children; caused by herpes zoster virus

5. Herpes simplex—viral infection that causes lesions on lips and oral mucosa that progress from vesicles to pustules, then crusts; can also occur in genitals

6. Herpes zoster—clusters of small vesicles that form on skin along sensory nerves; vesicles progress to pustules and then form crusts; results in intense pain and itching; more common and more severe in older adults; caused by eruption of dormant herpes zoster virus

7. Psoriasis—thickening of skin, resulting in dry, silvery, scaly patches; overproduction of skin cells results in buildup of cells faster than they can be shed; common areas include scalp, elbows, knees, lower back, and perineal area; caused by emotional stress or poor health

8. Contact dermatitis—inflammation of skin due to allergy to substance that comes into contact with skin (clothing, jewelry, plants, chemicals, or cosmetics); may progress from redness to hives, vesicles, or scales, which can result in intense itching; location of lesions may help identify allergen

9. Eczema—internally provoked inflammation of skin causing reddened papules and vesicles that ooze, weep, and progress to form crusts; common locations include scalp, face, elbows, knees, forearms, and wrists; usually causes intense itching

10. Impetigo—bacterial skin infection that usually appears on skin around nose and mouth; onset may begin with barely detectable patch of blisters that break, exposing red, weeping area beneath; tan crust forms and infection may spread from edges; contagious and common in children

F. **Malignant skin lesions (see attached Nursing Notes card for illustrations of malignant skin lesions); assessed for changes over time using ABCD mnemonic (A = appearance, B = border, C = color, D = diameter)**

1. **Basal cell carcinoma**—proliferation of cells of stratum basal into dermis and subcutaneous tissue; lesions begin as shiny papules that develop central ulcers with rounded, pearly edges; common areas include skin areas regularly exposed to sun; most common but least malignant type of skin cancer

2. **Squamous cell carcinoma**—develops from cells of stratum spinosum; lesions begin as reddened, scaly papule that forms shallow ulcer with clearly delineated, elevated border; common areas include scalp, ears, backs of hands, and lower lip; possible cause is exposure to sun; this type of cancer grows rapidly

3. **Malignant melanoma**—spreads rapidly to lymph and blood vessels; lesion contains areas of varied pigmentation ranging from black to brown, blue, or red; edges often irregular with notched borders and diameter greater than 6 mm; this type of cancer is least common but most serious type of skin cancer

4. **Kaposi's sarcoma**—malignant tumor of epidermis and internal epithelial tissues; lesions typically soft, blue to purple, and painless; other characteristics vary: may be macular or papular, and may resemble keloids or bruises; this type of sarcoma is common in HIV-positive people

G. **Skin lesions that result from alternative therapies (see Table 13-2)**

Table 13-2	Therapy Name	Results
Effects of Alternative Therapies on Skin Condition	Coining	Skin bruising from rubbing skin of back, upper chest, neck, and arms with coin in symmetrical patterns
	Cupping	Red circular lesions on forehead, upper chest, and back when glass cups are heated and placed on skin
	Pinching	Bruising from pulling upward on neck, back, and chest areas

H. Abnormalities of the hair

1. Seborrheic dermatitis (cradle cap)—appears as eczema of yellow-white, greasy scales on scalp and forehead; common in infants
2. Tinea capitis—patchy hair loss on head with pustules on skin; highly contagious fungal disease transmitted from soil, animals, or person to person
3. Alopecia areata—sudden loss of hair in a round, balding patch on scalp; no known cause
4. Folliculitis—infection of hair follicle that appears as pustules with underlying erythema
5. Furuncle/abscess—furuncle caused by infected hair follicle, appears as hard, erythematous, pus-filled lesions; abscesses caused by bacteria entering skin, and are larger than furuncles
6. Hirsutism—excess body hair in females on face, chest, abdomen, arms, and legs following male pattern; typically related to endocrine or metabolic dysfunction, but may be idiopathic

I. Abnormalities of the nails

1. Koilonychia (spoon nails)—concavity and thinning of the nails; caused by congenital condition
2. Paronychia—infection of skin adjacent to nail; area becomes red, swollen, and painful with pus that may ooze; caused by bacteria or fungi
3. Beau's line—linear depression that develops at base of nail and moves distally as nail grows; caused by trauma or illness
4. Splinter hemorrhage—reddish-brown spots in nails; caused by trauma or endocarditis
5. Clubbing—nail appears more convex and wide with increase in angle of nail greater than 180 degrees; caused by chronic respiratory and cardiac conditions in which oxygenation is compromised
6. Onycholysis—nail plate loosens from distal nail and proceeds to proximal portion

VIII. LIFESPAN CONSIDERATIONS

A. Infants and children

1. Vernix caseosa—white, cheese-like mixture of sebum and epidermal cells occurring at birth
2. Physiological jaundice—yellowing of skin, sclera, and mucous membranes that can occur within 24 hours to 7 days after birth; treatment includes fluids and phototherapy
3. Milia—tiny, white facial papules caused by collection of sebum in openings of hair follicles; spontaneously disappear within a few weeks of birth
4. Vascular markings—irregular red or pink patches on back of neck (stork bites)
5. Mongolian spots—gray, blue, or purple spots located in sacral and buttocks areas of newborns
6. Lanugo—fine, downy hair of newborns

B. Adolescent development

1. Increase in pigmentation, sweat and oil gland production, and appearance of pubic and axillary hair; in males this also includes facial and chest hair
2. Acne occurs as a result of increased production of sebum by oil glands

C. Pregnant female

1. Chloasma—hyper-pigmented patches on forehead ("mask of pregnancy"); may disappear after pregnancy
2. Linea nigra—dark line from umbilicus to pubic area and increased pigmentation of areolae and nipples, darkened moles and scars

D. Older adult

1. Decreased skin elasticity and increased skin wrinkling
2. Dryness of skin and hair due to decrease in sebum production
3. Decrease in perspiration due to decrease in sweat glands
4. Decrease in vascularity may cause paleness in light-skinned individuals, and a dull, gray, or darker appearance in dark-skinned elderly persons

Box 13–3	Senile lentigines (liver spots)—hyper-pigmented freckles on the backs of the hands and the arms
Common Lesions in Older Adults	Cherry angiomas—small, bright red spots that increase in number with age
	Cutaneous tags—skin tags that appear on the neck and upper chest
	Cutaneous horns—may occur on the face

5. Common lesions in older adults (see Box 13-3)

6. Hair thins and becomes gray as melanin production decreases; facial hair may become coarser

7. Nails may appear thicker, harder, more brittle, peeling, yellow or opaque, and oddly shaped

IX. DOCUMENTATION

A. Document findings obtained with inspection and palpation of the skin

1. Skin color

2. Skin temperature

3. Edema: location and characteristics

4. Lesions with description of location, size, and characteristics

5. Skin infections or infestations with description of location and characteristics

B. Document condition of hair (color, texture, amount, and location) and any abnormalities

C. Document condition of nails and any abnormalities

Case Study

During an annual physical examination, a 46-year-old client reports that she has noticed some recent changes in a mole located on her right shoulder.

1. What questions would be important for the nurse to ask first?

2. What other questions related to the client's past medical history would be important for the nurse to ask?

3. What questions would be important for the nurse to ask about skin care management?

4. What are the "ABCD" warning signs of skin cancer?

5. What should the nurse include in documentation of the mole?

For suggested responses, see page 311

POSTTEST

1 The nurse assessing a 2-day-old newborn notes a generalized yellow discoloration of the skin. After verifying that the medical record indicates physiologic jaundice, the nurse anticipates implementation of which prescribed treatment protocol?

1. Immunization
2. Electrolyte replacement
3. Fortified vitamins
4. Phototherapy

2 When assessing a pediatric client's skin rash, the nurse notes that the rash consists of small, red, fluid-filled vesicles that began on the trunk and progressed to the face, arms, and legs. The nurse concludes that the client most likely has which condition?

1. Chicken pox
2. German measles
3. Measles
4. Tinea capitis

3 Which finding would the nurse assess for in a client who has eczema?

1. Intense pain
2. Itching
3. Purple lesions
4. Thickening of the skin

4 A client who has a history of chronic obstructive pulmonary disease (COPD) has clubbing of the fingernails. The nurse explains to the client that this physical assessment finding has which etiology?

1. Anemia
2. Hypoxia
3. Iron deficiency
4. Trauma

5 In developing a plan of care to promote healthy skin for an adolescent client, the nurse considers that it is essential to consider which data regarding the client's skin?

1. Recent rashes
2. Skin infection
3. Pain assessment
4. Use of sunscreens

6 Based on the client's current symptoms, the nurse suspects an infectious process. What would be the most appropriate method for the nurse to use to determine the client's skin temperature as a follow-up assessment?

1. Inspect the face for redness
2. Assess for skin turgor
3. Use the dorsal surface of the hand to palpate the skin
4. Use the palm of the hand to palpate the skin

7 The nurse performs a skin turgor test on an older adult client and notes that the skin turgor is decreased. The next priority action of the nurse is to assess for which of the following?

1. Diaphoresis
2. Orientation
3. Signs of dehydration
4. Signs of vascular insufficiency

8 Which assessment data would the nurse consider to be an abnormal finding that warrants referral of the client to a healthcare provider for further evaluation?

1. Dark pigmented band on the nail bed
2. Beau's line at the nail base
3. Multiple nevi on the neck
4. Vitiligo

9 A nurse is assessing a client with a history of heart failure who presents with severe edema in the lower extremities. The nurse would document the presence of + 4 pitting edema after noting which finding?

1. Slight indentation, with no perceptible swelling of the leg
2. Moderate pitting, with indentation that subsides rapidly
3. Deep pitting, swollen leg, and indentation that remains for a short time
4. Very deep pitting, very swollen leg, and indentation that lasts for a long time

10 In monitoring a client's recent development of a skin lesion, which findings should alert the nurse to refer the client for further evaluation? Select all that apply.

1. Irregular borders
2. Yellow-white, greasy scales of the scalp
3. Change in pigmentation from brown to black
4. Diameter greater than 6 mm
5. Color of skin around the lesion is client's typical skin tone

➤ *See pages 262–264 for Answers and Rationales.*

ANSWERS & RATIONALES

Pretest

1 **Answer: 3** **Rationale:** "Can you tell me about any skin problems you have had?" is an open-ended question that allows the client the opportunity to provide information about specific skin problems or illness that may require further assessment and treatment (option 3). The other responses are closed questions that are focused on specific information and can be answered with a "yes" or "no" by the client.

Cognitive Level: Application **Client Need:** Physiological Integrity: Physiological Adaptation **Integrated Process:** Nursing Process: Assessment **Content Area:** Adult Health: Integumentary **Strategy:** Note the critical word *best* in the question. This tells you that more than one question could apply to the assessment being conducted, but that one is better than the others. Consider that during history taking broad questions are asked first and then followed by more specific questions as needed to gather a full set of data. With this in mind, you would eliminate each of the incorrect responses easily. **Reference:** D'Amico, D. & Barbarito, C. (2007). *Health & physical assessment in nursing.* Upper Saddle River, NJ: Pearson Education, Inc., p. 192.

2 **Answer: 2** **Rationale:** When evaluating a dark-skinned client for changes in skin color, it is recommended to inspect areas of the body with less pigmentation such as the lips, oral mucosa, sclera, palms of the hands, and conjunctivae of the inner eyelids (option 2). Assessing other areas of the body would make it more difficult for the nurse to detect color changes.
Cognitive Level: Comprehension **Client Need:** Health Promotion and Maintenance **Integrated Process:** Nursing Process: Assessment **Content Area:** Adult Health: Integumentary **Strategy:** Review each of the options in terms of expected skin tone. Consider which of the areas listed would have similar skin tones and use the process of elimination to choose the lips (option 2) as being close to mucous membranes, to choose correctly. **Reference:** D'Amico, D. & Barbarito, C. (2007). *Health & physical assessment in nursing.* Upper Saddle River, NJ: Pearson Education, Inc., p. 189.

3 **Answer: 1, 2, 4** **Rationale:** A warm, private environment will help to reduce the client's anxiety. It is important to be sensitive to cultural issues, as in some cultures touching or examination of the opposite sex is prohibited. It is recommended to use direct sunlight for assessment of the skin; if it is not available, lighting must be strong and direct. Tangential lighting may be helpful in assessment of dark-skinned clients (option 3). Standard precautions should be used throughout the assessment. It is not necessary to bathe the client prior to an assessment, although an assessment may be performed when providing hygiene (option 5).
Cognitive Level: Application **Client Need:** Health Promotion & Maintenance **Integrated Process:** Nursing Process: Assessment **Content Area:** Adult Health: Integumentary **Strategy:** Note that the question focuses on interventions that the nurse should incorporate when preparing the client for a skin, hair, and nail examination. Since this examination would require exposure of the body a private, warm environment would be more comfortable for the client. Both descriptors in this option are correct. Option 2 identifies cultural sensitivity, which should always be a consideration when providing nursing care. In some cultures, touching or examination by members of the opposite sex would be prohibited. An option that identifies a descriptor that suggests limitations would be an option to avoid. For example, in option 3, the option states to use tangential lighting only. To eliminate option 5 recall that it is not necessary to bathe the client prior to a skin assessment, although the nurse may perform a skin assessment when providing hygiene. **Reference:** D'Amico, D. & Barbarito, C. (2007). *Health & physical assessment in nursing.* Upper Saddle River, NJ: Pearson Education, p. 200.

4 **Answer: 4** **Rationale:** It would be very important for the nurse to determine whether the client is currently using any topical medications such as steroids, antibiotics, and medications for muscle pain, which may harm the developing fetus because they are absorbed through the skin (option 4). The other options are important for general assessment but are not directly related to preventing complications during pregnancy.
Cognitive Level: Application **Client Need:** Health Promotion and Maintenance **Integrated Process:** Nursing Process: Assessment **Content Area:** Maternal-Newborn **Strategy:** When a question involves a client who is pregnant, consider the safety of the fetus as a prime concern. In this question, evaluate each option in terms of the implications to the fetus and eliminate each of the incorrect options because medications, even topical ones, can cause harm to the fetus if absorbed. Confirm that this is the correct option after noting the words *first trimester* in the question—medications often cause greatest harm during the first trimester. **Reference:** D'Amico, D. & Barbarito, C. (2007). *Health & physical assessment in nursing.* Upper Saddle River, NJ: Pearson Education, Inc., p. 195.

5 **Answer: 1** **Rationale:** It is important for the nurse to explore the possibility of an allergic reaction or sensitivity to wearing gloves (option 1). Certain types of gloves, especially latex, can cause mild to severe allergic skin reactions. Stress levels, exposure to extreme temperatures, or excessive perspiration would not cause this type of skin reaction (options 2, 3, and 4).
Cognitive Level: Application **Client Need:** Physiological Integrity: Physiological Adaptation **Integrated Process:** Nursing Process: Assessment **Content Area:** Adult Health: Integumentary **Strategy:** A critical phrase in the question is *recently after starting a new job.* This suggests that the cause of the skin reaction could be environmental. With this in mind, evaluate each option in terms of its possible relationship to the work environment. Eliminate options 2 and 4 first because they relate to the client personally. Choose option 1 over option 3 because this is more likely to cause a skin reaction. **Reference:** D'Amico, D. & Barbarito, C. (2007). *Health & physical assessment in nursing.* Upper Saddle River, NJ: Pearson Education, Inc., p. 196.

6 **Answer: 2** **Rationale:** Skin tone varies according to the amount of melanin and carotene pigments, the oxygen level in the blood, and the level of exposure to the sun. Cyanosis or pallor usually indicates a low level of plasma oxygen, which places the client at risk for ineffective tissue perfusion (option 2). The question does not indicate any breaks in skin integrity (option 1). Signs of infection would include redness, heat, edema, and tenderness (option 3). There are no signs reported that the client is having difficulty breathing (option 4).
Cognitive Level: Application **Client Need:** Health Promotion and Maintenance **Integrated Process:** Nursing Process: Analysis **Content Area:** Adult Health: Integumentary **Strategy:** The critical words in the question are *highest priority* and *cyanosis.* The words *highest priority* indicate that one option is more important than the others and

the word *cyanosis* indicates that the client has insufficient circulating oxygen in the bloodstream. Eliminate options 1 and 3 first as least related to oxygenation concerns, and choose option 2 over 4 based on the information presented in the question without reading into it. **Reference:** D'Amico, D. & Barbarito, C. (2007). *Health & physical assessment in nursing.* Upper Saddle River, NJ: Pearson Education, Inc., p. 201.

7 Answer: 3 Rationale: A dark, pigmented band found in a single nail may be a sign of a melanoma in the nail matrix, and the client should be referred to a healthcare provider for further evaluation (option 3). A splinter hemorrhage would appear as reddish-brown spots in the nail, and occur as a result of trauma or in endocarditis (option 1). When clubbing occurs, the nail appears more convex and wide (option 2). Beau's line is a linear depression that develops at the base of the nail, usually caused by nail trauma (option 4), and moves distally as the nail grows. **Cognitive Level:** Analysis **Client Need:** Physiological Integrity: Physiological Adaptation **Integrated Process:** Nursing Process: Implementation **Content Area:** Adult Health: Integumentary **Strategy:** Review abnormalities of the nails. To answer this question accurately, it is necessary to understand the significance of the data in the question. Recall that coloration under the nails could indicate a cancerous growth to help you choose correctly. **Reference:** D'Amico, D. & Barbarito, C. (2007). *Health & physical assessment in nursing.* Upper Saddle River, NJ: Pearson Education, Inc., p. 228.

8 Answer: 2 Rationale: Metabolic disorders such as hypothyroidism and nutritional deficiencies may cause the hair to become very dull, coarse, dry, and brittle (option 2). Alopecia areata is widespread hair loss (option 1). Pediculosis capitis or head lice appear as oval bodies that would cause intense itching of the scalp (option 3). Seborrheic dermatitis or cradle cap, common in infancy, appears as thick, yellow-to-white, greasy scales (option 4). **Cognitive Level:** Application **Client Need:** Physiological Integrity: Physiological Adaptation **Integrated Process:** Nursing Process: Assessment **Content Area:** Adult Health: Integumentary **Strategy:** Eliminate option 1 first, recalling that the term *alopecia* is hair loss. Next eliminate option 3 because this option is referring to lice. Choose option 2 over option 4 either because metabolic factors can influence hair characteristics or because words ending in *–itis* indicate inflammation. **Reference:** D'Amico, D. & Barbarito, C. (2007). *Health & physical assessment in nursing.* Upper Saddle River, NJ: Pearson Education, Inc., p. 206.

9 Answer: 1 Rationale: Clubbing of the fingernails occurs when there is hypoxia or impaired peripheral tissue perfusion over a long period of time, as in conditions such as COPD (option 1). Onycholysis is a separation of the nail plate from the nail bed as a result of trauma, infection, or skin lesions (option 2). Paronychia is an infection of the cuticle (option 3). Spoon nails appear as a concave curve of the nail, and are associated with iron deficiency anemia (option 4).

Cognitive Level: Application **Client Need:** Physiological Integrity: Physiological Adaptation **Integrated Process:** Nursing Process: Assessment **Content Area:** Adult Health: Integumentary **Strategy:** Note that the critical words in the question are *enlarged nail beds and a spongy quality at the nail base.* Visualize this description and correlate it with the matching term to choose correctly. **Reference:** D'Amico, D. & Barbarito, C. (2007). *Health & physical assessment in nursing.* Upper Saddle River, NJ: Pearson Education, Inc., p. 208.

10 Answer: 2 Rationale: A trained medial interpreter will be able to obtain the necessary information needed without any bias (option 2). The family may need to be notified of the client's hospitalization but may not be able to communicate the data in a factual manner (option 1). A priority in caring for any client in which linguistic factors are a consideration is to establish a method of communication. Using sign language or a picture chart are other ways that the nurse can communicate with the client to identify specific client needs, but would not be the best method to use when obtaining the client's medical history (options 3 and 4). **Cognitive Level:** Application **Client Need:** Psychosocial Integrity **Integrated Process:** Communication and Documentation **Content Area:** Adult Health: Integumentary **Strategy:** Core concepts in this question are communication and cultural considerations for care. Focus on the critical words *avoid miscommunication or misinterpretation* to determine that the correct option is one that yields accurate and precise information. This will lead you to eliminate options 3 and 4 first. Choose option 2 over 1 as this person is trained in medical interpretation. **Reference:** D'Amico, D. & Barbarito, C. (2007). *Health & physical assessment in nursing.* Upper Saddle River, NJ: Pearson Education, Inc., pp. 73–76.

Posttest

1 Answer: 4 Rationale: Some newborns develop physiological jaundice 3–4 days after birth or as late as 7 days postnatally. Physiologic jaundice is a temporary condition that is treated with fluids and phototherapy (option 4). Treatment protocols aimed to assist with normal growth and development in infants and children would include immunizations and vitamin therapy (options 1 and 3). Electrolytes would only be replaced if there was an imbalance (option 2). **Cognitive Level:** Application **Client Need:** Physiological Integrity: Physiological Adaptation **Integrated Process:** Nursing Process: Planning **Content Area:** Child Health **Strategy:** Note the age of the client and the critical words *yellow discoloration of the skin* and *physiologic jaundice.* The word *physiologic* tells you that the condition is based in physiology and is temporary. Eliminate option 1 first since immunizations are used to prevent disease. Eliminate options 2 and 3 next (electrolytes and vitamins) since these are replacement therapies that do not have to do with the red blood cell breakdown leading to jaundice. **Reference:** D'Amico, D. & Barbarito, C. (2007). *Health & physical assessment in nursing.* Upper Saddle River, NJ: Pearson Education, Inc., p. 186.

2 Answer: 1 Rationale: Chicken pox or varicella begin as groups of small, red, fluid-filled vesicles usually on the trunk, and progress to the face, arms, and legs (option 1). German measles or rubella is a pale pink papular rash that begins on the face and spreads over the body, and may produce swollen glands (option 2). Measles or rubeola causes a red to purple rash composed of macules and papules that begin on the face and then progress over the neck, trunk, arms, and legs (option 3). Tinea capitis (option 4) is a fungal infection of the skin on the head. **Cognitive Level:** Application **Client Need:** Physiological Integrity: Physiological Adaptation **Integrated Process:** Nursing Process: Assessment **Content Area:** Child Health **Strategy:** First recall that tinea capitis is an infection of the scalp and eliminate option 4. Next recall that German measles and measles begin on the face (not the trunk) before spreading to other areas of the body, to help eliminate options 2 and 3, respectively. **Reference:** D'Amico, D. & Barbarito, C. (2007). *Health & physical assessment in nursing.* Upper Saddle River, NJ: Pearson Education, Inc., p. 221.

3 Answer: 2 Rationale: Eczema leads to development of red papules and vesicles that ooze, weep, and progress to form crusts. They are commonly located on the scalp, face, elbows, knees, forearms, and wrists and cause intense itching (option 2). Intense pain (option 1) and itching are associated with the herpes zoster virus. Purple lesions (option 3) are typical of Kaposi's sarcoma, which may resemble bruises. Thick skin (option 4) is consistent with psoriasis, which also involves dry, silvery, scaly patches. **Cognitive Level:** Application **Client Need:** Physiological Integrity: Physiological Adaptation **Integrated Process:** Nursing Process: Assessment **Content Area:** Adult Health: Integumentary **Strategy:** Specific knowledge is needed to answer this question. Recall first that eczema is a chronic condition that is intermittent with flare-ups. This will help you eliminate option 3 because a color change would not be intermittent. Eliminate option 1 next since viral infections typically cause the most pain. Choose option 2 (itching) over option 4 (thickening of the skin) because there is weeping and oozing of lesions with eczema but not thickening of skin. **Reference:** D'Amico, D. & Barbarito, C. (2007). *Health & physical assessment in nursing.* Upper Saddle River, NJ: Pearson Education, Inc., pp. 222, 223, 225.

4 Answer: 2 Rationale: Clubbing of the fingernails refers to changes in the structure of the nail beds, which become enlarged, soft, and spongy, and with a nail base greater than 160 degrees. These changes may occur due to hypoxia or impaired peripheral tissue perfusion over a long period of time (option 2). The nail beds of a client with anemia would appear pale and colorless (option 1). Nails that form a concave curve known as spoon nails are thought to be associated with iron deficiency (option 3).

Separation of the nail plate, or onycholysis, may occur with trauma, infection, or skin lesions (option 4). **Cognitive Level:** Application **Client Need:** Physiological Integrity: Physiological Adaptation **Integrated Process:** Nursing Process: Assessment **Content Area:** Adult Health: Integumentary **Strategy:** The core issue of the question is the etiology or cause of fingernail clubbing in clients with respiratory disease, such as COPD. To choose option 2, consider that a respiratory health problem would likely place the client at risk for hypoxia. Alternatively, eliminate options 1 and 3 because they are similar (iron deficiency is a type of anemia); then choose option 2 over 4 since trauma would result in tissue damage, not clubbing. **Reference:** D'Amico, D. & Barbarito, C. (2007). *Health & physical assessment in nursing.* Upper Saddle River, NJ: Pearson Education, Inc., pp. 207, 208.

5 Answer: 4 Rationale: In order to promote healthy skin in an adolescent client, it is essential for the nurse to instruct the client on using sunscreen in order to protect the skin from harmful sun rays that increase the risk of skin cancer (option 4). If a client is experiencing an infection, skin rash, or pain, an intervention would be required (options 1, 2, and 3). **Cognitive Level:** Application **Client Need:** Health Promotion and Maintenance **Integrated Process:** Nursing Process: Assessment **Content Area:** Adult Health: Integumentary **Strategy:** First note the age group of the client in the question, which is adolescent. A client's age in a question usually indicates the need to focus on age-specific characteristics, such as risk behaviors. Next note that the critical words in the question are *promote healthy skin.* With these two ideas in mind, consider that skin infections, rashes or pain may not be common in adolescents, while sun exposure is a common risk that can be reduced by the adequate use of sunscreens. **Reference:** D'Amico, D. & Barbarito, C. (2007). *Health & physical assessment in nursing.* Upper Saddle River, NJ: Pearson Education, Inc., p. 189.

6 Answer: 3 Rationale: The dorsal surface of the hand is most sensitive to the body's temperature (option 3), as opposed to the palms of the hand (option 4), which may not be as sensitive as the dorsum of the hand. The nurse should also compare both the right and left side of the body. Inspection of the face alone would not be definitive enough to determine if a client has an increase in temperature (option 1). Assessing for skin turgor is checking for the elasticity and mobility of the skin (option 2). **Cognitive Level:** Application **Client Need:** Health Promotion and Maintenance **Integrated Process:** Nursing Process: Assessment **Content Area:** Adult Health: Integumentary **Strategy:** To eliminate option 1, first note that skin temperature needs to be assessed by touching or palpating. Eliminate option 2 next since turgor is not a focus of the question. Specific knowledge of assessment technique is needed to discriminate between options 3 and 4. **Reference:** D'Amico, D. & Barbarito, C. (2007). *Health & physical assessment in nursing.* Upper Saddle River, NJ: Pearson Education, Inc., p. 202.

7 **Answer: 3** **Rationale:** When skin turgor is decreased, the skin fold "tents" or holds its pinched formation. A decrease in skin turgor can occur when a client is dehydrated or has lost large amounts of weight (option 3). It is not uncommon for elderly clients to become dehydrated, as their thirst mechanism and fluid intake is decreased. Diaphoresis, or profuse sweating, can be caused from exertion, fever, pain, and emotional stress, as well as some metabolic disorders such as hyperthyroidism (option 1). There are no other changes noted at this time that would necessitate the nurse to assess the client's level of orientation (option 2). Dry skin over the lower legs can be caused by vascular insufficiency (option 4). **Cognitive Level:** Application **Client Need:** Health Promotion and Maintenance **Integrated Process:** Nursing Process: Implementation **Content Area:** Adult Health: Integumentary **Strategy:** The critical words in the question are *next priority*. This tells you that the correct option is one that follows up on the original finding of decreased skin turgor. Recall that turgor is affected by hydration and age. This will help you to eliminate options 2 and 4 first as most unrelated. Choose option 3 over option 1 since diaphoresis could be a risk for dehydration, but not all clients who are diaphoretic become dehydrated if appropriate fluid replacement therapy is used. **Reference:** D'Amico, D. & Barbarito, C. (2007). *Health & physical assessment in nursing.* Upper Saddle River, NJ: Pearson Education, Inc., p. 203.

8 **Answer: 1** **Rationale:** A darkly pigmented band in a single nail may be a sign of a melanoma in the nail matrix and the client should be referred to a healthcare provider for further evaluation (option 1). A beau's line appears as a linear depression in the nail base, and is usually associated with trauma to the nail (option 2). Nevi are congenital pigmented marks that can occur in all people of various skin types (option 3). Vitiligo is a condition where patchy, depigmented areas occur over various parts of the body such as the face, neck, hands, feet, and body folds (option 4). These three conditions are variations of normal and do not require physician referral. **Cognitive Level:** Application **Client Need:** Physiological Integrity: Physiological Adaptation **Integrated Process:** Nursing Process: Assessment **Content Area:** Adult Health: Integumentary **Strategy:** The critical words in the question are *abnormal finding* and *warrants referral*. This tells you that the correct option is an abnormal finding that is serious enough to require follow-up assessment and care, instead of a condition that will resolve on its own. With this in mind, recall the definitions of the various items in the distracters. Choose option 1 over the others because it could indicate a form of cancer. **Reference:** D'Amico, D. & Barbarito, C. (2007). *Health & physical assessment in nursing.* Upper Saddle River, NJ: Pearson Education, Inc., pp. 207, 228.

9 **Answer: 4** **Rationale:** Edema is caused by fluid accumulation in the intercellular spaces, and is referred to as "pitting" edema if an indentation remains present after pressure is applied. To rate the severity of the edema a scale is used, which ranges from + 1 mild (2 mm depression in the skin), to + 2 moderate (4 mm depression), + 3 deep (6 mm depression), and + 4 very deep pitting edema (8 mm depression). **Cognitive Level:** Application **Client Need:** Physiological Integrity: Physiological Adaptation **Integrated Process:** Nursing Process: Assessment **Content Area:** Adult Health: Integumentary **Strategy:** To answer this question correctly, it is necessary to be familiar with the various ratings for depth of edema. First recall that the scale ranges from + 1 to + 4, with 4 being the deepest and most severe. Next, compare the adjectives used in the ratings in the various options. Select option 4 because the words *very deep* are consistent with the most significant or severe findings. **Reference:** D'Amico, D. & Barbarito, C. (2007). *Health and physical assessment in nursing.* Upper Saddle River, NJ: Pearson Education, Inc., p. 204.

10 **Answer: 1, 3, 4** **Rationale** A malignant melanoma can be described as a pigmented lesion than can vary from black to brown to blue or red, with edges or borders that are notched and irregular, and with a diameter greater than 6 mm (options 1, 3, and 4). Yellow-white, greasy scales that appear on the scalp and forehead are known as seborrheic dermatitis, which is very common in infants (option 2). Presence of the client's normal skin tone on skin surrounding the lesion would be an expected finding (option 5). **Cognitive Level:** Application **Client Need:** Physiological Integrity: Physiological Adaptation **Integrated Process:** Nursing Process: Assessment **Content Area:** Adult Health: Integumentary **Strategy:** The focus of the question is findings pertinent to a skin lesion. Note that the question indicates that the correct options will be abnormal or worsening findings for a lesion. With this in mind, recall that most dangerous changes in skin lesions are those compatible with skin cancer. From there, choose options 1, 3, and 4 as being consistent with skin cancer. **Reference:** D'Amico, D. & Barbarito, C. (2007). *Health & physical assessment in nursing.* Upper Saddle River, NJ: Pearson Education, Inc., pp. 224, 225.

References

Bickley, L. (2010). *Bates guide to physical examination and history taking* (10th ed.). Philadelphia: Lippincott Williams & Wilkins.

D'Amico, D. and Barbarito, C. (2007). *Health and physical assessment in nursing.* Upper Saddle River, NJ: Pearson Education, Inc., pp. 182–233.

Jarvis, C. (2008). *Physical examination and health assessment* (5th ed.). St. Louis, MO: Elsevier Saunders.

Zator Estes, M. (2009). *Health assessment and physical examination* (4th ed.). Clifton Park, NY: Delmar Cengage Learning.

Eye Assessment

14

Chapter Outline

Health History
Present Health History
Family History

Equipment, Preparation, and
Positioning
Examination Techniques
Expected Findings

Unexpected Findings
Lifespan Considerations
Documentation

Objectives

➤ Discuss questions utilized when obtaining a health history related to the eye.
➤ Describe the techniques used during the assessment of the eye.
➤ Describe normal and abnormal findings present during the assessment of the eye.
➤ Identify variations found during the assessment of the eye across the lifespan.

NCLEX-RN® Test Prep

Visit the Companion Website for this book at www.pearsonhighered.com/hogan to access additional practice opportunities and more.

Review at a Glance

astigmatism hereditary condition in which light rays with perpendicular planes have different foci on retina because cornea is not round in shape, but rather curves more in one direction than another

blepharitis inflammation of eyelid margins

cataract thickening and yellowish discoloration or opacity of lens or lens envelope, which reduces clarity of vision

convergence turning inward of eye toward the nose

cornea anterior outer layer of eye that is avascular, transparent, covers pupil, and contains nerves for pain; it provides most of the eye's focusing power

diplopia condition in which client sees double images

ectropion eversion or turning outward of edges of eyelid (usually lower eyelid) so that inner surface is exposed; usually results from muscle weakness, but may also result from trauma or nerve damage

entropion inversion or turning in of edges of eyelid (usually lower eyelid) so that lashes constantly rub against corneal surface of the eye

glaucoma a condition in which there is an increase in intraocular pressure (measured with tonometry) that adversely affects optic nerve and results in loss of retinal ganglion cells and peripheral vision

hyperopia a condition of eyeball that causes light to be focused behind retina, producing farsightedness; caused by eyeball being too short or a lens that is not round enough

iris a colored membrane responsible for controlling pupil diameter and size, thus controlling amount of light that reaches retina

iritis inflammation of iris of the eye

miosis constriction of the pupil

mydriasis dilation of the pupil

myopia condition in which light is distributed in front of retina, causing nearsightedness; caused by eyeball being too long or lens being overly round

nystagmus an involuntary oscillation of the eyeball due to muscle weakness, disorientation, a neurological disorder, or action of some medications

photophobia sensitivity to light; may or may not be associated with pain

presbyopia loss of elasticity of crystalline lens, possibly caused by loss of power of ciliary muscles and resulting in inability to focus on near objects

ptosis condition whereby eyelid droops, often because levator and Müller's muscles are too weak to raise eyelid properly

scotoma a blind spot or spots within or peripheral to visual field; peripheral presentation is called peripheral ring scotoma (may be caused by retinitis pigmentosa)

strabismus condition in which eyes cannot be focused on same object

tonometry a procedure that uses a device called a tonometer to measure intraocular pressure

PRETEST

1 The nurse assesses the client's visual acuity to be 20/25 using an eye chart. The client asks what that means. Which of the following is the nurse's best response?

1. "You can read at 25 feet what most people can read at 20 feet."
2. "Your left eye can see the chart at 20 feet while the right eye can see it at 25 feet."
3. "You can read at 20 feet what most people can read at 25 feet."
4. "You can read the chart perfectly with both eyes."

2 The nurse is preparing to assess extraocular eye movement (EOM). The nurse should select from which appropriate methods? Select all that apply.

1. Letter H method
2. Circular method
3. Wagon wheel method
4. Snellen eye chart
5. Shining light into pupils

3 The client's pupils are reactive to light and accommodation and appear normal. How would the nurse would best document this finding?

1. Pupils reactive to light and appear normal
2. Eye examination within normal limits
3. Pupils equal, round, reactive to light and accommodation (PERRLA)
4. Visual acuity within normal limits

4 The nurse is evaluating a client's pupils for consensual reaction to light. What is the most appropriate technique for the nurse to use?

1. Shine a light in one eye and observe that eye for reaction to light
2. Bring a penlight toward bridge of nose and observe for pupillary reaction to light
3. Bring a penlight toward bridge of nose and observe for convergence of eyes
4. Shine a light in one eye and observe the opposite eye for reaction to light

5 The nurse obtains a finding of 20/100 OS during a Snellen eye chart examination. The nurse should interpret these findings to mean that the client has which vision alteration?

1. Myopia in the right eye
2. Myopia in the left eye
3. Hyperopia in the right eye
4. Hyperopia in the left eye

6 A client presents to the emergency department with a report of something being in the eye. The nurse would conclude the client has a corneal abrasion when observing which clinical manifestation?

1. Bleeding from the lacrimal apparatus
2. Splintered look to the light reflecting off the cornea
3. Periorbital edema
4. Opacity of the lens

7 When an older adult client presents with periorbital edema the nurse would assess the client for which associated condition?

1. Facial and eye trauma
2. Congestive heart failure
3. Allergies to newly prescribed medications
4. Presbyopia

8 The client asks, "Am I going blind? I keep seeing black floating spots in front of my eyes." What is the nurse's best response to the client's question?

1. "You need a full evaluation of what is going on with your eyes before something develops."
2. "You will probably lose your sight."
3. "It is probably what we call floaters, which are pieces of vitreous humor."
4. "It is the result of hemorrhaging in the eye."

9 The client has just been diagnosed with hyperopia. The client asks what hyperopia is. What term should be included in the nurse's response?

1. Farsightedness
2. Nearsightedness
3. Emmetropia
4. Double vision

10 The nurse assesses the client's eyes and notes that the pupils are constricted despite being indoors without bright light in the room. How would the nurse document this finding?

1. Miosis
2. Mydriasis
3. Hyperopia
4. Myopia

➤ *See pages 281–283 for Answers and Rationales.*

I. HEALTH HISTORY

A. Purpose is to gather data related to the client's previous ocular problems; this provides information about the condition of the eye and vision over time

B. Eye examinations

1. "When was the last eye examination?" (regular visual examinations assist in maintaining visual health)
2. "What were the findings of the last eye exam?" (this may provide information related to problem that the client did not treat)
   a. Eye examination should be performed every two years
   b. If there is an acute finding, eye examinations may be performed more frequently
3. "What actions were taken for any problems?"
4. "Were medications prescribed for problems?"
5. "Did visual problems affect your activities of daily living (ADLs)?"
   a. Problems affecting ADLs usually prompt the client to seek treatment and follow a treatment plan
   b. Problems affecting ADLs may place the client at increased risk for injury
6. "How did the visual problems affect your ADLs?"

C. Vision correction

1. "Do you wear corrective glasses or contact lenses? If so, for how long?"
2. "Describe your vision with and without glasses or contact lenses."
3. Is the client wearing lenses or are the lenses accommodating for a decrease in vision?
4. Are there any problems with the corrective lenses?
5. "Do you wear the corrective lenses all the time or take them on and off for different activities?"

D. Eye disorders

1. "Have you been diagnosed with a disease of the eye?"
2. "Do you have **strabismus** (a condition of eye muscle weakness in which the eye turns in toward the client's nose, resulting in double vision)? If so, is it constant or does it come and go?"
3. "Have you ever had a **cataract** (thickening and yellowish discoloration or opacity of the lens or the lens envelope) corrected?" (cataracts decrease vision by causing opacity of the lens)
4. "Do you have **glaucoma** (a condition characterized by increased intraocular pressure that adversely affects the optic nerve)?" (increased intraocular pressure results in loss of retinal ganglion cells and peripheral vision)
5. "Do you have macular degeneration?"
6. "Have you experienced an eye injury? What type of eye injury did you experience?"
7. Have you had eye surgery? If so, what type of eye surgery did you have?" (this may provide information related to the current visual problem)
8. "What treatment or medication was prescribed for the eye disorder?"

9. "Has the visual problem reoccurred?"
10. "How are you managing the problem?"

E. **Miscellaneous questions related to eye health**

1. "Are you using over-the-counter eye medications or drops?"
2. "Do you have a history of allergies?" (this may cause the eye to appear red or swollen and cause it to burn or tear)
3. "Have you been diagnosed with diabetes? If so, is it type 1 or type 2?" (elevated blood glucose levels over time may cause loss of vision due to microvascular compromise, called retinopathy)
4. "Do you have hypertension? If so, how long have you had hypertension and how severe is it?" (if left untreated, hypertension ultimately causes vascular changes that may cause visual loss)

Practice to Pass

The nurse is taking a health history on a client. What previous health problems that either directly or indirectly affect eye health should the nurse inquire about?

II. PRESENT HEALTH HISTORY

A. **Current vision**

1. "Describe your vision."
2. "Describe any visual changes over the last few months."
3. "Are you able to read? If so, do you read accurately when the print is small or do you require extra large print?"
4. "Are your glasses or contact lenses working for you?"
5. "When was the last time you had a new set of glasses or lenses? Did your prescription change when you last ordered new glasses or lenses?"
6. "Do you have color blindness?"

B. **Blurred vision**

1. "Have you been experiencing blurred vision?"
2. "How long have you had blurred vision?"
3. "Is your vision blurred all the time? If not, does it occur in relation to certain times or events, such as at night, when tired, after medications, when hypoglycemic, or after exercising?"
4. "Describe your blurred vision."

C. **Eye pain**

1. "Have you been experiencing eye pain? If so, in which eye? When does the pain occur? Does eye pain occur in relation to something else, such as headaches or extended computer use?" (eye pain can accompany migraine headaches or excessive stress on the eyes)
2. If eye pain is present, ask questions to complete a full pain assessment
3. Sudden onset of pain needs immediate referral because it could indicate a condition that can result in loss of vision

D. **Miscellaneous eye symptoms**

1. "Are you experiencing any blind spots? If so, does the blind spot (**scotoma**) move with your gaze?" (discriminate between blind spots that have developed versus the blind spot that occurs naturally in each eye of all persons)
2. "Do you have sensitivity to light (**photophobia**)?" (this may be the result of a condition or side effect of medication; may be associated with pain)
3. "Do you experience itching of the eyes?" (this may be associated with allergies or irritation)
4. "Do you have burning of the eyes? If so, have you been rubbing the eyes?" (burning may be associated with allergies, irritation, or infection; rubbing the eyes may increase irritation and/or transfer an infection from one eye to the other)
5. "Are you experiencing redness or swelling of the eyes?" (this may indicate a condition or may be a clinical manifestation of a condition)

6. "Do you have watering or discharge from the eyes?" (tearing or lacrimation may be the result of allergens, irritation, or obstruction of lacrimal apparatus)
   a. "Describe the discharge. Is the discharge present upon wakening?"
   b. "Is it hard to open eyelids in the morning because of the discharge?"
   c. "How do you remove discharge from the eyes?"

7. "Are you experiencing double vision (**diplopia**)?" (perception of two images of a single object due to strabismus or other conditions)
8. "Do you see black floaters?" (occasional floaters usually present in people with myopia due to compression of vitreous humor; sudden onset of floaters may indicate retinal detachment)
9. "Do you see halos?" (usually indicative of narrow angle glaucoma)
10. "Are you experiencing trouble seeing at night?" (night vision decreases with age, and difficulty may also result from a vitamin A deficiency)
11. "Do you have tearing or dry eyes?" (decreased lacrimation occurs with aging)
12. "Have you had any eye infections?"
13. "What activities do you participate in daily?"
    a. "Does your vision problem affect your ability to participate in your activities?"
    b. "Does your visual problem limit your ability to exercise?"
    c. "Does your visual problem affect your ability to use computers?"
    d. "Does your visual disorder affect your ability to sleep?"
    e. "Does your visual disorder affect your social interactions?"

E. **Current environmental risks to eyes**
   1. "Are you exposed to toxic chemicals, bright light, or high temperatures?"
   2. "Are you exposed to environmental irritants such as pollutants, tobacco, or allergens?"
   3. "Do you have any current allergies that result in eye symptoms such as redness or tearing?"

F. **Current health problems that could affect vision**
   1. "Do you have multiple sclerosis?"
   2. "Do you have headaches?"
   3. "Have you been diagnosed with a neurological condition such as Bell's palsy or trigeminal neuralgia?"
   4. "Are you immunocompromised?"

Practice to Pass

The client reports having difficulty seeing at night and has stopped driving at night because of this. What nutritional assessment should the nurse make?

III. FAMILY HISTORY

A. **Provides information about the client's risk factors for eye diseases**
B. **Family history of disorders that could affect vision**
   1. "Do you have a family history of diabetes?"
   2. "Do you have a family history of hypertension?"
   3. "Do you have a family history of cardiovascular disease?"
C. **Family history of eye disorders**
   1. "Do you have a family history of glaucoma?"
   2. "Does anyone in your family have color blindness? If so, have you ever had an Ishihara test to determine if you have color blindness?"
   3. "Does anyone in your family have cataracts?"

IV. EQUIPMENT, POSITIONING, AND PREPARATION

A. **Equipment**
   1. Gloves for use when palpating eye
   2. Small hand-held eye chart
   3. Snellen eye chart

4. Index card to cover eye

5. Penlight

6. Cotton-tipped applicator or cotton ball to make wisps of cotton

7. Ophthalmoscope

8. Tonometer pen

B. Positioning; chart should be fixed at eye level on the wall without objects near the chart

1. Position the client 20 feet from the eye chart

2. Client may be seated or standing

3. Provide adequate lighting

C. Preparation; provide the client with instruction

1. Near and distance vision are being tested

2. Explain that the client will read the chart from top to bottom until he or she cannot see a line or read from left to right

D. After testing visual acuity, explain to the client that extraocular eye movements (EOMs) will be tested

1. Position the client in a sitting position

2. Explain that assessment of eye movement will involve keeping the head still and following an object or the examiner's finger

E. Assessment of the corneal light reflex is completed after assessing extraocular eye movements

1. Position the client in a sitting position

2. Inform the client that light will be shone onto the **cornea** (anterior outer layer of eye that is avascular, transparent, covers pupil, and contains nerves for pain; it provides most of the eye's focusing power)

F. Assessment of pupils

1. Position the client in a sitting position

2. Inform the client about inspection of the client's eyes for pupil characteristics: size, shape, and coloration

  a. Miosis is the constriction of pupils

  b. Mydriasis is the dilation of pupils

3. To test for reaction to light, darken the room and have the client look into the distance to increase the dilation of pupils

4. Inform the client that after inspection a light will be shone into the eyes to evaluate pupillary reaction to light

5. While being assessed for pupillary reaction to light the client will be evaluated for accommodation (constriction of the pupil when an object is brought toward the eye)

6. If the client does not have a blink reflex, stroke the cornea with a wisp of cotton to evaluate the corneal reflex, blinking of the eye when the cornea is touched

7. Palpate the eyelid; completed with gloves on to assess for pain and edema

8. Last step is evaluation with an ophthalmoscope, an instrument used to inspect inner eye structures; inform the client that it will not be painful

V. EXAMINATION TECHNIQUES

A. Examination of distance visual acuity is achieved by positioning the client in front of a Snellen eye chart (see Figure 14-1)

1. Client covers one eye with an eye cover or index card and then reads the chart from left to right, top to bottom, down to the lowest line that he or she can read

2. Repeat the procedure, assessing the other eye while covering the eye that was examined first

Figure 14-1

Testing distance vision

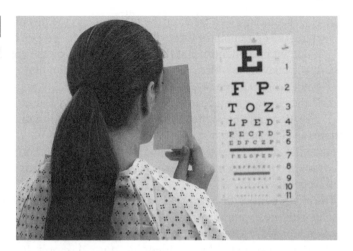

3. If the client is wearing corrective lenses, vision is assessed both with and without them
   a. Record findings as a fraction; the numerator is the distance of the client from the eye chart; the denominator is the distance from which a person with normal vision can read that line (identified at the end of each line on the chart the client reads from)
   b. If the client makes more than two mistakes on a line, record vision as the score from the line above
   c. If the client cannot read letters or is a small child, use a chart with Es in various directions and have the client point in the direction that each E is facing
B. **Assessment of near vision is accomplished by using a handheld eye chart held 12–14 in. from the eyes (see Figure 14-2)**
   1. Client covers one eye with an eye cover or index card and then reads the chart from left to right, top to bottom, down to lowest line he or she can read, maintaining an arm's distance of 12–14 in.
   2. Repeat the procedure, assessing the other eye while covering the eye that was examined first
      a. If the client is wearing corrective lenses, vision is assessed with the lenses in place

Figure 14-2

Testing near vision

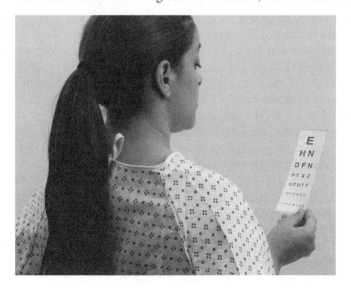

!

    b. Record findings as a fraction; the numerator is the distance of the client from the eye chart; the denominator is the distance from which a person with normal vision can read that line (identified at the end of each line on the chart the client reads from)

    c. If the client is unable to read half the letters on a line, record vision as the distance from the line above

    d. If the client cannot read letters or is a small child, use a chart with Es in various directions and have the client point in the direction that each E is facing

C. Performing confrontation test

!

    1. Have the client cover the right eye with a cover or index card while the examiner covers his or her own left eye with a cover or index card; this test measures gross peripheral vision

    2. The examiner positions him- or herself at the client's level two feet apart; start distally with the examiner wiggling fingers and moving inward; have the client state when a finger is seen; both the examiner and the client should see fingers at the same time (assuming the examiner has normal peripheral vision)

    3. Repeat the procedure by having the client cover the left eye with a cover or index card while the examiner covers his or her own right eye

D. Testing cardinal fields of gaze (see Figure 14-3)

    1. Tests extraocular eye movements, motor function of eye, and peripheral vision

    2. Have the client sit in front of the examiner at eye level; instruct the client to keep eyes still

    3. The examiner stands two feet in front of the client; starting at midline move a penlight or pencil in the shape of a capital letter H

    4. Repeat the procedure, making the letter H in the extreme right and then left

    5. This test can be performed using a wagon wheel or star instead of the letter H; start at midline and move a pen or light in the direction of the star or wheel

    6. Repeat the procedure to the extreme right or left

E. Assessment of corneal light reflex (Hirschberg test)

    1. Have the client sit in front of the examiner and inform him or her that the cornea will be examined

    2. Holding a penlight about 12 in. from the client, assess where the reflection of the light is in the eyes (whether symmetrical, in approximately same location in each eye)

F. Performing cover test

    1. Sit in front of the client

    2. Explain that the test evaluates the fusion reflex, which keeps both eyes parallel

    3. Have the client stare at a fixed point; cover one eye

    4. Observe the uncovered eye; it should remain fixed on the object

G. Assessing pupils

    1. Sit at eye level with the client

    2. Inform the client that the shape and size of the pupils will be assessed

    3. Inspect the pupils by looking for roundness, equality, and position within the eye

H. Assessing pupillary response

    1. Sit at eye level with the client

    2. Instruct the client that pupillary response to light will be assessed by shining a light into each eye while the client is looking straight ahead

    3. Move the light from a penlight onto the right eye from the lateral side of the eye

    4. Observe the pupil with light on it for constriction; if the pupil constricts, this is a direct reaction to light; observe the pupil without light shining on it for an equal reaction; this is a consensual reaction to light

    5. Repeat the procedure by shining a light onto the left eye

I. Assessing eye for accommodation

    1. Sit opposite the client at eye level

Practice to Pass

The nurse working on a neuroscience unit needs to perform a routine assessment of the client's pupils during the neurological assessment. What should the nurse do to perform the pupil check correctly?

!

Figure 14-3

Testing six fields of gaze

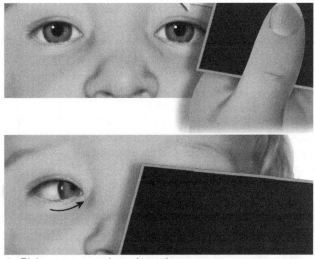

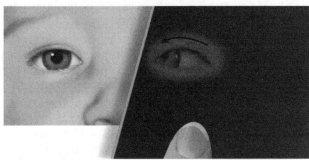

A Right, or uncovered eye, is weaker.

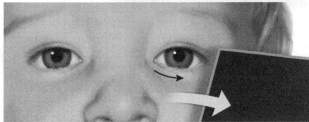

B Left, or covered eye, is weaker.

    2. Explain to the client that you will be evaluating the muscles of eye while the client is staring at the wall

    3. Hold a penlight or pencil 4 in. from the client's nose and bring the object close to the bridge of the nose

    4. Observe pupils for constriction as the object is brought close to the bridge of the nose; observe for **convergence** (turning inward of the eye toward the nose)

J. Testing of the corneal reflex

    1. Inform the client that you will be assessing corneal reflex by touching the eye with a wisp of cotton; tell the client he or she will react either by blinking or having tearing of the eye

    2. With a sterile wisp of cotton, approach the eye from the lateral side and gently touch the sclera

    3. Observe the eyes for a blink or tearing response

K. Inspection of external eye

    1. Tell the client you will be assessing the external eye and will be providing directions throughout the assessment

2. While sitting in front of the client, observe the client's eyebrows for symmetry of shape, quantity, and distribution

3. With the client's eyes open, assess for equality of palpebral fissures

4. Upper eyelid should cover a small part of the **iris** (colored membrane responsible for controlling pupil diameter and size, and amount of light that reaches the retina)

5. Evaluate conjunctiva and sclera for consistency of color, smoothness of surfaces, and whether they are clear and moist

6. Observe the iris and cornea to determine whether they are clear or have opacity, and whether there is presence or absence of inflammation

7. Ask the client to close both eyes and observe for complete closure of both lids

L. **Palpation of eye**

1. Apply gloves and have the client close both eyes

2. Using the first two fingers, palpate the lacrimal sacs, eyelids, and globe

3. Using a cotton-tipped applicator, invert the upper lid for the purpose of inspecting the conjunctiva

M. **Inspection of internal eye with ophthalmoscope**

1. Instruct the client that an ophthalmoscope will be used to inspect the fundus after the room is darkened; tell the client that he or she will need to stare at a fixed point in the room

2. Begin inspecting the client's right eye by holding the ophthalmoscope in your right hand with the index finger on the wheel and with the zero diopter against your right eye

3. Make sure the ophthalmoscope is at a 15-degree angle as you approach the client's eye

4. Direct light into the client's pupil and see a red reflex (light's reflection off the retina)

5. Wheel may need to be rotated to bring structures into focus
    a. If the client is myopic, rotate the wheel toward the minus numbers to focus structures
    b. If the client is hyperopic, rotate the wheel toward the plus numbers

6. Find a blood vessel and trace it to the optic disc on the nasal side of the retina

7. Follow the vessel to the lateral side to see the macula

8. Inspect the internal eye structures systematically

9. Use the optic disc as clock for describing any finding

10. Inspect blood vessels for color, size, and crossing of any vessels; inspect retinal fields for any dark areas or presence of white areas (scarring from retinal hemorrhage)

11. Repeat the procedure to assess the internal structures of the left eye; hold the ophthalmoscope in your left hand and use your left eye to assess the client's left eye

N. **Measuring intraocular pressure with *tonometry* (a procedure that uses a device called a tonometer to measure intraocular pressure)**

1. Explain the procedure to the client, indicating that it will not be painful but may startle the client

2. Use a tonometer pen to measure intraocular pressure

3. Hold the pen to the cornea and tap gently to release a burst of air to obtain the reading

VI. EXPECTED FINDINGS

A. **Testing visual acuity involves having the client read the smallest line possible and comparing it to a person with normal vision**

1. Distance vision testing
    a. Normal result is 20/20; the numerator indicates the distance of the client from the chart (20 feet), whereas the denominator indicates the distance at which a person with normal vision can read that line
    b. If the client is unable to read at least half of the numbers on a line, document the result as the score from the line above

2. Near vision testing
   a. Completed with corrective lenses if worn
      1) Normal finding is 14/14
      2) If the client is unable to read a line on the card, document the result as the score from the line above
3. Confrontation test
   a. Client should be able to see the object or the examiner's fingers at the same time examiner does
   b. Test requires the examiner to have peripheral vision
   c. Both eyes should have symmetrical peripheral vision
4. Cardinal fields of gaze
   a. Client should be able to follow with the eyes all movements of the examiner's hand
      1) Test of visual fields is a test of peripheral vision
      2) There should be no loss of peripheral vision; eyes should be able to move through all visual fields
   b. Eye movements should be steady; there should be no oscillation or rapid movements of the eyeball (**nystagmus**)
5. Corneal light reflex: reflection of light on the cornea should be symmetrical
6. Cover test
   a. Client should have fusion reflex; fusion reflex is documented when there is no shift in gaze
   b. Eyes should have parallel eye movement
7. Pupils should be round, symmetrical, and of equal size and shape; no opacity of the lens should be noted
8. Pupillary response
   a. Pupils should constrict in direct response to light
   b. Pupils should have consensual response to light; when light illuminates the right pupil, the left pupil should constrict in consensual response to the light
9. Accommodation
   a. When an object is brought toward the bridge of the nose, the eyes should constrict and converge toward the nose
   b. During assessment the pupils should be equal, round, reactive to light, and show accommodation
10. Assessment of the corneal reflex; the client should blink or tear when the cornea is touched with a wisp of cotton
11. External eye
    a. Eyebrows and eyelids should be symmetrical and hair should be equally distributed; there should be no flaking or drainage
    b. Palprebral fissures should be equal; the eyelid should cover the upper aspect of the iris
    c. Eyelids should close entirely and no iris should be visible; an open eye is more susceptible to injury
    d. Conjunctiva should be pink, moist, and clear; dry eyes or discoloration are indicative of an underlying condition
    e. Irises should be round and of equal color
    f. Pupils should be equal, round, and reactive to light
12. Palpation of eyes
    a. Eyes should have no swelling
    b. Eyes should have no drainage from the eyelids or lacrimal ducts
    c. Eyeballs should feel firm
    d. Eyelids should not be tender to the touch

Practice to Pass

The nurse has completed an inspection of internal eye structures using an ophthalmoscope. What would be the nurse's findings if the client's results were within normal limits?

13. Internal eye structures
    a. When examining the internal eye structures, red reflex should be noted
    b. There should be visible blood vessels that are fairly straight in contour
    c. Optic disk should be round or oval and of a reddish or yellowish-orange color
    d. Dark circle (macula) should be present
    e. Retina should be free of spots
14. Intraocular pressure: normal intraocular pressure is 12–21 mmHg

VII. UNEXPECTED FINDINGS

A. Distance vision
1. The higher the denominator, the poorer the vision
2. If the client's vision is 20/200 with best correction, the client is considered legally blind
3. If the client is unable to see objects in the distance, his or her condition is described as **myopia** (nearsightedness)
   a. Myopia is a genetic condition in which the eye is longer than expected
   b. In myopia, light rays focus in front of the retina

B. Near vision
1. Client should be able to read a card at a distance of 14 in.
2. If the client unable to see near objects, his or her condition is termed **hyperopia** (farsightedness)
   a. Hyperopia is an inherited disorder in which the eye is shorter than expected
   b. In hyperopia, light is focused behind the retina

C. Other visual conditions
1. As the client ages he or she may not be able to accommodate (focus); this is known as **presbyopia**
   a. The lens and supporting musculature lose elasticity and are unable to accommodate
   b. When light is focused behind the retina the client will lose the ability to focus on near objects
2. **Astigmatism** is an inherited condition in which light is refracted over a large area of the retina rather than a single point
   a. The cornea is elongated in one direction, thus causing a distortion of vision because of altered light refraction
   b. Light focused on two points near or on the retina will cause double vision or blurred vision
3. Night blindness may be produced by retinal disorders or cataracts

D. Confrontation: if the client is not able to see the object or finger at the same time as the examiner then the client is experiencing loss of peripheral vision

E. Cardinal fields of gaze
1. Client should be able to move his or her eyes in all directions
2. Strabismus is a condition in which the eyes cannot focus on one object
   a. Can be classified as exotropia or endotropia
   b. *Exotropia* is condition in which the eye deviates outward
   c. *Esotropia* is condition in which the eye deviates inward
3. There should be no eye oscillation or abnormal eye movements
4. Loss of peripheral vision may be caused by vascular damage to the retina, increased intraocular pressure, or a lesion of the optic nerve (see Figure 14-4)

F. Corneal light reflex: light should be reflected symmetrically off the cornea

G. Cover test
1. There should be no weakness of the eyes; they should be able to be held parallel
2. There should be no abnormal eye movements

Figure 14-4

Client's view with visual field loss

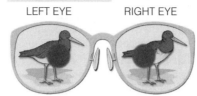

Retinal Damage

LEFT EYE   RIGHT EYE

Blind spots—in localized damaged areas.

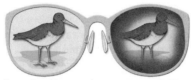

Increased intraocular pressure resulting in decreased peripheral vision.

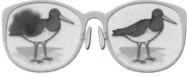

Retinal detachment—vision diminishes in affected area.

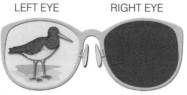

LEFT EYE   RIGHT EYE

Optic nerve or globe lesion results in unilateral blindness.

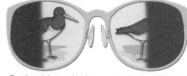

Optic chiasm lesion—results in bilateral heteronymous hemianopsia (loss of temporal visual fields).

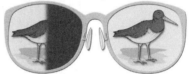

Lesion occurs in uncrossed fibers of optic chiasm resulting in left hemianopsia (nasal).

Right optic tract or optic radiation lesion resulting in loss of right nasal and left temporal fields. Homonymous hemianopsia.

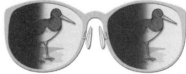

H. Pupils
  1. Pupils not equal in size and shape are usually considered abnormal; note that a small percentage of the population may have unequal pupil size (anisocoria)
  2. Clients should be able to verify that finding
I. Pupillary response (see Table 14-1)
  1. There is an abnormal finding if the pupil does not constrict when light is reflected on it
  2. There is an abnormal finding if opposite pupil does not have a consensual response to light
J. Accommodation: lack of constriction and convergence when an object is brought close to the bridge of the nose is considered abnormal
K. Corneal reflex: if the client does not blink or tear when the cornea is touched with a wisp of cotton, the client may have impairment of cranial nerve (CN), V (trigeminal nerve), or VII (facial nerve)
L. Inspection of external eye
  1. Absence of eyelashes or eyebrow hair is considered abnormal
  2. Eyelid should not droop (**ptosis**)
  3. Inflammation of the eyelid is known as **blepharitis**
    a. Presents as red, scaly, crusted lids
    b. Is caused by a staphylococcus infection, which causes the eye to burn, itch, and tear
  4. Iritis is inflammation of the iris and cornea associated with pain, decreased vision, and an irregularly shaped pupil
  5. Protrusion of the eye beyond the supraorbital ridge is considered abnormal

Table 14-1	Abnormal Pupil Condition	Description
Abnormal pupils	Miosis	Constricted pupils that may be the result of a lesion, glaucoma, or a normal response to bright light
	Mydriasis	Dilated pupils that may be due to a brain lesion, glaucoma, or a normal response to a dark environment
	Adie's pupils	Unilateral slow pupillary response
	Argyll Robertson pupils	Small, irregularly shaped pupils due to a tumor or syphilis; it may also be the result of narcotic use
	Anisocoria	Pupils that are unequal in size due to a central nervous system disorder
	Cranial Nerve III damage	Unilaterally unequal pupil due to a brain lesion or head trauma
	Horner's syndrome	Unilateral small nonreactive pupil associated with ptosis (drooping of the eyelid) on the affected side

6. Edema of the eyelids may be the result of heart disease, allergies, or renal failure, known as periorbital edema
7. Paralysis of the facial nerve may inhibit the client from opening an eye
8. In a client experiencing glaucoma the pupil becomes oval-shaped and is dilated
   a. In a client with glaucoma the cornea becomes cloudy
   b. There is pain with a decrease in vision and the client sees halos around lights
9. In a client experiencing cataracts, the lens will have opacity
10. Presence of a papule on the lower lid and medial canthus is usually indicative of basal cell carcinoma
11. Inversion of the lower eyelid is caused by muscle weakness and is known as **ectropion**
12. Eversion of the eyelid is caused by muscle spasms and is known as **entropion**; if untreated it will cause corneal irritation
13. A chalazion is an infection of the meibomian gland that produces a nodule on the upper eyelid that is not tender unless the nodule becomes inflamed
14. Conjunctivitis is inflammation of the eyelid caused by bacteria, virus, or foreign substance
15. A hordeolum or stye is a staphylococcal infection of the follicles of the eyelashes, producing redness, pain, and edema
16. Trauma or injury is considered an abnormal finding
    a. Determine the type of injury because that would provide information as to treatment
    b. Splashes require copious irrigation, whereas perforations may necessitate surgery

M. Palpation of eye
1. Eyeballs and eyelids should be free of edema; swelling may be the result of cardio-vascular or renal disease, or may also indicate allergies or infection
2. Sunken, less firm eyeballs may be the result of dehydration

N. Inspection of internal eye structures
1. Lack of a red reflex indicates opacity of the lens
2. Splitting of light reflected on the cornea may indicate a corneal abrasion
3. Spots on the macula may be the result of a hemorrhage or cyst
4. Dark or opaque spots on the retina may indicate scarring as a result of an old hemorrhage or laser or coagulation therapy
5. Absence of blood vessels is considered abnormal
6. Arteries that are smaller than veins may be the result of constriction
7. Tortuous blood vessels are considered abnormal

8. Macular degeneration produces degenerative patches on the retina; causes loss of central vision
9. Retinopathy produces changes in the retina
   a. Diabetic retinopathy causes microaneurysms, macular edema, and retinal exudates
   b. Hypertensive retinopathy is due to elevated blood pressure producing changes in vasculature of retina
10. Glaucoma produces an increase in intraocular pressure (IOP); tonometer readings are high (normal 12–21 mmHg)
11. Papilledema is elevation of the optic disc, which is indicative of increased IOP

VIII. LIFESPAN CONSIDERATIONS

A. Infants

Practice to Pass

The nurse is examining the external eyes of a client. How would the nurse be able to differentiate the presence of cataracts from the presence of glaucoma using visual inspection? What questions would the nurse ask the client to gather further supportive data?

1. At birth the eyes should be symmetrical; pupils should be equal and respond to light
2. Iris is brown in dark-skinned people and blue in light-skinned people; at approximately three months of age the iris takes on its permanent color
3. At birth the eyes may be swollen or edematous due to trauma during the birthing process; tears will not be present for the first month
4. For the first six weeks of life the infant only has monocular vision; during this period the infant will fixate on a bright light or moving objects
5. Infants are born farsighted and remain so until approximately 8 years of age
6. Strabismus and nystagmus are normal in newborns but should resolve by 6–8 weeks of age

B. Children

1. Eyes reach adult size by age 8
2. Children should have regular eye examinations; if the child is unable to read, assess vision with a Snellen picture chart
3. Assess eye muscle function very early in the child's development to prevent permanent vision damage

C. Older Adults

1. By the mid-forties the lens of the eye begins to lose elasticity, which in turn weakens the musculature of the eyes, resulting in decreased near vision; condition is known as presbyopia
2. With aging there is decreased tear production, resulting in dry eyes and uncomfortable eye sensations
3. White-yellow discoloration may appear around the cornea, known as arcus senilis
4. Cataract formation begins to occur due to plaque formation on the lens
5. Macular degeneration is a cause of blindness associated with aging; produces loss of central vision
6. Periorbital edema may develop if the client develops congestive heart failure

IX. DOCUMENTATION

A. Visual acuity using a Snellen eye chart
B. Visual fields tested using a confrontation test
C. Muscle function and external eye structures
D. Pupillary function (evaluated to provide valuable neurological data)
E. Optic disc color, size, and shape as well as condition of vessels in eye (as seen using an ophthalmoscope)

Case Study

An African-American client presents to the emergency department with severe eye pain in the right eye. When assessing the client, the nurse gathers the following data: decreased visual acuity, all objects are blurry, decreased peripheral vision, sudden onset of pain with no precipitating factors or interventions that relieve the pain, and an opaque appearance of the cornea. The client has had yearly eye examinations and denies any health problems.

1. What additional data should the nurse gather?

2. What risk factors may contribute to the development of this condition?

3. What is the priority nursing diagnosis for this client?

4. What diagnostic tests should be performed on this client?

5. If left untreated what condition may this progress to?

For suggested responses, see page 311

POSTTEST

1 Upon assessment of the client, the nurse notes increased intraocular pressure (IOP). The nurse should develop a plan of care for this client using the diagnosis visual impairment related to which etiology?

1. Mydriasis
2. Miosis
3. Cataract
4. Glaucoma

2 A client has experienced a head injury. The nurse is assessing the client and observes papilledema. Based on this finding, the nurse concludes that the finding is consistent with which condition?

1. Glaucoma
2. Increased intracranial pressure
3. Hyperopia
4. Iritis

3 The client presents with a complaint of seeing halos around objects. The nurse would prepare the client for eye evaluation to detect which condition?

1. Glaucoma
2. A head injury
3. Miosis
4. Hordeolum

4 The nurse is reviewing the past medical history of a client. The nurse notes that the client has strabismus. The nurse would expect to see what clinical manifestation?

1. One pupil nonreactive to light
2. Redness and inflammation around the iris and cornea
3. Convergence of eyes toward the bridge of the nose
4. Drooping of the eyelid

5 The nurse is caring for a client who sustained eye injury because of a pencil in the eye, which was removed 4 days ago. The pupil is unresponsive to light and the client has no blink response when the nurse's finger is brought toward the eye. The client is crying and asks, "Am I blind?" What is the nurse's best initial response to the client?

1. "You will get your sight back."
2. "It is likely that you will get all your sight back eventually."
3. "You will be a candidate for a prosthetic."
4. "It seems you are upset. I can sit with you and talk for awhile."

6 During assessment of the external eye, the nurse should inspect which structures of the eye? Select all that apply.

1. Eyebrows and lashes
2. Pupillary reaction to light
3. Sclera and irises
4. Cornea
5. Conjunctiva

7 The nurse assesses the vision of an older adult client and finds that the client has no central vision but has peripheral vision. The nurse concludes that this is consistent with which disorder?

1. Blepharitis
2. Hypertensive retinopathy
3. Diabetic retinopathy
4. Macular degeneration

8 When taking a health history of an older adult client, the nurse would inquire about a history of which eye conditions? Select all that apply.

1. Cataracts
2. Macular degeneration
3. Discharge from the eyes
4. Presbyopia
5. Glaucoma

9 To evaluate for the presence of a foreign body in the client's eye, the nurse would perform which assessment?

1. Test for extraocular movement to visualize all areas of the sclera
2. Evert the eyelid to assess the sclera
3. Palpate the puncta
4. Inspect the cornea and lens

10 The nurse is evaluating the red reflex and observes white spots on the lens along with a diminished red reflex. What would the nurse do next?

1. Refer the client for evaluation of cataracts
2. Assess the client for increased intraocular pressure
3. Assess the client for extraocular movement and reevaluate the reflex
4. Assess the fundus for color

➤ *See pages 283–284 for Answers and Rationales.*

ANSWERS & RATIONALES

Pretest

1 **Answer: 3** **Rationale:** The numerator represents the distance the client is standing from the chart and the denominator denotes the distance at which most people can see the object. The expected result is 20/20 for visual acuity. The numerator and denominator reflect visual acuity in one eye. Two readings are needed: one for each eye (options 3 and 4). This client can read at 20 feet what most people can see at 25 feet, making the client nearsighted or myopic (option 2). **Cognitive Level:** Analysis **Client Need:** Health Promotion and Maintenance **Integrated Process:** Teaching/Learning **Content Area:** Adult Health: Eye, Ear, Nose, & Throat **Strategy:** Recall that with "20-20 vision" the numerator indicates the client's distance from the chart and the denominator represents the distance of a person with no loss of visual acuity (normal vision). From there, consider that the number 25 for this client must indicate the distance at which a client with normal vision can see the object on the eye chart. **Reference:** D'Amico, D. & Barbarito, C. (2007). *Health & physical assessment in nursing.* Upper Saddle River, NJ: Pearson Education, Inc., p. 277.

2 **Answer: 1, 3** **Rationale:** The letter H method and the wagon wheel method are both used to evaluate EOM (options 1 and 3). The nurse should instruct the client to keep the head still and follow the penlight with his or her eyes only. EOM is not assessed using a circular method (option 2). The Snellen eye chart is used to assess visual acuity (option 4). Shining the light in the pupils assesses reaction to light (option 5).

Cognitive Level: Application **Client Need:** Health Promotion and Maintenance **Integrated Process:** Nursing Process: Assessment **Content Area:** Adult Health: Eye, Ear, Nose, & Throat **Strategy:** Recall that the nurse positions the client in a sitting position and instructs him or her to keep the head still and follow the penlight with his or her eyes. From there, visualize the options that will assess EOM. Eliminate options 2, 4, and 5, realizing that options 4 and 5 will not assess eye movements and that option 2 is not proper technique. **Reference:** D'Amico, D. & Barbarito, C. (2007). *Health & physical assessment in nursing.* Upper Saddle River, NJ: Pearson Education, Inc., pp. 279–280.

3 **Answer: 3** **Rationale:** The pupils should be equal, round, and reactive to light and accommodation (option 3). Option 1 does not address accommodation. An eye examination (option 2) constitutes more than just a pupillary assessment. Visual acuity (option 4) requires assessment of vision using a Snellen eye chart (option 4). **Cognitive Level:** Application **Client Need:** Health Promotion and Maintenance **Integrated Process:** Communication and Documentation **Content Area:** Adult Health: Eye, Ear, Nose, & Throat **Strategy:** Recall that an examination of the eye requires a visual acuity assessment as well as an assessment of the internal eye structures. Next recall that a pupillary assessment is documented as pupils being equal, round, and reactive to light and accommodation (PERRLA). **Reference:** D'Amico, D. & Barbarito, C. (2007). *Health & physical assessment in nursing.* Upper Saddle River, NJ: Pearson Education, Inc., p. 282.

4 **Answer: 4** **Rationale:** Consensual reaction is assessed by shining a light in one eye and observing the opposite eye for a reaction to the light (option 4). Shining the light in one eye and observing that eye for a reaction to the light is assessing for direct reaction to light (option 1). It is normal for the eyes to turn inward when an object is brought toward the nose, but accommodation is when the object comes toward the nose and the pupils constrict (options 2 and 3).
Cognitive Level: Application **Client Need:** Health Promotion and Maintenance **Integrated Process:** Nursing Process: Assessment **Content Area:** Adult Health: Eye, Ear, Nose, & Throat **Strategy:** Recall that the nurse should position the client in a sitting position and shine the light in one eye while observing the opposite eye for constriction to evaluate consensual reaction to light. **Reference:** D'Amico, D. & Barbarito, C. (2007). *Health & physical assessment in nursing.* Upper Saddle River, NJ: Pearson Education, Inc., pp. 281–282.

5 **Answer: 2** **Rationale:** The abbreviation OS refers to the left eye, and the larger the denominator the more myopic the client is (option 2). The abbreviation for the right eye is OD (options 1 and 3). Hyperopia is difficulty with near vision (options 3 and 4).
Cognitive Level: Analysis **Client Need:** Health Promotion and Maintenance **Integrated Process:** Nursing Process: Assessment **Content Area:** Adult Health: Eye, Ear, Nose, & Throat **Strategy:** Recall that myopia (nearsightedness) is reflected by a large denominator; this will help eliminate options 3 and 4. Next recall that the abbreviation OD (from the Latin *os dextra*) indicates the right eye to eliminate option 1, or recall that the abbreviation OS (from the Latin *os septra*) indicates the left eye to choose option 2 over option 1. **Reference:** D'Amico, D. & Barbarito, C. (2007). *Health & physical assessment in nursing.* Upper Saddle River, NJ: Pearson Education, Inc., pp. 277–278.

6 **Answer: 2** **Rationale:** A corneal abrasion causes light reflecting off of the cornea to split or look splintered (option 2). The lacrimal duct bleeds when it is obstructed with calculi (option 1). Periorbital edema, swelling of the tissue surrounding the eye, may be due to congestive heart failure or allergens (option 3). Opacity of the lens is consistent with a cataract (option 4).
Cognitive Level: Application **Client Need:** Health Promotion and Maintenance **Integrated Process:** Nursing Process: Analysis **Content Area:** Adult Health: Eye, Ear, Nose, & Throat **Strategy:** Recall that corneal abrasion is extremely painful and produces a splintered-appearing light reflecting off of the cornea. Alternatively, associate the critical words *something being in the eye* in the question with the word *abrasion* to choose correctly.
Reference: D'Amico, D. & Barbarito, C. (2007). *Health & physical assessment in nursing.* Upper Saddle River, NJ: Pearson Education, Inc., p. 283.

7 **Answer: 2** **Rationale:** In the older adult client periorbital edema usually reflects congestive heart failure (option 2).

While facial and eye trauma may cause edema, trauma usually does not cause edema surrounding the entire eye (option 1). Allergies may cause edema, but this is not usually the cause of edema in the older adult client (option 3). Presbyopia is the loss of elasticity and weakening of the eye muscle, producing difficulty seeing near objects (option 4).
Cognitive Level: Application **Client Need:** Health Promotion and Maintenance **Integrated Process:** Nursing Process: Analysis **Content Area:** Adult Health: Eye, Ear, Nose, & Throat **Strategy:** Note the age of the client in the question as being an older adult. Then evaluate each option in terms of its frequency in older adult clients. Recall that periorbital edema is a sign of congestive heart failure to choose correctly. Alternatively, associate the word *edema* in the question with *heart failure* in the correct option to make the same selection. **Reference:** D'Amico, D. & Barbarito, C. (2007). *Health & physical assessment in nursing.* Upper Saddle River, NJ: Pearson Education, Inc., p. 298.

8 **Answer: 3** **Rationale:** Floaters occur due to vitreous humor. The floaters are not usually significant (option 3). It is not therapeutic to tell the client something may happen (option 1). It is inappropriate to tell the client he or she will lose his or her eyesight (option 2). Hemorrhaging usually causes the visual fields to darken (option 4).
Cognitive Level: Application **Client Need:** Health Promotion and Maintenance **Integrated Process:** Teaching/Learning **Content Area:** Adult Health: Eye, Ear, Nose, & Throat **Strategy:** First eliminate options that contain non-therapeutic statements, such as those in options 1 and 2. Next recall that floaters are pieces of vitreous humor that are not significant to choose option 3 over option 4. **Reference:** D'Amico, D. & Barbarito, C. (2007). *Health & physical assessment in nursing.* Upper Saddle River, NJ: Pearson Education, Inc., p. 272.

9 **Answer: 1** **Rationale:** When the client is farsighted (hyperopia) the light rays focus behind the retina (option 1). Emmetropia is normal refraction (option 3). Double vision is diplopia in which two objects are seen (option 4). Nearsightedness (myopia) occurs when the light rays are focused in front of the retina (option 2).
Cognitive Level: Application **Client Need:** Health Promotion and Maintenance **Integrated Process:** Nursing Process: Implementation **Content Area:** Adult Health: Eye, Ear, Nose, & Throat **Strategy:** Eliminate option 3 first because emmetropia has the same suffix as hyperopia, and thus must be a different term. Recall the term *diplopia* as meaning double vision to eliminate option 4. Finally, recall that hyperopia is farsightedness, or that myopia is nearsightedness, to make the correct selection from the remaining options. **Reference:** D'Amico, D. & Barbarito, C. (2007). *Health & physical assessment in nursing.* Upper Saddle River, NJ: Pearson Education, Inc., p. 289.

10 **Answer: 1** **Rationale:** Miosis is pupillary constriction (option 1), while mydriasis is pupillary dilation (option 2).

Hyperopia is farsightedness (option 3), while myopia is nearsightedness (option 4).
Cognitive Level: Application **Client Need:** Health Promotion and Maintenance **Integrated Process:** Communication and Documentation **Content Area:** Adult Health: Eye, Ear, Nose, & Throat **Strategy:** First eliminate the terms ending in *-opia* (options 3 and 4) because they have to do with vision. Next recall either that miosis is pupillary constriction or that mydriasis is pupillary dilation to choose option 1 over option 2. **Reference:** D'Amico, D. & Barbarito, C. (2007). *Health & physical assessment in nursing.* Upper Saddle River, NJ: Pearson Education, Inc., p. 294.

Posttest

1 **Answer: 4** **Rationale:** Glaucoma is an increase in IOP from either excess production of aqueous humor or blockage to aqueous outflow from the anterior chamber (option 4). A cataract is opacity of the lens that is prevalent in older adults (option 3). Mydriasis (option 1) is dilation of the pupil, whereas miosis (option 2) is constriction of the pupil.
Cognitive Level: Application **Client Need:** Health Promotion and Maintenance **Integrated Process:** Nursing Process: Analysis **Content Area:** Adult Health: Eye, Ear, Nose, & Throat **Strategy:** Recall that a cataract is opacity of the lens; none of the other conditions produces a cloudy lens. **Reference:** D'Amico, D. & Barbarito, C. (2007). *Health & physical assessment in nursing.* Upper Saddle River, NJ: Pearson Education, Inc., p. 295.

2 **Answer: 2** **Rationale:** Papilledema is a sign of increased intracranial pressure (option 2). Glaucoma is caused by an increase in intraocular pressure (option 1). Hyperopia is the term to describe farsightedness (option 3). Iritis is an infection of the iris and cornea (option 4).
Cognitive Level: Application **Client Need:** Health Promotion and Maintenance **Integrated Process:** Nursing Process: Evaluation **Content Area:** Adult Health: Eye, Ear, Nose, & Throat **Strategy:** Select the option that is a clinical manifestation or sign of a condition, as all the other options are actual disease processes. **Reference:** D'Amico, D. & Barbarito, C. (2007). *Health & physical assessment in nursing.* Upper Saddle River, NJ: Pearson Education, Inc., p. 297.

3 **Answer: 1** **Rationale:** Glaucoma is an increase in intraocular pressure that produces halos around objects (option 1). A head injury would manifest as papilledema (option 2). In miosis the nurse would observe pinpoint pupils (option 3). A hordeolum is a stye that manifests as a swollen, red, and painful infection of the eyelid (option 4).
Cognitive Level: Application **Client Need:** Health Promotion and Maintenance **Integrated Process:** Nursing Process: Planning **Content Area:** Adult Health: Eye, Ear, Nose, & Throat **Strategy:** Recall that the symptoms of glaucoma are pain, a cloudy cornea, poor vision, and halos around objects and lights. **Reference:** D'Amico, D. & Barbarito, C.

(2007). *Health & physical assessment in nursing.* Upper Saddle River, NJ: Pearson Education, Inc., pp. 294, 297.

4 **Answer: 3** **Rationale:** Strabismus is a condition in which weakened eye muscles produce convergence of the eye toward the nose (option 3). A non-reactive pupil may be indicative of conditions such as increased intracranial pressure or monocular blindness (option 1). Iritis produces redness and inflammation around the iris and cornea (option 2). Drooping of one eyelid is known as ptosis (option 4).
Cognitive Level: Analysis **Client Need:** Health Promotion and Maintenance **Integrated Process:** Nursing Process: Assessment **Content Area:** Adult Health: Eye, Ear, Nose, & Throat **Strategy:** To eliminate option 2, recall that disorders characterized by inflammation often end in *-itis.* To eliminate option 4, recall that drooping of one eyelid is called ptosis. Choose option 3 over option 1, recalling either that strabismus is a condition caused by weakened eye muscles, or that a non-reactive pupil reflects an underlying neurological condition and is not itself a condition that has a name. **Reference:** D'Amico, D. & Barbarito, C. (2007). *Health & physical assessment in nursing.* Upper Saddle River, NJ: Pearson Education, Inc., pp. 282–283.

5 **Answer: 4** **Rationale:** The client who is upset should have his or her feelings acknowledged. Option 4 is therapeutic. Options 1 and 2 may provide false reassurance. A prosthetic eye will not offer the client sight; it is cosmetic (option 3). Options 1, 2, and 3 do not address the client's feelings.
Cognitive Level: Application **Client Need:** Health Promotion and Maintenance **Integrated Process:** Caring **Content Area:** Adult Health: Eye, Ear, Nose, & Throat **Strategy:** Note the critical word *initial* in the question and recall that the first step in communication is to acknowledge the client's feelings. Eliminate options that do not address the client's feelings, which would then eliminate options 1, 2, and 3. **Reference:** D'Amico, D. & Barbarito, C. (2007). *Health & physical assessment in nursing.* Upper Saddle River, NJ: Pearson Education, Inc., p. 275.

6 **Answer: 1, 3, 4, 5** **Rationale:** Inspection of the external eye includes evaluating the eyebrows, which should be symmetrical, and eyelashes, which should be similar in quantity bilaterally. The sclera should be white and the iris should be round and of equal color. The cornea should be clear and the conjunctiva should be pink, moist, and free of drainage. The assessment of the pupils for reaction to light is an evaluation of the neurological system (option 2).
Cognitive Level: Application **Client Need:** Health Promotion and Maintenance **Integrated Process:** Nursing Process: Assessment **Content Area:** Adult Health: Eye, Ear, Nose, & Throat **Strategy:** Eliminate options that are not an external structure of the eye. Pupillary assessment provides data related to the functioning of the neurological system. The structures of the external eye include the

eyebrows, eyelashes, sclera, conjunctiva, and irises. **Reference:** D'Amico, D. & Barbarito, C. (2007). *Health & physical assessment in nursing.* Upper Saddle River, NJ: Pearson Education, Inc., p. 283.

7 **Answer: 4** **Rationale:** Macular degeneration is a condition that affects central vision and the client is left with peripheral vision due to degeneration of the retina (option 4). Diabetic retinopathy is changes in the retina and its vasculature (option 3). Hypertensive retinopathy is changes (hemorrhages) in the retina due to high blood pressure (option 2). Blepharitis is an inflammation of the eyelid (option 1).
Cognitive Level: Application **Client Need:** Health Promotion and Maintenance **Integrated Process:** Nursing Process: Analysis **Content Area:** Adult Health: Eye, Ear, Nose, & Throat **Strategy:** Eliminate any option ending in *-itis* due to the fact that the question asks for a condition of vision loss, not inflammation. Retinopathies are conditions where there is retinal hemorrhaging. Macular degeneration is a condition of central vision loss.
Reference: D'Amico, D. & Barbarito, C. (2007). *Health & physical assessment in nursing.* Upper Saddle River, NJ: Pearson Education, Inc., pp. 295–296.

8 **Answer: 1, 2, 4, 5** **Rationale:** As the client ages, cataracts (opacity of the lens), macular degeneration (loss of central vision), glaucoma (increased ocular pressure), and presbyopia (the inability to accommodate for near vision) may develop. There should be no discharge from the eyes at any age, as this indicates an infection or inflammation (option 3).
Cognitive Level: Application **Client Need:** Health Promotion and Maintenance **Integrated Process:** Nursing Process: Evaluation **Content Area:** Adult Health: Eye, Ear, Nose, & Throat **Strategy:** Eliminate an infection signaled by discharge from the eye, recalling that an infection can be present in all age groups. **Reference:** D'Amico, D. & Barbarito, C. (2007). *Health & physical assessment in nursing.* Upper Saddle River, NJ: Pearson Education, Inc., p. 295.

9 **Answer: 2** **Rationale:** When the client presents with a complaint of a foreign body in the eye the nurse would invert the lid to assess for the object (option 2). Assessing for extraocular movement evaluates neurological and motor function (option 1). Palpating the puncta will evaluate the lacrimal duct for blockage (option 3). The cornea and lens are evaluated for abrasions (option 4).
Cognitive Level: Application **Client Need:** Health Promotion and Maintenance **Integrated Process:** Nursing Process: Assessment **Content Area:** Adult Health: Eye, Ear, Nose, & Throat **Strategy:** The extraocular movements are part of the assessment of the cranial nerves. The puncta are evaluated when a blockage of the lacrimal duct is suspected. The cornea and lens are assessed for irregularities, opacities, or abrasions. **Reference:** D'Amico, D. & Barbarito, C. (2007). *Health & physical assessment in nursing.* Upper Saddle River, NJ: Pearson Education, Inc., p. 292.

10 **Answer: 1** **Rationale:** If a finding is abnormal it requires referral to a healthcare provider who can diagnose eye disorders. Opacity may indicate a cataract (option 1). Intraocular pressure indicates glaucoma (option 2). Extraocular movement is performed to evaluate cranial nerve function (option 3). Abnormal color of the fundus may indicate hemorrhage and exudates (option 4).
Cognitive Level: Application **Client Need:** Health Promotion and Maintenance **Integrated Process:** Nursing Process: Assessment **Content Area:** Adult Health: Eye, Ear, Nose, & Throat **Strategy:** Recognize that three of the options have assessment as the action. The first option is *refer*, implying the finding is in need of further evaluation. If a finding is abnormal it requires further assessment. **Reference:** D'Amico, D. & Barbarito, C. (2007). *Health & physical assessment in nursing.* Upper Saddle River, NJ: Pearson Education, Inc., p. 286.

References

Bickley, L. (2010). *Bates guide to physical examination and history taking* (10th ed.). Philadelphia: Lippincott Williams & Wilkins.

D'Amico, D. & Barbarito, C. (2007). *Health & physical assessment in nursing.* Upper Saddle River, NJ: Pearson Education, Inc., pp. 348–396.

Jarvis, C. (2008). *Physical examination and health assessment* (5th ed.). St. Louis, MO: Elsevier Saunders.

Zator Estes, M. (2009). *Health assessment and physical examination* (4th ed.). Clifton Park, NY: Delmar Cengage Learning.

Ears, Nose, and Throat Assessment

15

Chapter Outline

Health History
Present Health History
Family History

Equipment, Preparation, and
  Positioning
Examination Techniques
Expected Findings

Unexpected Findings
Lifespan Considerations
Documentation

Objectives

➤ Identify the anatomy and physiology of the ears, nose, and throat.
➤ Conduct a health history regarding the ears, nose, and throat.
➤ Prepare the client for an ears, nose, and throat assessment.
➤ Utilize the techniques needed for an ears, nose, and throat assessment.
➤ Describe expected and unexpected findings associated with the ears, nose, and throat.

NCLEX-RN® Test Prep

Visit the Companion Website for this book at www.pearsonhighered.com/hogan to access additional practice opportunities and more.

Review at a Glance

air conduction transmission of sound through tympanic membrane to auditory nerve
auricle (or pinna) external portion of ear
bone conduction transmission of sound through bones of skull to auditory nerve

frontal sinus air filled cavities above eyebrows
maxillary sinus air filled cavities beside nares

tragus projection at anterior meatus of auditory canal of ear
tympanic membrane thin transparent membrane that separates middle from external ear, also known as the eardrum

PRETEST

1 During the assessment of an adult client's ear the nurse should expect to document that the tympanic membrane will have which characteristics?

1. Pink and shiny in appearance
2. Pearly gray with a cone of light near the five or seven o'clock position
3. Covered with a thin to moderate layer of cerumen
4. Beefy red in color across the tympanic membrane

2 When obtaining a health history a 38-year-old client states a need to keep turning up the television to hear. Based on this data the nurse would conclude that the client's symptom is consistent with which ear condition?

1. Infection of the inner ear
2. Presbycusis
3. Otosclerosis
4. Labyrinthitis

3 The nurse is to perform an otoscopic examination on an adult client. The nurse plans to perform this assessment by utilizing which technique?

1. Pull the pinna up and back
2. Pull the pinna down and back
3. Tilt client's head backward to increase client comfort
4. Use the largest speculum possible to maximize inner ear visualization

4 The nurse is performing the Weber test on an adult client who can only hear the tuning fork in the left ear. What is the appropriate conclusion the nurse would draw from this assessment?

1. Client has poorer hearing in left ear
2. Client has poorer hearing in right ear
3. Client is developing presbycusis
4. Client has inner ear infection

5 When assessing the tympanic membrane of a client with an otoscope the nurse finds many scars. The nurse would conclude that these scars are the result of which etiological problem?

1. Conductive hearing loss
2. Sensorineural hearing loss
3. Middle ear infections
4. Sticking an object in the ear as a child

6 During a hearing assessment the nurse should ask which questions to gather data about the client's hearing? Select all that apply.

1. "Have you ever had external otitis?"
2. "What changes have you noticed in your hearing?"
3. "When was your last hearing test?"
4. "Is your hearing better in one ear than the other?"
5. "Tell me about your hearing."

7 The nurse would test the client's nose for patency by performing which action?

1. Occlude right naris and ask the client to breathe through the left naris and then repeat procedure by occluding left naris
2. Occlude one naris and ask the client to state if there is pain and then repeating procedure on the other side
3. Palpate each naris one at a time for tenderness and swelling
4. Inspect the nasal cavity using a speculum

8 The nurse has transilluminated the sinuses and found that there is no red glow. How should the nurse interpret this finding?

1. Expected and document it as such
2. Inflammation of the sinuses
3. Mass blocking the light
4. Result of a conductive hearing problem

9 The nurse is assessing the client's lips and notes a bluish tinge. This finding would indicate to the nurse that the client may be experiencing which problem?

1. Beginning of a fever blister
2. Lack of dental care
3. Inflammation of the lips
4. Hypoxia

10 The nurse assesses a child's mouth and notes that tip of the tongue is fixated to the floor of the mouth. How should the nurse document this finding?

1. Ulceration
2. Ankyloglossia
3. Carcinoma
4. Leukoplakia

➤ *See pages 300–301 for Answers and Rationales.*

I. HEALTH HISTORY

 A. Information gained from health history provides necessary information about risks for hearing loss, both currently and in future

! **B. Begin assessing hearing with first a health history question; if client hears and answers the first question, begin gathering data about client's ability to hear**

 C. Assessment of ears; ask the client the following questions:

  1. "Describe your ability to hear."

  2. "Are you experiencing changes in your hearing? If so, please describe the changes."

   a. "Were the changes sudden or gradual?"

   b. "When do you experiencing these changes? All of the time? Just on the phone? During conversation?"

   c. "Do you hear better in one ear than the other? If so which ear?"

  3. "When was your last hearing test? What were the results of the hearing test?"

  4. "Do you have vertigo?"

  5. "Do you have Ménière's disease?"

  6. "Do you have an acoustic neuroma?"

  7. "Do you have a history of ear infection or inflammation? If so, what type of infection do you get?"

   a. External otitis (outer ear canal infection)

   b. Otitis media (middle ear infection)

   c. Labyrinthitis (inner ear)

  8. "Do you have mastoiditis?"

  9. "Do you have ear drainage?"

  10. "Are you experiencing dizziness, nausea, vomiting, or tinnitus (ringing in the ears)?"

  11. "Do you have pain in your ears? If so, describe."

  12. "How do you clean your ears?"

  13. "Do you use a hearing aid?"

  14. "Are you taking any medications? If so, what are you taking?"

  15. "Are you exposed to excessive noise?"

 D. Assessment of the nose; ask the client the following questions:

  1. "Are you experiencing any problems with your nose and sinuses? If so, please describe."

  2. "Are you having any nasal discharge?"

  3. "Do you have nosebleeds?"

  4. "Have you had any nasal injuries?"

  5. "Have you had any nose surgery? If so, please describe."

  6. "Describe your sense of smell."

  7. "Do you use over-the-counter medications to relieve nasal congestion? If so, what do you take and how often?"

  8. "Do you use recreational drugs? If so, what are you taking and how often?"

 E. Assessment of mouth and throat; ask the client the following questions:

  1. "Please describe the condition of your mouth and teeth."

  2. "Are you experiencing any difficulty swallowing?"

  3. "Do you have any lesions in your mouth?"

  4. "Do your gums bleed?"

Practice to Pass

The nurse has found several lesions in the client's mouth. The nurse should ask the client which assessment questions?

5. "Have you experienced any change in your sense of taste? If so, please describe."
6. "What dental conditions have you experienced?"
7. "Do you wear dentures, partial plates, retainers, or any other dental appliance?"
8. "When was your last dental examination?"
9. "How often do you floss?"
10. "How often do you brush your teeth?"
11. "Do you experience sore throats?"
12. "Have you experienced any changes in your voice? If so, please describe."
13. "Do you use tobacco? If yes, what type?"

II. PRESENT HEALTH HISTORY

A. Ask client more detailed questions about symptoms the client is currently experiencing regarding ear, mouth, nose, and throat problems

B. Follow-up with detailed questions about the ear and hearing loss as needed (see Box 15-1 for common reasons for hearing loss)
   1. "How would you describe the condition of your ears?"
   2. "How would you describe your hearing?"
   3. "Are you experiencing hearing difficulty?"
      a. "What sounds are you not hearing?"
      b. "Are you experiencing difficulty hearing on the phone?"
      c. "Are you having trouble hearing a conversation?"
      d. "Are there any other symptoms associated with the hearing loss?"
      e. "Does the hearing loss affect your activities of daily living (ADLs)?"
   4. "Are you experiencing chronic illness? Please tell me what illnesses you are being treated for."
   5. "Are you currently taking any medications? If so, please tell me what they are."
   6. "Are you experiencing ringing in your ears (tinnitus)?"
      a. "Describe the characteristics of the ringing."
      b. "Is it constant or does it come and go?"
      c. "Is it associated with any activity?"
      d. "What medications are you taking to treat this ringing?"
   7. "Have you had your hearing tested? If so, when was the last time you had your hearing tested?"
   8. "What were the results of your most recent hearing test?"
   9. "Do you use any devices to improve or enhance your hearing?"
      a. "What devices do you use?"
      b. "Does the hearing device improve your hearing?"
      c. "Do you wear the device all the time?"
      d. "Are you experiencing any difficulty with the device?"
   10. "What noises are you exposed to at work, school, or in your environment?"
   11. "Do you ever wear ear plugs, ear buds, or other hearing protection devices?"
   12. "Do you listen to loud music or participate in loud activities?"
   13. "Do you stick anything in your ears?"
   14. "How do you clean your ears?"

!

Practice to Pass

What should the nurse assess for regarding the ears of a client who is taking diuretics for hypertension?

Practice to Pass

What should the nurse evaluate for with the client who has a history of tinnitus?

Box 15-1 **Common Causes of Hearing Loss**	Heredity—family history of loss Congenital hearing loss—due to maternal exposure to toxins Environmental chemicals—butyl nitrite, mercury, carbon disulfide, styrene, carbon monoxide, tin, hexane, toluene, lead, trichloroethylene, manganese, and xylene Side effects of medication—some medications such as aspirin and aminoglycosides cause ringing in the ears or problems with balance

15. "Do you have any difficulty with your balance?"
16. "Are you experiencing dizziness? If so, are you experiencing the dizziness with your eyes open or closed?"
17. "Are you experiencing ear pain?"
    a. "Describe the pain."
    b. "Where is the pain? Is it inside the ear or outside?"
    c. "Is the pain constant or does it come and go?"
    d. "Describe the characteristics of the pain."
    e. "Does it hurt when you touch the ear?"
    f. "Are you experiencing drainage from the ear?"
    g. "Is there anything that precipitates the pain?"
    h. "Is there anything that relieves the pain?"

C. **Follow-up with detailed questions about the nose and sinuses**
    1. "Are you having any trouble at this time with your nose or sinuses? If so, can you describe the problem?"
        a. "Can you breathe through both nostrils or is one side blocked or obstructed?"
        b. "How long has this been a problem?"
        c. "Are you experiencing seasonal allergies? If so, how do you treat the problem?"
    2. "Do you have any discharge from your nose?"
        a. "If so, is it constant or occasional? Can you describe the discharge?"
        b. "Have you taken any medications to treat this and did it work?"
    3. "Do you have nosebleeds? How often?"
        a. "What do you do to treat nosebleeds when they occur?"
        b. "What is your typical blood pressure?"

D. **Follow-up with detailed questions about the mouth and throat if client answered affirmatively to general screening questions in health history, such as the following:**
    1. "Can you describe the lesion(s) on your tongue or in your mouth?"
    2. "Do these mouth and/or tongue lesions come and go or are they present constantly?"
    3. "Do you experience bleeding of the gums? If so, how often and how do you treat it?"
    4. "Has your sense of taste changed recently? If so, how?"
    5. "If you wear dentures, partial plates, retainers or another dental appliance, does it fit well and comfortably? Has it resolved the problem for which it was prescribed?"
    6. "Do you have caps on any of your teeth?"

III. FAMILY HISTORY

A. **Obtain a family medical history to determine client's risk factors**
    1. "Does anyone in your family have a hearing disorder?"
    2. "Does anyone in your family have a history of tumors of the ear?"
    3. "Does anyone in your family have Ménière's disease?"
    4. "Has anyone in your family been diagnosed with cancer of the mouth or throat (larynx)?"
B. **Have client review as many family generations as possible to provide maximal data**
C. **Information about adopted family members does not provide genetic information for client; however, it does provide information about environmental factors, since all individuals residing in the home will share exposure to same toxins**

IV. EQUIPMENT, PREPARATION, AND POSITIONING

A. **Gather equipment to perform an assessment of ears, nose, and throat**
B. **Explain equipment and examination techniques to client**
    1. Examination gown
    2. Non-sterile gloves

3. Otoscope
4. Tuning fork
5. Nasal speculum
6. Penlight
7. Gauze pads
8. Tongue blade
C. Use standard precautions
D. Position client sitting with his or her head midline until Romberg test is performed and then client will stand for that aspect of assessment
E. Provide adequate light

V. EXAMINATION TECHNIQUES

A. Assessment of the ear
   1. With client sitting, explain that you will be touching his or her ear and there should not be any pain or discomfort
   2. Evaluate client's hearing with every question; is the client responding appropriately to each question?

   3. Inspect external ear for symmetry and proportion
      a. Inspect ear for drainage, redness, nodules, swelling, or lesions
      b. Assess color of ear

Practice to Pass

How should the nurse assess a client who is experiencing otitis externa?

   4. Palpate auricle and **tragus** (projection at anterior meatus of auditory canal of ear) for lesions, nodules, and swelling (Figure 15-1A)
   5. Palpate mastoid process for lesions, pain, and swelling (see Figure 15-1B)
   6. Inspect auditory canal with an otoscope using largest speculum that fits into auditory canal
      a. Have client tilt head to opposite shoulder
      b. Hold otoscope in the dominant hand using thumb and first two fingers with handle upward or downward (Figure 15-2)
      c. Use non-dominant hand to straighten auditory canal
      d. In an adult client pull pinna up and back; in a child pull pinna down and back
      e. Instruct client to hold head still and to state if assessment produces discomfort

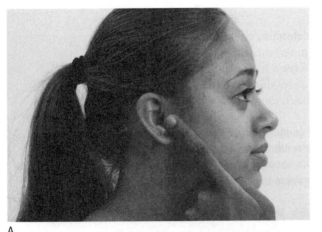
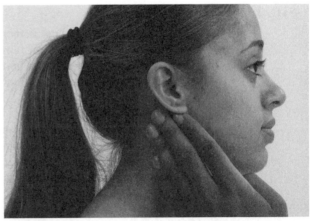

A   B

Figure 15-1

Palpation of the ear. A. Palpation of the tragus. B. Palpation of the mastoid process.

Figure 15-2

Two correct techniques for
using an otoscope

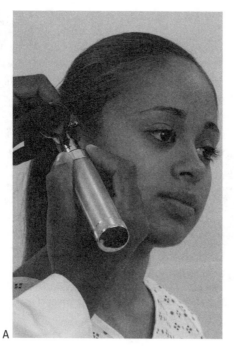
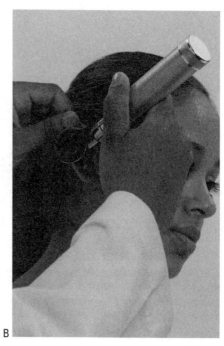

A   B

Practice to Pass

In order to inspect the
tympanic membrane
the nurse would use
what equipment?

f. Insert otoscope into auditory canal and inspect for characteristics of cerumen and foreign body; if a foreign body is in canal, do not insert scope any further into auditory canal because object should be removed prior to continuing the examination

g. Inspect **tympanic membrane** (thin transparent membrane that separates middle from external ear, also known as the eardrum) for contour, color, and translucency using otoscope

h. Perform whisper test to evaluate hearing acuity by having client hold heel of hand over the left ear; cover your own mouth so the client cannot see your lips; state a phrase and have client repeat phrase back to you

i. Use tuning forks to evaluate hearing acuity; the size of the tuning fork determines the number of vibrations per second; strike, squeeze, or tap the tuning fork to generate sound

   1) Perform Rinne test by striking handle of tuning fork and placing tuning fork on mastoid process (see Figure 15-3A); ask client when sound is no longer heard, noting number of seconds (tests bone conduction), then place tuning fork in front of external ear about 1–2 cm in front of ear (Figure 15-3B); ask client to say when the sound is no longer heard (tests air conduction); repeat sequence on other ear

   2) Perform Weber test (which compares equality of hearing in both ears) by striking tuning fork, placing it on head in midline of skull, and asking the client if sound is heard equally on both sides (Figure 15-4); if so, document as no lateralization; if heard better in one ear or the other document as lateralizes to one side or other

j. Perform Romberg test to assess equilibrium by having client stand with feet together, arms at his or her side with eyes open and then with eyes closed; observe client for 20 seconds; client should be able to maintain position for 20 seconds with minimal swaying; if there is swaying document as such

B. Assessment of the nose and sinuses

   1. Inspection

      a. Inspect nose for shape, symmetry, and lesions and for signs of infection

      b. Test for nasal patency by occluding one naris and asking client to breathe through opposite naris; repeat procedure with opposite naris

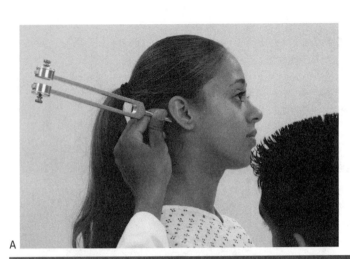

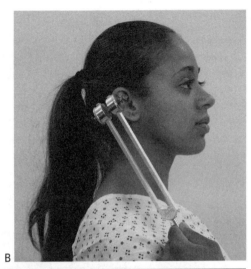

A

B

Figure 15-3

Using the Rinne test to compare bone and air conduction in the ear. A. Bone conduction. B. Air conduction.

2. Palpation

  a. Palpate external nose for tenderness, swelling, and stability by using two fingers to palpate nose, noting consistency and stability of underlying tissue

  b. Inspect nasal cavity using a nasal speculum by stabilizing client's erect head with non-dominant hand and inserting speculum with blades closed, then open blades to inspect nasal cavity; repeat procedure with head tilted backward (Figure 15-5)

  c. Palpate sinuses by pressing thumbs over frontal sinuses and maxillary sinuses and ask client if this produces pain (Figure 15-6)

Practice to Pass

To assess the nasal cavity the nurse should place the client in what position?

Figure 15-4

Performing the Weber test to compare bone conduction in each ear

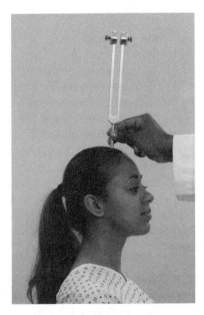

Figure 15-5

Proper use of a nasal speculum

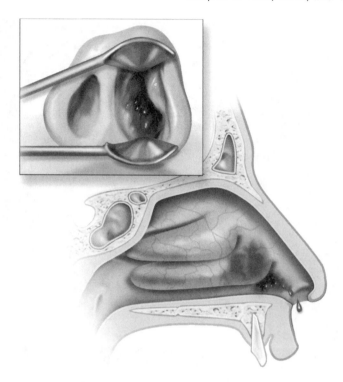

3. Percussion
   a. Percuss **frontal sinus** (air-filled cavities above the eyebrows) and ask client if he or she is experiencing pain
   b. Percuss **maxillary sinus** (air-filled cavities beside the nares) and ask client if he or she is experiencing pain

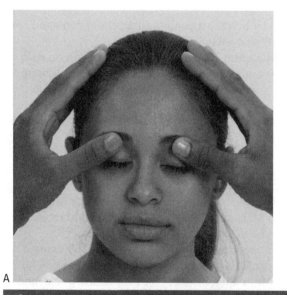
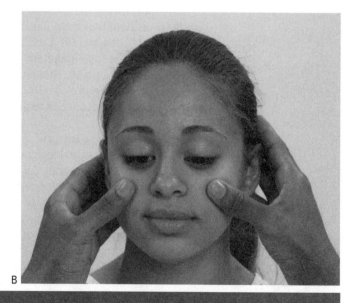

A   B

Figure 15-6

Palpation of sinuses. A. Frontal sinuses. B. Maxillary sinus.

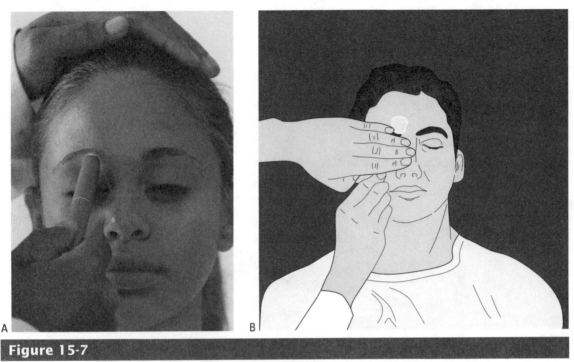

Figure 15-7

Transillumination of frontal sinuses. A. Placement of penlight. B. Covering area with non-dominant hand.

4. Transillumination
   a. Transilluminate frontal sinuses by holding a penlight under the supraorbital ridge (see Figure 15-7A) and covering with non-dominant hand (Figure 15-7B); observe for a red glow
   b. Transilluminate maxillary sinuses by holding a penlight over cheekbone and covering it; observe for a red glow on hard palate (Figure 15-8A)
   c. Transilluminate maxillary sinus by shining a penlight in client's mouth on each side of hard palate (one at a time) and observing for a red glow on cheekbone of same side (Figure 15-8B)

C. **Assessment of the mouth and throat**
   1. Inspection
      a. Inspect lips and observe for symmetry, color, moistness, and lesions
      b. Inspect teeth by asking client to smile while observing the mouth
      c. Inspect buccal mucosa, gums, and tongue using a penlight to assess inside of client's mouth for lesions, color, and continuity of mucosa; assess for movement
      d. Inspect salivary glands by assessing Wharton gland located in submandibular space close to frenulum as well as Stenson glands located near second molars; these glands should be without redness, swelling, or edema
      e. Inspect throat by asking client to open mouth and say "Aahh," while using a tongue blade; depress middle of arched tongue enough so that throat can be visualized; observe for rising of soft palate; inspect color of tonsils, uvula, and pharynx; observe for swelling, lesions, or inflammation, and for odors associated with mouth

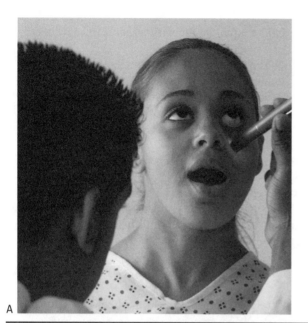
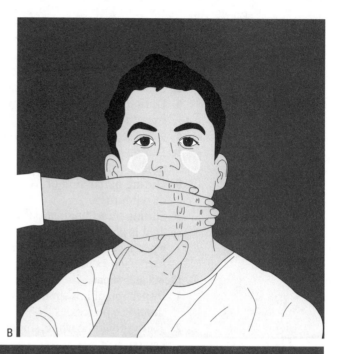

Figure 15-8

Transillumination of maxillary sinuses. A. Shining flashlight onto cheek. B. Shining flashlight onto hard palate.

VI. EXPECTED FINDINGS

A. Ear

1. Ear should be of same color as client's skin without redness, discharge, or swelling; there should be no nodules, lesions, or pain
2. The **auricle** (or **pinna**) (external ear) and tragus should be movable and pain should not be elicited
3. During examination of mastoid there should be no lesions, pain, or swelling
4. When using an otoscope to visualize auditory canal it should be patent without tenderness, inflammation, lesions, discharge, or foreign substances
5. Tympanic membrane should be flat, pearly gray, intact, and translucent with no scars; a cone-shaped reflection of otoscope light should be visible at the five o'clock position in right ear and seven o'clock position in left ear
6. When using an otoscope have client perform a valsalva maneuver and tympanic membrane should flutter
7. During a whisper test the client should be able to hear and be able to repeat back phrases whispered
8. Expected result of Rinne test is that **air conduction** (transmission of sound through tympanic membrane to auditory nerve) should be twice as long as **bone conduction** (transmission of sound through bones of skull to auditory nerve)
9. Expected result of the Weber test is that client should be able to hear sound bilaterally in both ears
10. During Romberg test client should be able to maintain position and balance with minimal swaying

B. Noses and sinuses
1. Nose should be straight; nares should be equal in size with intact skin; and there should not be drainage, tenderness, or swelling
2. During a test for patency, client should be able to breathe through each naris
3. During inspection of nares with speculum, mucous membranes should be pink and smooth without swelling, discharge, bleeding, or foreign bodies
4. Nasal septum should be midline, straight, and intact
5. During palpation of frontal and maxillary sinuses there should be no discomfort or tenderness
6. During percussion of frontal and maxillary sinuses there should be no pain or tenderness
7. During transillumination of sinuses there should be a red glow over frontal sinus if light is placed on the superior orbital ridge; maxillary sinuses should transilluminate when a penlight is placed in client's mouth; if maxillary sinus is illuminated then hard palate should transilluminate

C. Mouth and throat
1. Inspection of lips should reveal symmetrical, smooth, pink, moist membranes; there should be no lesions
2. Teeth should be white, smooth, and free of debris; there should be no loose or broken teeth
3. Gums should be pink and moist without redness, swelling, or edema
4. Tongue should be pink, moist, and smooth; there should be no lesions or nodules
5. Hard and soft palate should appear to have a consistent appearance

D. Salivary glands
1. Salivary glands should be visible with no pain, tenderness, redness, or swelling when palpated
2. When area around gland is touched saliva should be produced

E. Throat
1. During inspection of throat, the tonsils (if present) should be pink, without redness edema or swelling; there should be no odor
2. Uvula should be midline and rise when client says "aah"
3. Soft palate should rise when client says "aah"

Practice to Pass

What should the nurse expect to find during an otoscopic examination of the tympanic membrane or ears?

VII. UNEXPECTED FINDINGS

A. Ear
1. Drainage or foreign bodies should not be present during inspection of external ear; redness, presence of nodules or lesions, and swelling are unexpected findings; drainage may indicate an infection or allergy
2. Otitis externa is evident by observing redness and swelling on external ear and may be associated with itching, swelling, fever, and enlarged lymph glands; may also be indicated by tenderness elicited by pulling on pinna
3. When palpating auricle and tragus, presence of nodules, redness, lesions, or swelling is an unexpected finding
4. Pain is an unexpected finding during palpation of tragus as it may indicate otitis media or temporomandibular joint dysfunction (TMJ); nodules on external ear are known as tophi and are due to uric acid crystal formation as result of gouty arthritis
5. Lesions on external ear may be cancerous due to sun exposure
6. Pain on palpation of mastoid process could indicate mastoiditis, or a throat or inner ear infection; this finding should prompt immediate attention as it could lead to an infection of the brain
7. During an otoscopic examination, it is unexpected to find impacted cerumen; tympanic membrane should not have scars or white patches as this indicates a history of

infections; redness or a yellow tympanic membrane may indicate a prior infection; bulging of the tympanic membrane may indicate increased inner ear pressure whereas a retracted tympanic membrane may indicate eustachian tube blockage

8. Rigidity of tympanic membrane is considered abnormal
9. Blood or a bluish tint on tympanic membrane indicates blood in middle ear; otitis media is evidenced by a red, bulging tympanic membrane that does not reflect light
10. A perforated tympanic membrane is found on otoscopic examination as a dark spot on tympanic membrane
11. A scarred tympanic membrane usually produces white patches on tympanic membrane and is a result of inner ear infections
12. If client is unable to repeat words during a whisper test, this indicates a loss of high frequency hearing
13. During Rinne test, bone conduction of sound should be longer then air conduction; if not, then it may indicate conductive hearing loss
14. During Weber test it is considered abnormal to lateralize sound; sound should be heard equally in both ears
15. If client is unable to maintain balance or needs to move his or her feet apart during Romberg test, then this is considered an abnormal finding indicating a neuro-vestibular problem

B. Nose and sinuses
1. Client should not have noisy breathing; breathing should be effortless; noisy breathing may indicate airway obstruction or inflammation
2. Presence of discharge may indicate infection or allergies
3. Deviation or asymmetry during inspection of nose could indicate nasal trauma
4. During an inspection of nasal mucosa, red and swollen tissue indicates inflammation or infection; if nasal mucosa is pale, boggy, or swollen, client may be experiencing allergies
5. Epistaxis is an abnormal finding associated with rhinitis, hypertension, trauma, or a bleeding disorder
6. A deviated septum is an unexpected finding during an inspection of the nares as this usually is the result of trauma; there should not be a perforated septum as this is associated with infection, trauma, or substance inhalation
7. Rhinitis is inflammation of nares due to allergy or infection; associated with watery discharge, sneezing, and congestion
8. Sinusitis is inflammation of sinuses associated with facial pain, discharge, fever, chills, and a throbbing pain in face
9. In a client with chronic allergies, nasal polyps may develop; polyps are pale benign growths
10. It is abnormal to have tenderness or pain during palpation of sinuses
11. Transillumination of sinuses will not occur if the sinuses are fluid filled or inflamed

C. Mouth and throat
1. During inspection of lips, there should be no lesions as this may indicate a viral infection or cancer
2. There should be no cyanosis or pallor of lips or mucosa as this indicates hypoxia
3. Loose, broken, or misaligned teeth; or inflamed gums indicate a lack of dental care and warrants further attention and evaluation
4. Hyperplasia of gums is the result of pregnancy, phenytoin (Dilantin) use, or leukemia
5. A smooth or coated tongue may indicate dehydration or an underlying disease process such as iron or vitamin B deficiency; tongue should not have tremors as this indicates a problem with the hypoglossal cranial nerve
6. A small tongue can indicate malnutrition; it can also be a sign of several other abnormal conditions
7. Lesions on tongue may indicate a cancerous condition; white patches on tongue are known as leukoplakia

Practice to Pass

The client has a history of seizures, which are controlled by medication. Based on this information the nurse should perform what assessment?

8. Hairy tongue can be caused by a fungal infection and is associated with prolonged antibiotic use, smoking, and tea drinking; it can also result from poor oral hygiene

9. Ankyloglossia is a finding in which tip of tongue is fixated to floor of mouth

10. Aphthous ulcers or canker sores are small white lesions that result from trauma, food irritants, stress, exhaustion, and allergies

D. **Salivary glands: pain, redness, or tenderness indicates an obstruction or infection of salivary glands**

E. **Throat**

1. Mucosa of throat should be pink as redness indicates infection

2. Odors are considered abnormal

3. A red and swollen throat usually indicates pharyngitis; white spots usually indicate infection

VIII. LIFESPAN CONSIDERATIONS

A. **Infants**

1. Salivation begins around three months of age; teeth begin to erupt between six months and two years; mucous membranes of nose and mouth should be pink and without lesions

2. Do not use a nasal speculum on an infant as nares are too small for speculum

3. External ear should be well formed and should not be low set as this may indicate Down's Syndrome; until six months of age the tympanic membrane may diffuse light; infant should startle at a loud sound

B. **Older adult**

1. Older adults may have hair in auditory canal; ears become more prominent and thicker in appearance as part of aging process due to cartilage growth

2. Ability to hear high-frequency sounds is decreased and eventually ability to hear low-pitched sounds is lost; this is known as presbycusis

3. Lips and mucosa of mouth become thinner and less vascular; tongue develops fissures

4. An older adult client may develop a decreased sense of taste and smell, which may lead to poor appetite; gums may recede and tooth loss may occur

IX. DOCUMENTATION

A. **Document condition of external ear such as color and presence of lesions, discharge, and edema**

B. **Describe findings of an otoscopic examination such as condition of tympanic membrane, presence of discharge, color, and light reflex**

C. **Hearing acuity and balance should also be included**

Case Study

An adult client presents in the clinic with pain in the left ear since yesterday. Vital signs are within normal limits except for a temperature of 100.6° F. The external ear is without redness, swelling, or lesions. Otoscopic examination reveals discharge and a red tympanic membrane with a cone of light at seven o'clock. No perforation is found. Mouth, gums, and nose findings are within normal limits.

1. What other assessments should be performed?

2. What other health history should the nurse obtain?

3. What is the most appropriate nursing diagnosis for the nurse to develop a plan of care?

4. What will the nurse expect to happen to the tympanic membrane?

5. What assessment technique will the nurse use to perform the otoscopic assessment?

For suggested responses, see page 311

POSTTEST

1 The nurse performing the Rinne test on a client would expect to document which finding if the client's result is normal?

1. Bone conduction is greater than air conduction
2. Air conduction is greater than bone conduction
3. The client can hear a whispered voice
4. Sound is lateralized in one ear

2 To assess the sinuses, the nurse would perform the following assessments in what order?

1. Inspect nasal cavity with speculum
2. Palpate sinuses for tenderness
3. Transilluminate the sinuses
4. Percuss the sinuses

3 The nurse assesses the nasal turbinates and observes a pale, boggy, swollen mucosa. To what problem would the nurse most likely attribute these findings?

1. Allergies
2. Infection
3. Nasal polyps
4. Pharyngitis

4 The nurse would palpate the tongue to evaluate for which oral health problem?

1. Infection
2. Lesions or nodules
3. Allergic reaction
4. Polyps

5 To assess the maxillary sinus the nurse should use which technique(s)? Select all that apply.

1. Shine the light on each side of the hard palate and observe for red glow on cheeks
2. Shine the light above the eyebrow
3. Shine the light below the eyebrow and cover it with hand while observing sinus for glow
4. Shine the light on the cheek and observe for glow on the hard palate
5. Palpate sinuses with one finger

6 To assess the mastoid process, the nurse would perform which technique?

1. Palpate the external ear
2. Use an otoscope to examine the inner ear
3. Palpate behind the ear
4. Inspect the external ear

7 When teaching a middle-aged client about hearing screening or testing the nurse includes that hearing should be evaluated how often?

1. Every six months
2. Annually
3. Every two years
4. Every five years

8 To gather data about a client's report of tinnitus the nurse would ask the client about which factor that could be the etiology of the symptom?

1. Loud noise
2. Previous infections
3. Medication use
4. Ear drainage

9 When the client presents to the clinic with a problem related to the sinuses, the nurse should gather data about which possible related problem?

1. Respiratory system infection
2. Humming in the ears
3. Difficulty swallowing
4. Hearing loss

10 If the client reports dizziness and a loss of hearing, the nurse should perform which test to further evaluate the problem?

1. Rinne
2. Weber
3. Romberg
4. Whisper

➤ *See pages 301–303 for Answers and Rationales.*

ANSWERS & RATIONALES

Pretest

1 **Answer: 2** **Rationale:** The pearly gray tympanic membrane reflects the otoscope light at the five or seven o'clock position (option 2). "Pink and shiny in appearance" does not describe any ear structure (option 1). Cerumen is a yellow waxy substance that lubricates and protects the ear but does not cover the entire tympanic membrane (option 3). A beefy red color to the tympanic membrane usually reflects an inflammation of the structure (option 4).
Cognitive Level: Application **Client Need:** Health Promotion and Maintenance **Integrated Process:** Communication and Documentation **Content Area:** Adult Health: Eye, Ear, Nose, and Throat **Strategy:** Eliminate option 3, containing the words "covered with...cerumen," as not all people produce cerumen to cover their tympanic membrane. Eliminate option 4 next because a beefy red color usually indicates inflammation. Finally, eliminate option 1 as the tympanic membrane should not be shiny.
Reference: D'Amico, D. & Barbarito, C. (2007). *Health & physical assessment in nursing.* Upper Saddle River, NJ: Pearson Education, Inc., p. 322.

2 **Answer: 3** **Rationale:** Otosclerosis, an abnormal growth of bone of the middle ear that prevents structures within the ear from working properly, is a conductive hearing loss that results in the client needing increased volume to hear (option 3). For some people with otosclerosis, the hearing loss may become severe. Infections do not usually cause a hearing deficit (option 1). Presbycusis is hearing loss associated with aging (option 2). Labyrinthitis is an inflammation or infection of the labyrinth causing the sensation of spinning but not hearing loss (option 4).
Cognitive Level: Analysis **Client Need:** Health Promotion and Maintenance **Integrated Process:** Nursing Process: Assessment **Content Area:** Adult Health: Eye, Ear, Nose, and Throat **Strategy:** Eliminate options 1 and 4 first as these are infection processes. Eliminate option 2 next as presbycusis is a hearing loss associated with aging.
Reference: D'Amico, D. & Barbarito, C. (2007). *Health & physical assessment in nursing.* Upper Saddle River, NJ: Pearson Education, Inc., pp. 311, 325.

3 **Answer: 1** **Rationale:** For the adult client the nurse should pull the pinna up and back to visualize the inner ear (option 1). For a child client the nurse should pull the pinna down and back (option 2). Tilting the head backward may not increase client comfort (option 3). Tilting the head to the opposite shoulder when the ear is being examined will make assessment easier. The nurse should select the smallest speculum that will afford maximum visualization (option 4).
Cognitive Level: Application **Client Need:** Health Promotion and Maintenance **Integrated Process:** Nursing Process: Implementation **Content Area:** Adult Health: Eye, Ear, Nose, and Throat **Strategy:** Remember adults are tall so pull the pinna up and back, whereas children are short so pull the pinna down and back. **Reference:** D'Amico, D. & Barbarito, C. (2007). *Health & physical assessment in nursing.* Upper Saddle River, NJ: Pearson Education, Inc., p. 321.

4 **Answer: 1** **Rationale:** During the Weber test the client hears the sound from a tuning fork in the ear with the poorer hearing (option 1). The right ear would not hear the sound better because it is the poorer ear in which the sound is heard (option 2). Presbycusis is a decrease in hearing that is associated with aging (option 3). Inner ear infections should not cause hearing loss (option 4).
Cognitive Level: Application **Client Need:** Health Promotion and Maintenance **Integrated Process:** Nursing Process: Assessment **Content Area:** Adult Health: Eye, Ear, Nose, and Throat **Strategy:** Eliminate the inner ear infection option 4 as this does not involve hearing loss. Eliminate option 3 as the client is not specified as an older adult, and presbycusis affects older adults. Recognize that in options 1 and 2, the client will hear the tuning fork in the ear with the poorer hearing due to background noise. **Reference:** D'Amico, D. & Barbarito, C. (2007). *Health & physical assessment in nursing.* Upper Saddle River, NJ: Pearson Education, Inc., pp. 324 and 325.

5 **Answer: 3** **Rationale:** Middle ear infections cause scarring of the tympanic membrane (option 3). Conductive hearing loss is usually due to trauma or infection (option 1). Sensorineural hearing loss is the result of nerve degradation (option 3). Sticking an object in the ear would produce a puncture scar and not scarring (option 4).
Cognitive Level: Application **Client Need:** Health Promotion and Maintenance **Integrated Process:** Nursing Process: Assessment **Content Area:** Adult Health: Eye, Ear, Nose, and Throat **Strategy:** Recall that conductive hearing loss is

due to trauma or infection, whereas sensorineural deficits are due to nerve damage. Recognize that sticking an object in the ear would cause a conductive hearing deficit as it is a traumatic injury. **Reference:** D'Amico, D. & Barbarito, C. (2007). *Health & physical assessment in nursing.* Upper Saddle River, NJ: Pearson Education, Inc., p. 325.

6 **Answers: 2, 3, 4, 5** **Rationale:** To gather data about the client's hearing the nurse should ask about the ability to hear, changes in hearing, the client's last hearing test, and whether hearing is better in one ear than the other. External otitis is also known as swimmer's ear (option 1). It is an inflammation of the outer ear canal and does not affect hearing.
Cognitive Level: Analysis **Client Need:** Health Promotion and Maintenance **Integrated Process:** Nursing Process: Assessment **Content Area:** Adult Health: Eye, Ear, Nose, and Throat **Strategy:** Eliminate option 1 as external otitis is not a middle or inner ear problem that will affect hearing. **Reference:** D'Amico, D. & Barbarito, C. (2007). *Health & physical assessment in nursing.* Upper Saddle River, NJ: Pearson Education, Inc., p. 313.

7 **Answer: 1** **Rationale:** The nares are assessed by occluding one naris and having the client breathe through the opposite naris and then repeating the procedure (option 1). Pain in the nares may indicate infection or inflammation (option 2). Palpation of the nares may indicate infection or inflammation (option 3). Inspection with a speculum will provide visualization of the inner nares (option 4).
Cognitive Level: Application **Client Need:** Health Promotion and Maintenance **Integrated Process:** Nursing Process: Assessment **Content Area:** Adult Health: Eye, Ear, Nose, and Throat **Strategy:** Eliminate option 4 first as that is a technique for inspection of the inner nares. Recall that palpation is used to detect pain, which helps to eliminate option 3. Finally, eliminate option 2 as it is not an assessment technique. **Reference:** D'Amico, D. & Barbarito, C. (2007). *Health & physical assessment in nursing.* Upper Saddle River, NJ: Pearson Education, Inc., p. 326.

8 **Answer: 2** **Rationale:** Transillumination of the sinuses that results in no red glow usually indicates an inflammation of the sinuses (option 2). Transillumination of the sinuses normally results in a red glow of the sinuses (option 1). A mass, such as a large number of polyps filling the sinuses, are visualized with a nasal speculum (option 3). Hearing is assessed through the technique of the Weber test or the whispered hearing test (option 4).
Cognitive Level: Application **Client Need:** Health Promotion and Maintenance **Integrated Process:** Nursing Process: Assessment **Content Area:** Adult Health: Eye, Ear, Nose, and Throat **Strategy:** Eliminate option 4 as the hearing is not usually affected by the sinuses. Next recall that polyps are assessed by the use of a nasal speculum and not a flashlight to eliminate option 3. Recall that sinuses should transilluminate to choose option 2 over option 1.

Reference: D'Amico, D. & Barbarito, C. (2007). *Health & physical assessment in nursing.* Upper Saddle River, NJ: Pearson Education, Inc., pp. 392.

9 **Answer: 4** **Rationale:** Blue-tinged lips or cyanotic lips usually indicate hypoxia (option 4). A fever blister is due to stress and is a blister-like lesion (option 1). A lack of dental care would result in loose painful teeth or inflamed gums (option 2). An inflammation of the lips would produce redness, swelling, or tenderness (option 3).
Cognitive Level: Application **Client Need:** Health Promotion and Maintenance **Integrated Process:** Nursing Process: Assessment **Content Area:** Adult Health: Eye, Ear, Nose, and Throat **Strategy:** Eliminate option 2 as a lack of dental care causes inflammation of the mouth and poor dentition. Eliminate options 3 and 4 as inflammation would produce redness and swelling. **Reference:** D'Amico, D. & Barbarito, C. (2007). *Health & physical assessment in nursing.* Upper Saddle River, NJ: Pearson Education, Inc., pp. 330–331.

10 **Answer: 2** **Rationale:** Ankyloglossia is a term used to describe a fixation of the tongue (option 2). Ulcerations are lesions due to trauma, stress, or allergies (option 1). Carcinoma is a non-healing lesion that can result from alcohol, smoking, using a pipe, or chewing tobacco (option 3). Leukoplakia is a precancerous condition in which the tongue or mucous membranes develop a whitish thickening that is non-removable (option 4).
Cognitive Level: Application **Client Need:** Health Promotion and Maintenance **Integrated Process:** Communication and Documentation **Content Area:** Adult Health: Eye, Ear, Nose, and Throat **Strategy:** Recall that the prefix *anky-* means fixation and the suffix *-glossia* indicates tongue to select option 2. **Reference:** D'Amico, D. & Barbarito, C. (2007). *Health & physical assessment in nursing.* Upper Saddle River, NJ: Pearson Education, Inc., p. 339.

Posttest

1 **Answer: 2** **Rationale:** The Rinne test consists of striking the tuning fork and placing it on the mastoid process. When the client can no longer hear the sound the tuning fork is placed in front of the mastoid process and air conduction should be heard for twice as long as it was felt on the mastoid process (option 2). Bone conduction should be shorter than air conduction (option 1). If bone conduction is longer than air conduction then the client is experiencing a conductive hearing loss. The whispered voice test is performed by having the client cover one ear while the nurse whispers and evaluates if the client can hear it (option 3). When sound lateralizes to one ear after a tuning fork is placed on the center of the head, this indicates conductive hearing loss (option 4).
Cognitive Level: Application **Client Need:** Health Promotion and Maintenance **Integrated Process:** Communication and Documentation **Content Area:** Adult Health: Eye, Ear, Nose, and Throat **Strategy:** The test taking strategy that

can be applied here is the rule of opposites as options 1 and 2 are opposites. Whispered voice and the Weber test also evaluate hearing but are not associated with the Rinne test. **Reference:** D'Amico, D. & Barbarito, C. (2007). *Health & physical assessment in nursing.* Upper Saddle River, NJ: Pearson Education, Inc., p. 324.

2 Answers: 1, 2, 4, 3 Rationale: The correct order of the assessment of the sinuses should be inspection of the nasal cavity (option 1), then palpation of the sinuses for tenderness (option 2), percussion of the sinuses (option 4), and finally transillumination of the sinuses (option 3). **Cognitive Level:** Application **Client Need:** Health Promotion and Maintenance **Integrated Process:** Nursing Process: Assessment **Content Area:** Adult Health: Eye, Ear, Nose, and Throat **Strategy:** Recall that the order of assessment is usually inspection, palpation, percussion, and auscultation. Then recall that the sinuses are not auscultated but rather transilluminated. **Reference:** D'Amico, D. & Barbarito, C. (2007). *Health & physical assessment in nursing.* Upper Saddle River, NJ: Pearson Education, Inc., pp. 327–332.

3 Answer: 1 Rationale: Allergies cause the nasal turbinates to become pale, swollen, and boggy (option 1). Infection produces red, inflamed mucosa (option 2). Nasal polyps are small growths in the nasal cavity (option 3). Pharyngitis is an inflammation of the pharynx (option 4). **Cognitive Level:** Application **Client Need:** Health Promotion and Maintenance **Integrated Process:** Nursing Process: Assessment **Content Area:** Adult Health: Eye, Ear, Nose, and Throat **Strategy:** Recognize that options 2 and 4 would produce redness and not pale membranes. Polyps are growths so the only viable option is 1 to produce paleness. **Reference:** D'Amico, D. & Barbarito, C. (2007). *Health & physical assessment in nursing.* Upper Saddle River, NJ: Pearson Education, Inc., p. 327.

4 Answer: 2 Rationale: The nurse should palpate the tongue for lesions and nodules to evaluate for possible malignant growths (option 2). Infection would leave the tongue red (option 1). Allergic reactions will produce a swollen tongue if the client is experiencing an allergic reaction (option 3). Polyps are not found on the tongue but rather in the nasal cavity (option 4). **Cognitive Level:** Application **Client Need:** Health Promotion and Maintenance **Integrated Process:** Nursing Process: Assessment **Content Area:** Adult Health: Eye, Ear, Nose, and Throat **Strategy:** Eliminate options in which palpation would not elicit the findings. Infection and a swollen tongue are assessed by inspection. Polyps are not found in the oral cavity but rather the nasal cavity. **Reference:** D'Amico, D. & Barbarito, C. (2007). *Health & physical assessment in nursing.* Upper Saddle River, NJ: Pearson Education, Inc., p. 331.

5 Answers: 1, 4, 5 Rationale: The maxillary sinuses are assessed by shining a light on the hard palate and inspecting for a red glow on the cheeks, or shining a light on the cheeks and observing a glow on the hard palate, or by palpating the sinuses with one finger. Shining the light above the eyebrow (option 2) or shining

the light below the eyebrow and covering it with the hand while observing the sinus for a glow (option 3) will not achieve the desired result of accurate assessment of the maxillary sinus. **Cognitive Level:** Application **Client Need:** Health Promotion and Maintenance **Integrated Process:** Nursing Process: Assessment **Content Area:** Adult Health: Eye, Ear, Nose, and Throat **Strategy:** Recall that the frontal sinuses are located under the eyebrow so eliminate options 2 and 3. The maxillary sinuses are located on either side of the nose. **Reference:** D'Amico, D. & Barbarito, C. (2007). *Health & physical assessment in nursing.* Upper Saddle River, NJ: Pearson Education, Inc., pp. 328–330.

6 Answer: 3 Rationale: The nurse would palpate behind the external ear to determine if there are lesions, pain, or swelling (option 3). Palpating the external ear will provide data about the tragus and auricle (option 1). Using an otoscope will provide information about the auditory canal (option 2). Inspecting the external ear should provide information about problems such as redness, nodules, swelling, or lesions (option 4). **Cognitive Level:** Application **Client Need:** Health Promotion and Maintenance **Integrated Process:** Nursing Process: Assessment **Content Area:** Adult Health: Eye, Ear, Nose, and Throat **Strategy:** Eliminate option 2, as the otoscope is used to assess the auditory canal. Options 1 and 4 will provide data about the external ear. The mastoid process could become inflamed from a middle ear or throat infection. **Reference:** D'Amico, D. & Barbarito, C. (2007). *Health & physical assessment in nursing.* Upper Saddle River, NJ: Pearson Education, Inc., p. 320.

7 Answer: 2 Rationale: Hearing should be assessed annually in children, middle-aged adults, and older adults (option 2). The other options are not recommended. **Cognitive Level:** Application **Client Need:** Health Promotion and Maintenance **Integrated Process:** Teaching and Learning **Content Area:** Adult Health: Eye, Ear, Nose, and Throat **Strategy:** Recall that hearing should be evaluated every year in children, middle-aged adults, and older adults who are subjected to noise. **Reference:** D'Amico, D. & Barbarito, C. (2007). *Health & physical assessment in nursing.* Upper Saddle River, NJ: Pearson Education, Inc., p. 313.

8 Answer: 3 Rationale: Many medications such as aspirin and furosemide (Lasix) can cause tinnitus so the nurse should always assess medication use in the client who reports ringing in the ears (option 3). Loud noise can cause hearing loss but not tinnitus (option 1). Infections will produce pain, ear drainage, or fever. Infections may cause hearing loss but are usually not associated with tinnitus (option 2). Ear drainage is a sign of an infection and is not associated with tinnitus (option 4). **Cognitive Level:** Application **Client Need:** Health Promotion and Maintenance **Integrated Process:** Nursing Process: Assessment **Content Area:** Adult Health: Eye, Ear, Nose, and Throat **Strategy:** Eliminate options 2 and 4 as ear drainage is a symptom of infection. Recall that loud noise does not cause tinnitus. **Reference:** D'Amico, D. & Barbarito, C. (2007). *Health & physical assessment in nursing.* Upper Saddle River, NJ: Pearson Education, Inc., pp. 315–317.

9 **Answer: 1** **Rationale:** A history of respiratory problems or the presence of a current respiratory infection may be related to a client's current sinus infection (option 1). Humming in the ear is associated with hypertension during pregnancy (option 2). Difficulty swallowing (dysphagia) is associated with a tooth problem, ill fitting dentures, cancer, or esophageal problems but is not associated with sinus problems (option 3). Hearing loss is not a symptom of a sinus problem but a neurological or sensory problem (option 4).
Cognitive Level: Application **Client Need:** Health Promotion and Maintenance **Integrated Process:** Nursing Process: Assessment **Content Area:** Adult Health: Eye, Ear, Nose, and Throat **Strategy:** Recall that when evaluating a sinus problem, the nurse should gather data about ability to breathe, discharge, nosebleeds, injuries, or surgeries.

Reference: D'Amico, D. & Barbarito, C. (2007). *Health & physical assessment in nursing.* Upper Saddle River, NJ: Pearson Education, Inc., pp. 316–317.

10 **Answer: 3** **Rationale:** The Romberg test evaluates equilibrium and balance (option 3). The Rinne test compares air to bone conduction of sound (option 1). The Weber test evaluates bone conduction in the client who states he or she hears better in one ear than the other (option 2). The whisper test evaluates hearing acuity with higher frequency sounds (option 4).
Cognitive Level: Application **Client Need:** Health Promotion and Maintenance **Integrated Process:** Nursing Process: Assessment **Content Area:** Adult Health: Eye, Ear, Nose, and Throat **Strategy:** Recognize that the Rinne, Weber, and Whisper tests all evaluate hearing whereas the Romberg test is the only test that evaluates balance. **Reference:** D'Amico, D. & Barbarito, C. (2007). *Health & physical assessment in nursing.* Upper Saddle River, NJ: Pearson Education, Inc., pp. 323–325.

References

Bickley, L. (2010). *Bates guide to physical examination and history taking* (10th ed.). Philadelphia: Lippincott Williams & Wilkins.

D'Amico, D. & Barbarito, C. (2007). *Health and physical assessment in nursing.* Upper Saddle River, NJ: Pearson Education, Inc.

Jarvis, C. (2008). *Physical examination and health assessment* (5th ed.). St. Louis, MO: Elsevier Saunders.

Brown, P. (2008). Vertigo. *Pulse, 682,* 35–38.

Zator Estes, M. (2009). *Health assessment and physical examination* (4th ed.). Clifton Park, NY: Delmar Cengage Learning.

Appendix

➤ **Practice to Pass Suggested Answers**

Chapter 1

Page 3: *Answer* — The nurse should provide for privacy, maintain a comfortable temperature, ensure adequate lighting, and sit at eye level with the client.

Page 5: *Answer* — The nurse should use the client's own words to document the chief complaint.

Page 6: *Answer* — The nurse should include the client's history of immunizations, allergies, illnesses, mental health history, and any substance use.

Page 6: *Answer* — The nurse should include information about the health of the client's relatives incorporating chronic illnesses, relationships to the client, causes of death, occupations, and status of health.

Page 10: *Answer* — The nurse should make sure that documentation is clear, concise, timely, legible, and confidential.

Chapter 2

Page 18: *Answer* — To provide privacy before a physical exam, the nurse drapes the client, offers a blanket, closes doors, draws curtains, makes sure conversations can not be overheard and makes sure only one body part is examined at a time.

Page 19: *Answer* — Because the liver is a dense organ that does not lie near the surface of the thorax, the liver is assessed using deep palpation, which is also the skill used to palpate other internal organs.

Page 21: *Answer* — The nurse would expect to hear tympany when percussing an empty bladder.

Page 21: *Answer* — The earpieces of a stethoscope should be positioned toward the nares to maximize sound.

Page 22: *Answer* — Physical assessment of a client is systematically performed beginning with the skill of inspection.

Chapter 3

Page 40: *Answer* — Genetics is an important component of a psychosocial assessment since genetics has an influence on every health problem (except trauma) that people can have throughout their lifetime. A person's genetic makeup influences physical and psychosocial health, so it is important to document relevant genetic influences such as a family history of hypertension, diabetes, mental illness, and other illnesses to indicate some features the person may have or could inherit from his or her parents.

Page 41: *Answer* — The nurse is gathering information about relationships and trying to establish the client's ability to engage in or form bonds with others in his or her life.

Page 41: *Answer* — In order to gather the most significant information about a client, the nurse includes in a psychosocial assessment the client's personal and family beliefs, values, morals and customs that provide a pattern of living. This helps to design and implement a more individualized plan of care for the client.

Page 43: *Answer* — The nurse understands that client safety is the most important consideration for a client in any situation. The nurse does not begin an admission process if the client's physical condition is not stable.

Page 44: *Answer* — The nurse must use listening and observation skills to gather valuable data from the client. These cues can include the client's posture, grooming, speech pattern, eye contact, and verbalization methods.

Chapter 4

Page 59: *Answer* — Excess caloric intake, excessive alcohol intake, and lack of knowledge about food consumption and preparation are common causes of overnutrition.

Page 59: *Answer* — Food intolerances or allergies may cause nutrient deficiencies. Food allergies may cause abdominal discomfort, skin rash or hives, nausea, vomiting or diarrhea. Severe allergic reactions will cause anaphylaxis.

Page 61: *Answer* — [(165 − 143) / 165] × 100 = 13.3%. The client lost 13.3% of his or her body weight.

Page 62: *Answer*—A client with a BMI of 16 would be classified as being moderately malnourished.

Page 62: *Answer*—A female client with a waist circumference of 96 cm is at risk for cardiovascular disease because women should have a waist circumference less than 88 cm.

Page 62: *Answer*—The nurse should teach the client that skinfold measurements provide data about subcutaneous fat stores. This information can then be used as part of the overall assessment of nutritional status.

Chapter 5

Page 79: *Answer*—The nurse should ask about a history of congenital heart disease, childhood rheumatic fever, repeated sore throat or tonsillitis, unexplained joint pains, or anemia.

Page 81: *Answer*—The nurse should determine how long the client has had the edema; whether it decreases with rest, elevation, or after sleep; whether the client needs to get up at night to urinate (and if so, for how long); if the edema is accompanied by other symptoms such as shortness of breath; and whether the client has noticed any weight gain or loss that corresponds to the amount of edema present.

Page 82: *Answer*—The nurse should gather an examination gown and a drape for the client, as well as a stethoscope with a diaphragm, a bell, and a flashlight. The nurse should also ensure that the room chosen has adequate lighting, preferably with a natural light source.

Page 85: *Answer*—The nurse would expect to use palpation to locate the point of maximal impulse on the anterior chest (usually 5th intercostal space, mid-clavicular line) and to assess the adequacy of the carotid, brachial, radial, femoral, popliteal, dorsalis pedis, and posterior tibial pulses.

Page 87: *Answer*—The nurse should detect whether the client has a systolic or diastolic murmur (or both), how loud it is (grade 1 to 6), whether it is continuous during systole or diastole (or only for part of the cycle), the sound configuration of the murmur (gets softer or louder, is continuous, or has a crescendo/decrescendo pattern), the quality (blowing, harsh, musical, raspy, or rumbling) and pitch (low, medium or high) of the murmur, where it is best heard using the cardiac landmarks, whether it radiates to the throat or axilla, whether the pattern increases or decreases during inspiration and expiration, whether it is associated with variations in heart sounds, and if the intensity of the murmur changes when the client changes position (squatting, left lateral position).

Chapter 6

Page 101: *Answer*—The health history will provide information about age, symptoms, and exposure to environmental toxins.

Page 101: *Answer*—The past medical history is used to identify predisposing factors and previous medical problems.

Page 104: *Answer*—The nurse should document respiratory inspection findings related to symmetry, color, contour, anterior posterior diameter, respiratory rate, and use of accessory muscles.

Page 105: *Answer*—When assessing for fremitus the nurse should palpate for vibration on the chest when the client speaks. The nurse asks the client to say "99" or "1, 2, 3."

Page 110: *Answer*—During the assessment for bronchophony, the nurse should hear muffled sounds.

Page 111: *Answer*—The client who has a dusky color would require assessment of oxygen saturation via pulse oximeter, should be positioned upright, and he or she should be further evaluated.

Page 111: *Answer*—The respiratory pattern that the nurse would expect to observe in a client who has fever and is experiencing anxiety is tachypnea.

Page 112: *Answer*—The nurse should expect crackles to be heard on expiration, since this is the usual presentation.

Page 113: *Answer*—The infant should be held by the parent.

Chapter 7

Page 122: *Answer*—The nurse should ask if the client is intentionally dieting or if the client has an idea about what is causing the weight change. The nurse should also assess for any other associated symptoms. Next the nurse should conduct a dietary history, including foods eaten in the last 24 hours, routine food intake from each of the food groups, and ask if the client's current diet is customary for him.

Page 126: *Answer*—The nurse will need to gather a gown (as the client will need to undress), a drape or blanket to cover the client, examination gloves, a light source, stethoscope, skin marker, metric ruler, tissues, and a tape measure. The nurse should explain the procedure to the client, provide a warm and well lit environment, and place all equipment within easy reach. The nurse should position the client supine with a pillow under his or her head and knees to ensure the abdominal muscles are relaxed.

Page 127: *Answer*—The nurse should first note the contour of the abdomen between the costal margins and the symphysis pubis, noting whether it is flat, rounded or protuberant, or, scaphoid or concave. The nurse next observes the umbilicus and notes whether it is centrally located, and whether it is inverted or protruding. General observations of abdominal skin include color, texture, lesions, scars or other markings. The nurse also looks for symmetry side to side and for the presence of any bulges or masses. Finally the nurse inspects whether peristalsis is visible, or whether there are any pulsations in the abdomen.

Page 129: *Answer*—The nurse should auscultate all four quadrants of the abdomen to assess for bowel sounds. The nurse should complete auscultation after inspection and before percussion and palpation to avoid altering characteristics of bowel sounds, which may correspond to the client's abdominal problem and source of pain. The nurse auscultates in each quadrant, one at a time, usually beginning in the right lower quadrant, and listening for 60 seconds in each quadrant as needed for accurate assessment.

Page 131: *Answer*—The nurse should palpate for rebound tenderness by holding his or her hand on the abdomen at a 90-degree angle to the abdominal wall and pressing deeply into abdomen, then withdrawing the fingers quickly and asking the client if he or she experiences pain with this maneuver (most clients will show visible signs of pain if positive).

Chapter 8

Page 144: *Answer*—A client who experienced frontal lobe injury would exhibit alterations in any of the following areas of function: skeletal movement, speech, emotions, and intellectual activities such as the following: intellect, reasoning, judgment, and ability to learn and think abstractly.

Page 144: *Answer*—A client who develops a fever immediately on arrival to the Emergency Department following a motor vehicle accident most likely has suffered damage to the hypothalamus.

Page 144: *Answer*—The function of CSF is to act as a shock absorber to protect the spinal cord and brain.

Page 145: *Answer*—When assessing the gag reflex, the nurse is evaluating the function of the glossopharyngeal nerve.

Page 146: *Answer*—Questions to ask include the following:

- Do you experience headaches?
- Tell me about the frequency of your headaches?
- Where is the headache located?
- Is the headache associated with anything?

Page 147: *Answer*—To conduct a neurological exam, the nurse should position the client in a sitting position, but the client may lie supine if his or her condition does not allow the client to tolerate sitting.

Page 148: *Answer*—If the client does not respond when his or her name is called, the nurse should gently shake the client, such as on the shoulder area, to try to arouse the client.

Page 149: *Answer*—The most appropriate method for assessing the corneal reflex is to use a wisp of cotton to touch the cornea.

Page 150: *Answer*—Air conduction is longer than bone.

Page 152: *Answer*—The nurse would need a Snellen eye chart to test a client's vision.

Page 152: *Answer*—The nurse should have the client puff out his or her cheeks to evaluate CN VII.

Page 153: *Answer*—False—A reflex is involuntary.

Page 153: *Answer*—No, the Babinski should not be evaluated during every assessment; rather, it should only be assessed when a deficit is suspected.

Page 154: *Answer*—The medical term for edema of the optic disk is papilledema.

Page 155: *Answer*—The nurse would evaluate for cerebellar disease by performing the Romberg test, and would assess the acoustic nerve using the Rinne and Weber Tests.

Chapter 9

Page 168: *Answer*—The nurse should assess for the common symptoms of pain; stiffness in the knee joint; the presence of any swelling, heat, or redness; and any limitation of movement.

Page 169: *Answer*—To complete a musculoskeletal assessment, the nurse needs a tape measure, goniometer, and skin marking pen. The client should be given an examination gown, and the examiner explains that part of the exam will be done with the client standing and other parts will be done with the client sitting.

Page 174: *Answer*—The nurse should ask the client to do each of the following movements: Make a tight fist with each hand with fingers folded into palm and thumb across knuckles (thumb flexion); open fist and stretch fingers (extension); point fingers downward toward forearm, then back as far as able; spread fingers far apart and then together; move thumb toward ulnar side of hand and then away from hand to extent possible; touch thumb to tip of each finger and to base of little finger.

Page 176: *Answers*—The nurse should note that the client's legs are slightly apart and the toes are pointed toward the ceiling with the client lying on an examination table. The hip joints should be firm, stable, and nontender.

Page 179: *Answers*—An enlarged or swollen TMJ appears as a rounded protuberance and is accompanied by pain or discomfort in TMJ area. Swelling, limited movement, or crackling sounds may be associated findings.

Chapter 10

Page 192: *Answer*—An early age at onset of menstruation has been associated with cancer.

Page 193: *Answer*—The nurse should recall that breast cancer is characterized by dimpling of the skin on the breast. The nurse should realize that this finding requires further assessment and examination by a healthcare provider, along with possible mammography for further diagnosis.

Page 194: *Answer*—Factors related to breast cancer include infertility, not having children, being pregnant for the first time after age 30, and taking oral contraceptives or hormone replacement therapy.

Page 194: *Answer*—The nurse should look for close relatives who may have a history of breast cancer such as mother, sisters, or aunts.

Chapter 11

Page 208: *Answer*—The nurse should ask, "When was the abnormal Pap smear?" "What did the abnormal Pap smear show?" "What treatment was recommended?" "Did you complete the treatment?"

Page 208: *Answer*—It is important that the nurse ask the client about rashes, lesions, ulcerations, sores, or warts on the tissues of the genitalia.

Page 209: *Answer*—The nurse should ask when the discharge began, how much discharge the client is experiencing, what color the discharge is, and whether there is an odor associated with the discharge.

Page 210: *Answer*—The nurse should ask the client about what chronic illness she is experiencing, what medications are currently being taken, and what over-the-counter medications or herbal preparations are being taken.

Page 217: *Answer*—The nurse would document the position of the uterus by using the following terms: anteversion, which is a normal variation of position in which the uterus is tilted forward and the cervix is tilted downward; midposition, which is a normal variation of position in which the uterus lies parallel to the tailbone and the cervix points straight; and retroversion, which is a normal variation of position in which the uterus is pointed backward and the cervix is pointed upward.

Chapter 12

Page 230: *Answer*—The nurse should provide privacy for the interview and take a nonjudgmental approach when questioning the client and listening to the client's responses.

Page 231: *Answer*—Use standard precautions by applying gloves prior to examining the client.

Page 233: *Answer*—The nurse should assess the client for lice and scabies.

Page 234: *Answer*—Dry the area well, do not scratch, and wash hands thoroughly.

Page 234: *Answer*—The nurse should next illuminate the area with a penlight because a hydrocele will transilluminate.

Page 235: *Answer*—The nurse would document a tender, warm, painful mass upon rectal examination. The client may also have a fever.

Chapter 13

Page 245: *Answer*—The nurse should include a history of yeast infections in the past medical history. If the client stated that he or she currently has a yeast infection then the nurse should document this information in the present medical history.

Page 246: *Answer*—The nurse should ask where the rash is, when it started, whether there are any additional symptoms, whether the client used any new products, and whether the rash is painful.

Chapter 14

Page 268: *Answer*—The nurse should inquire about eye disorders such as strabismus, vision impairment, glaucoma, cataracts, macular degeneration, eye injury or surgery, or disorders that affect the eye such as hypertension, diabetes, or allergies.

Page 269: *Answer*—The nurse should assess the client's diet for adequate intake of vitamin A. Deficiency of this vitamin could be responsible for decreased night vision in the client. If dietary intake is adequate, other causes may be investigated.

Page 272: *Answer*—The nurse should dim the lights in the room to prevent ambient room light from affecting the amount of pupillary response possible. The nurse should assess each eye, one at a time, by moving a penlight from the lateral side of the client's vision onto the pupil. The nurse should observe for constriction of the pupil in response to the light (direct reaction) and for constriction of the pupil of the opposite eye (consensual reaction). The assessment is then repeated with the other pupil.

Page 275: *Answer*—The nurse should find that the red reflex is present, blood vessels are fairly straight, and the optic disk should be round or oval in shape and have a yellow-orange color. The macula should be seen as a dark circle and the retina should be free of spots on examination.

Page 279: *Answer*—With cataracts the lens would have opacity instead of being clear. The nurse could ask the client about decreasing visual acuity over time. With glaucoma, the nurse would note that the pupil is dilated and is more oval-shaped than round. The cornea may be cloudy and the client may have eye pain and/or see halos around lights.

Chapter 15

Page 288: *Answer*—To assess for the risk of cancer, the nurse could ask questions such as, "Do you use tobacco? Do you smoke?" The nurse could then ask follow-up questions about oral hygiene (frequency of tooth brushing, flossing, and dental exams). Finally the nurse could ask what medications the client is taking—chemotherapy drugs used to treat cancer frequently cause problems with oral mucosa.

Page 288: *Answer*—Because diuretics used for hypertension can be ototoxic, the nurse should assess for hearing loss as well as for intended effects of this class of medication.

Page 288: *Answer*—The nurse should ask whether the client currently is experiencing tinnitus (ringing in the ears). If the client answers affirmatively, the nurse should assess the characteristics of the ringing, whether it is constant or intermittent, whether it is associated with any particular activity, and whether the client is taking any medications for this problem.

Page 290: *Answer*—The nurse should inspect the external auditory canal to be sure it is patent and to assess for drainage, redness, swelling, lesions, or nodules. The nurse would then palpate the tragus at the medial side of the ear canal, which may cause pain if the client has otitis externa.

Page 291: *Answer*—The nurse would need to use an otoscope, a device with a light and a speculum that can be inserted gently into the outer ear canal to visualize the tympanic membrane.

Page 292: *Answer*—For optimal assessment the nurse should ask the client to sit with head tilted back.

Page 296: *Answer*—The tympanic membrane should be flat, pearly, gray, intact, and translucent with no scars; a cone-shaped reflection of an otoscope light should be visible at a five o'clock position in the right ear and a seven o'clock position in the left ear.

Page 297: *Answer*—A common side effect of phenytoin (Dilantin), a medication used to control seizures, is gingival hyperplasia. For this reason, the nurse should ask the client specifically about what medications the client is taking to control seizure activity and should inspect the client's gums for hyperplasia.

➤ Case Study Suggested Answers

Chapter 1

1. In preparing to interview the client, the nurse should ensure privacy and adequate room temperature and lighting. The nurse should also decrease external stimuli in the room, maintain a distance of 4 to 5 feet from the client, and arrange to sit at eye level.
2. The nurse should introduce him or herself by stating his or her name and role, address the client using the client's surname, and include the reason for the interview.
3. The nurse should use open-ended questions during the nurse–client interview because open-ended questions will allow the client to communicate more data. Closed-ended questions requiring a "yes" or "no" response limit the information that the client is able to share.
4. In obtaining information related to the client's chief complaint of abdominal pain, the nurse should ask questions that include the onset, location, duration, and frequency of the current symptoms; the description and quality of pain; alleviating and aggravating factors; and other associated symptoms.
5. During the closing phase of the nurse–client interview, the nurse should summarize the important aspects of the interview, and always allow an opportunity for the client to ask questions. The client may be more comfortable at this time to ask questions.

Chapter 2

1. The nurse should see if a nurse of the same sex is available to perform the physical assessment. If there is no other nurse of the same sex available the nurse should ask the client if she wishes a family member or female staff member to be present in the room.
2. The factors to be considered include cultural and religious beliefs of the client.
3. The common cultural beliefs include having same sex practitioners. Having family members care for the ill in the home environment. Family support systems are extremely important. Illness may be viewed as God's will.
4. The nurse should inform the client that he will see if a female nurse is available to conduct the physical assessment.
5. The nurse should respect the client's wishes and not perform the physical assessment with or without family members present. Proceeding with the examination could be considered battery.

Chapter 3

1. The nurse should ask if the client drinks alcohol.
   a. If yes, how much and how often. And also ask when he last had a drink.
   b. If no, then ask the wife if she has ever seen her husband acting this way before and if yes, when and what were the circumstances.
2. The nurse should conduct a mental status exam as soon as possible. The client may be demonstrating a hallucination. If he is, then he will need a thorough assessment and care. He may just be apprehensive about his surgery; however, if he has demonstrated this behavior on other occasions, physical diagnoses, psychiatric diagnoses, or alcohol/other drug abuse should all be ruled out before the surgery is performed.
3. The major nursing diagnosis for the client at this moment is Disturbed Sensory Perception related to unknown etiology as evidenced by his conversing with words and gestures while alone.
4. The client should have tests to rule out brain trauma, brain tumors, electrolyte imbalance, multiple sclerosis, psychiatric or alcohol and other drug history or abuse or any other physiological causes for his behavior. He should also have a focus interview to help determine the level of impairment.
5. The client's surgery should be postponed until the client's psychological and physiological health status can be determined.

Chapter 4

1. The client is experiencing weight loss, inappropriate diet for disease process, and social isolation at meal times.
2. The client's previous weight was 200 pounds, for a weight loss of 28 pounds. After dividing 28 by 200, the client has lost 14% of body weight.

3. The current BMI is 24, while the previous one was 28. The client has changed from overweight status to healthy or normal weight status. However, if the client continues to lose weight, the client is at risk for being undernourished.

4. The nurse should provide instruction about congestive heart failure, medication teaching related to hydro-chlorothiazide (a diuretic requiring increased intake of high potassium foods). The nurse should teach the client that orange juice, bananas, potatoes, strawberries, and melons are high potassium foods. The client is currently consuming a high-sodium diet and is prescribed a low-sodium diet, so instruction about low-sodium foods is also needed, as well as instruction to avoid foods high in sodium such as canned goods, processed foods, frozen meals, and soda bread. The nurse may suggest that the client join a dinner club for companionship during dinner or arrange to dine with friends, if this is possible, to reduce social isolation.

5. The nurse should document that the client had a 28-pound weight loss in four months, his past medical history, objective findings such as skin turgor, ill fitting dentures, all subjective statements, dietary recall, medication history, and all teaching.

Chapter 5

1. Chest pain can be related to a variety of conditions, but when unrelieved by rest, the client may be experiencing a heart attack or myocardial infarction. This may occur as a result of coronary artery occlusion, which causes a disruption in blood flow to the heart. If blood flow is not restored to the heart within a few hours, the heart muscle dies. Classic symptoms of a myocardial infarction include a gradual onset of pain or pressure felt most intensely in the center of the chest, sometimes radiating into the neck, jaw, shoulders, or arms, and lasting more than a half hour. With early intervention, the survival rate increases, so it would be imperative for the client to seek early intervention.

2. Pain assessment should include the following elements:
   - Onset, such as when the pain began and whether the client has had the pain before
   - Location of the pain and whether or not it radiates to other areas, such as neck, jaw, shoulder, or arm
   - Character, including a description of the pain (crushing, stabbing, burning, pressure, etc.), and intensity (on a scale of 1 to 10 ranging from minimal to maximal discomfort)
   - Precipitating factors, such as activity or emotional stress, and whether pain was relieved when precipitating factor is removed (such as resting or stopping activity)
   - Associated symptoms such as dizziness, shortness of breath, nausea, or vomiting
   - Alleviating factors that relieved the pain or whether nitroglycerin was effective, if taken

3. The nurse should ask questions related to history of hypertension, diabetes, thyroid disorders, high cholesterol or triglyceride levels, heart murmur, and previously diagnosed heart disease to get information that could relate to the current problem. The nurse should also inquire about past history, such as congenital heart disease, rheumatic fever, unexplained joint pains as a child, recurrent tonsillitis, and anemia; these could be responsible for cardiac problems later in adulthood.

4. Examination of the heart would include visual inspection of the chest, palpation of the point of maximal impulse (PMI), possible percussion of heart borders, and auscultation of heart sounds (S1 and S2 normal; S3 and S4 would be abnormal in an adult presenting with a cardiac complaint; murmurs or pericardial friction rub would be abnormal).

5. Examination of the vascular system should include visual inspection of the skin, palpation of peripheral pulses (carotids in the neck; brachial, radial, and ulnar in the arms; femoral, popliteal, dorsalis pedis, and posterior tibial in the legs), and evaluation of peripheral edema if present.

Chapter 6

1. The nurse should document the shortness of breath as subjective data.

2. The nurse should assess this client in an upright sitting position. This position is appropriate for the client to assist with breathing and it facilitates the assessment for the nurse.

3. The nurse should assess for expansion of the thorax.

4. Hyperresonance is usually heard on percussion.

5. The most appropriate nursing diagnosis for this client would be Ineffective Breathing Pattern.

Chapter 7

1. The diet of the client is high in fat, does not include selections from all food groups, and is low in fiber. A high fat diet contributes to acid reflux.

2. The diet is high caloric and the client performs very little exercise.

3. The nurse should inspect, auscultate, percuss, and then palpate the abdomen to decrease the risk of increasing abdominal sounds.

4. The nurse should develop a plan of care based on the nursing diagnosis Imbalanced Nutrition: More than Body Requirements.

5. Driving a truck is a sedentary profession that may contribute to his excessive weight.

Chapter 8

1. Safety is a key concern for the client and the priority nursing diagnosis is Risk for Falls.

2. The nurse should provide information to keep the client safe. Low vision interventions such as instructing the client to keep the furniture in the same place as well as frequently used items. Medication teaching and conservation of energy strategies would be needed.

3. The nurse should assess the visual system, musculoskeletal system, and urinary system.
4. Subjective information is information that the client states but the nurse cannot objectively see. In this case study, fatigue is subjective.
5. This client is going to need a magnetic resonance imaging (MRI) study or a computerized tomography (CT) scan.

Chapter 9

1. The nurse should ask questions such as the following:
   - "Do you have any pain, stiffness, swelling, heat, redness, or limitation of movement in any of your joints?"
   - "Do you have any pain, cramping, or weakness in any muscles?"
   - "Do you have any bone pain or have you recently sustained any injuries that may affect your bones?"
   If the client has any positive responses, the nurse would then follow up with a full symptom analysis of each symptom.
2. The nurse may position the client in either a standing or a sitting position to begin conducting the examination; however, with the client's age, and without knowing further details of the client's health, the sitting position is likely to be better to conserve energy because of age-related musculoskeletal changes.
3. During an assessment of each joint, the nurse should inspect the joint, palpate the joint, assess the range of motion of the joint, and test the strength of the muscles surrounding the joint.
4. Age-related musculoskeletal changes that are likely to be present in this 72-year-old client are the following:
   - Decreased bone density and possible osteoporosis, especially in vertebrae and long bones
   - A decrease in height and kyphosis
   - Slight flexion of the hips and knees when the client is standing, altering the center of gravity and placing the client at increased risk for falls
   - A decrease in size and quantity of muscle fibers and increased connective tissue, resulting in fibrous or stringy muscles; less elastic tendons; and reduced reaction time, speed of movement, agility, and endurance
   - Changes in synovial fluid, fragmentation of connective tissue, and scarring and calcification in joint capsules
   - Frayed, thin, and cracked joint cartilage, with possible underlying bone erosion, less shock absorbency of joints, and decreased flexibility and range of motion (if osteoarthritis is present)
   - A bowlegged stance caused by reduced muscle control, which alters the normal angle of the hip
5. General recommendations to promote musculoskeletal health and reduce safety risks would include the following:
   - Eat a well-balanced diet and engage in regular exercise
   - Beware of and eliminate factors that can increase risk of falls, such as loose carpeting or throw rugs, walking on wet surfaces, and having objects on floor or other clutter

Chapter 10

1. The nurse should ask the following questions:
   a. "Do you have a family history of breast cancer? If so, what family members have the cancer?"
   b. "What type of cancer did they have?"
   c. "Do you have any children? If so, how old were you when you had the first?"
   d. "At what age was your first period?"
   e. "Do you take oral contraceptives or hormone replacement therapy?"
   f. "Besides the lump do you have any other manifestations such as swelling, edema, node enlargement in the axillae, discharge, nipple or breast changes, or nipple retraction? When was your last mammogram? (This will help establish a baseline for any possible changes). Have you had any recent breast injury or trauma? What medications are you taking?"
2. Multiple positions will be used for the breast examination. The breasts should be examined with the client sitting, and also standing and leaning forward with hands over head or on hips to assist in detecting dimpling or a change in contour of the breasts. Next, a supine position permits breast tissue to be evenly distributed over the chest wall and will be used when doing breast palpation.
3. The nurse can use a warm soap lather or powder to facilitate the hands gliding over the breasts.
4. When the client presents with a lump the nurse should evaluate the client for the size, shape, and location of the lump, as well as thickening in the axillae or nodal enlargement; nipples that are red, dimpled, or retracted; skin that is scaly; or any discharge.
5. The nurse should document any findings noted during the interview, inspection, or palpation.

Chapter 11

1. The nurse should position the client in the lateral position when the client is unable to assume the lithotomy position.
2. The nurse should explain to the client that she is experiencing a prolapsed uterus, which is due to musculature weakness causing the uterus to fall into the vagina.
3. The most appropriate nursing diagnosis is Impaired Comfort as the client states she is uncomfortable and has a heavy feeling.
4. The nurse should moisten the uterus with saline and attempt to reinsert the uterus to keep it moist. The client should be referred to her physician if the prolapsed uterus persists.
5. The nurse should instruct the client to perform Kegel exercises to prevent urinary incontinence by contracting and relaxing the pelvic muscles.

Chapter 12

1. The nurse should evaluate the client for other sexually transmitted diseases.
2. The nurse should provide information on medication purpose, action, dosage, nursing considerations, and should stress the importance of taking all of the medications. The nurse should stress abstinence from intercourse until the client's treatment is complete. The nurse should provide information on condom use and about other types of sexually transmitted infections.
3. The nurse should implement case notification and arrange for the client's girlfriend to come to the center for testing, education, and treatment.
4. The client and his girlfriend should return to the clinic within one week for follow-up.
5. The most important diagnosis for this client is Deficient Knowledge related to medication use as manifested by re-infection of a sexually transmitted disease.

Chapter 13

1. Important questions for the nurse to ask would include the following:
   • "What type of change did you notice?"
   • "When did you first notice the change?"
   • "Have you noticed any bleeding or discharge?"
   • "Have you experienced any itching?"
   • "Are you having any pain?"
   • "Have you initiated any treatment for the symptoms?"
   • "Have you obtained any relief from the treatment?"
2. Other questions related to the client's past medical history would include the following:
   • "Have you ever had any skin problems?"
   • "If so, describe them."
   • "What type of treatment did you receive?"
   • "Was the treatment effective?"
   • "Has the problem ever recurred?"
   • "How are you managing the problem now?"
3. Important questions about skin care management should include the following:
   • "Do you sunbathe?"
   • "Do you go to the tanning salon?"
   • "Have you ever sunbathed?"
   • "Do you work outdoors?"
   • "How does your skin react to sun exposure?"
   • "Do you remember having any sunburn that left blisters?"
   • "How do you care for your skin?"
   • "Have you ever reacted to any skin products? If so, in what way?"

4. The "ABCD" warning signs of skin cancer include the following:
   • Asymmetry—any changes in the symmetry of a lesion need to be evaluated further.
   • Border—changes in the border of a lesion from smooth to rough and jagged need to be evaluated further.
   • Color—changes in the color of a lesion to a darker color, or more than one color, need to be further evaluated.
   • Diameter—lesions that enlarge in size need to be evaluated further.
5. The nurse would document the current status of the lesion, including a description of the size, shape, color and other characteristics of the lesion. The lesion should be measured for accuracy. The nurse should also document how the lesion has changed according to the description given by the client.

Chapter 14

1. The nurse should obtain a medication history.
2. The major risk factor is that the client is African-American. African Americans have an increased incidence of glaucoma.
3. The priority nursing intervention for this client is pain related to increased intraocular pressure as manifested by decreased visual acuity and blurred vision.
4. The nurse should prepare the client for tonometry. Tonometry is a diagnostic study whereby a puff of air is used to measure eye pressure. The test is painless.
5. If left untreated this condition may lead to blindness

Chapter 15

1. The nurse should perform the Rinne, Weber, and whisper tests to evaluate hearing and balance.
2. The nurse should ask the client about his or her ability to hear, if he or she has a history of infections, to describe pain, to give a medication history, about recent illnesses, and about any problems with his or her nose and throat.
3. The most appropriate diagnosis for the nurse to use in developing a plan of care is Risk for Infection related to inflammation and redness of the tympanic membrane.
4. The tympanic membrane may become scarred as evidenced by the development of white patches.
5. In the adult client the nurse will pull the ear up and back to facilitate visualization of the inner ear.

Index

Abdominal Assessment

Order of Physical Assessment Skills in Abdominal Assessment

Inspection
Auscultation
Percussion
Palpation
Note: always assess painful area last; use abdominal quadrants or regions as needed to aid in documenting assessment findings.

Nine Regions of the Abdomen

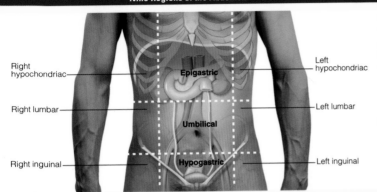

Right hypochondriac
Epigastric
Left hypochondriac
Right lumbar
Left lumbar
Umbilical
Right inguinal
Hypogastric
Left inguinal

Quadrants of the Abdomen

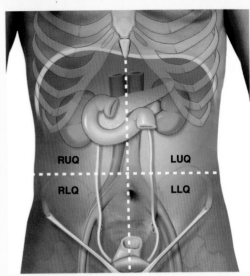

RUQ
LUQ
RLQ
LLQ

Skin Assessment

Malignant Skin Lesions

Basal Cell Carcinoma

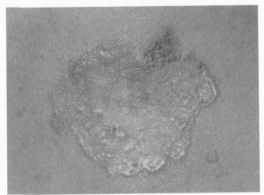

Source: Dr. Jason L. Smith. Used by Permission.

Squamous Cell Carcinoma

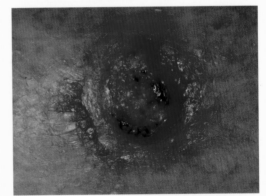

Source: Photo Researchers, Inc. Used by Permission.

Malignant Melanoma

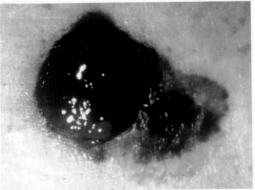

Source: Elizabeth A. Abel, M.D. Used by Permission.

Kaposi's Sarcoma

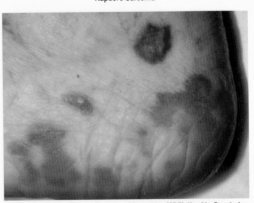

Source: Centers for Disease Control and Prevention (CDC). Used by Permission.

Tinea (fungal infection)

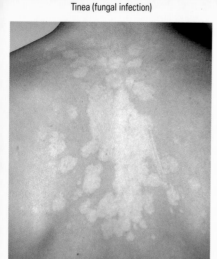

Source: Logical Images, Inc. Used by Permission.

Measles (Rubeola)

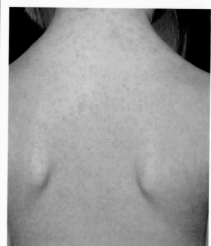

Source: Custom Medical Stock Photo, Inc. Used by Permission.

German Measles (Rubella)

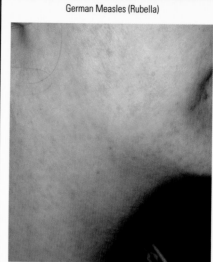

Source: Custom Medical Stock Photo, Inc. Used by Permission.

Chickenpox (Varicella)

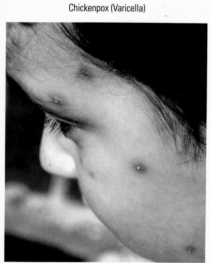

Herpes Simplex (viral infection)

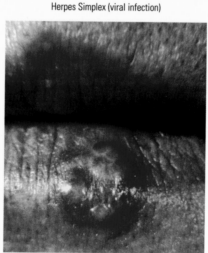

Source: National Archives and Records Administration. Used by Permission.

Herpes Zoster

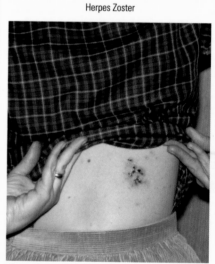

Source: Custom Medical Stock Photo, Inc. Used by Permission.

Psoriasis

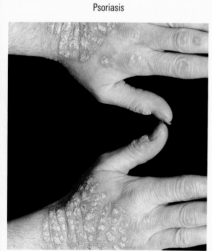

Source: Custom Medical Stock Photo, Inc. Used by Permission.

Contact Dermatitis

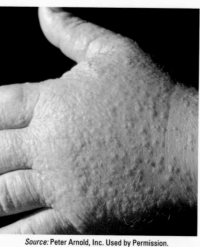

Source: Peter Arnold, Inc. Used by Permission.

Eczema (Atopic Dermatitis)

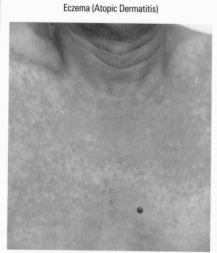

Source: Peter Arnold, Inc. Used by Permission.